Third Edition

Nursing Ethics

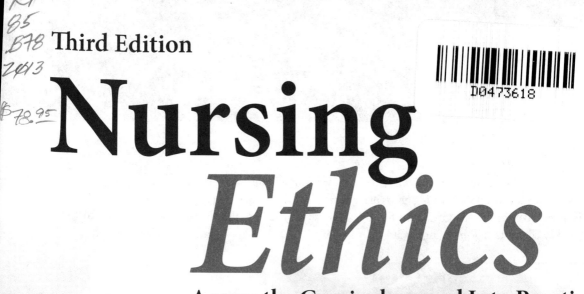

Across the Curriculum and Into Practice

Welcome to *Nursing Ethics: Across the Curriculum and Into Practice, Third Edition!*

The Pedagogy

Nursing Ethics: Across the Curriculum and Into Practice, Third Edition drives comprehension through various strategies that meet the learning needs of students, while also generating enthusiasm about the topic. This interactive approach addresses different learning styles, making this the ideal text to ensure mastery of key concepts. The pedagogical aids that appear in most chapters include the following:

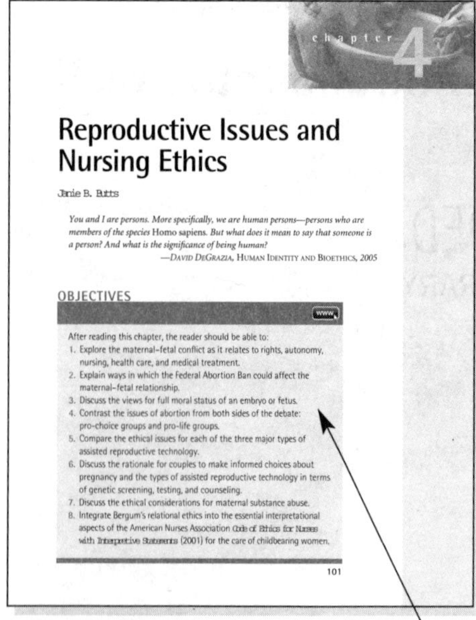
chapter 4

Reproductive Issues and Nursing Ethics

Janie B. Butts

You and I are persons. More specifically, we are human persons—persons who are members of the species Homo sapiens. *But what does it mean to say that someone is a person? And what is the significance of being human?*

—David DeGrazia, *Human Identity and Bioethics*, 2005

OBJECTIVES

www

After reading this chapter, the reader should be able to:

1. Explore the maternal-fetal conflict as it relates to rights, autonomy, nursing, health care, and medical treatment.
2. Explain ways in which the Federal Abortion Ban could affect the maternal-fetal relationship.
3. Discuss the views for full moral status of an embryo or fetus.
4. Contrast the issues of abortion from both sides of the debate: pro-choice groups and pro-life groups.
5. Compare the ethical issues for each of the three major types of assisted reproductive technology.
6. Discuss the rationale for couples to make informed choices about pregnancy and the types of assisted reproductive technology in terms of genetic screening, testing, and counseling.
7. Discuss the ethical considerations for maternal substance abuse.
8. Integrate Bergum's relational ethics into the essential interpretational aspects of the American Nurses Association *Code of Ethics for Nurses with Interpretive Statements* (2001) for the care of childbearing women.

101

Ethical Reflections

Develop your critical thinking skills with these discussion-based activities that revolve around nursing ethics. The "www" icon directs students to the companion website **http://go.jblearning.com/butts** to delve deeper into concepts by completing these exercises online.

Objectives

These objectives provide instructors and students with a snapshot of the key information they will encounter in each chapter. They serve as a checklist to help guide and focus study. Objectives can also be found on the companion website at **http://go.jblearning.com/butts**.

Key Terms

Key Terms are in bold throughout the text, and are included in an Interactive Glossary at the companion website at **http://go.jblearning.com/butts**. Quickly search for key terms and definitions, or preview a definition of key terms from the book in the Animated Flashcards and respond with an answer. You'll immediately see if you are correct!

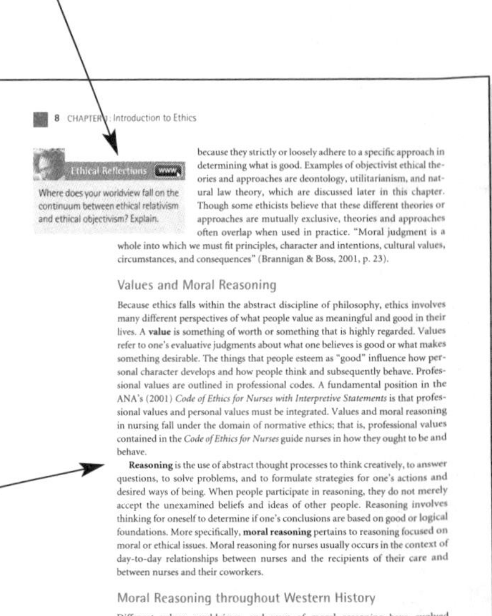
8 CHAPTER [illegible]: Introduction to Ethics

Ethical Reflections www

Where does your worldview fall on the continuum between ethical relativism and ethical objectivism? Explain.

because they strictly or loosely adhere to a specific approach in determining what is good. Examples of objectivist ethical theories and approaches are deontology, utilitarianism, and natural law theory, which are discussed later in this chapter. Though some ethicists believe that these different theories or approaches are mutually exclusive, theories and approaches often overlap when used in practice. "Moral judgment is a whole into which we must fit principles, character and intentions, cultural values, circumstances, and consequences" (Brannigan & Boss, 2001, p. 23).

Values and Moral Reasoning

Because ethics falls within the abstract discipline of philosophy, ethics involves many different perspectives of what people value as meaningful and good in their lives. A **value** is something of worth or something that is highly regarded. Values refer to one's evaluative judgments about what one believes is good or what makes something desirable. The things that people esteem as "good" influence how personal character develops and how people think and subsequently behave. Professional values are outlined in professional codes. A fundamental position in the ANA's (2001) *Code of Ethics for Nurses with Interpretive Statements* is that professional values and personal values must be integrated. Values and moral reasoning in nursing fall under the domain of normative ethics; that is, professional values contained in the *Code of Ethics for Nurses* guide nurses in how they ought to be and behave.

Reasoning is the use of abstract thought processes to think creatively, to answer questions, to solve problems, and to formulate strategies for one's actions and desired ways of being. When people participate in reasoning, they do not merely accept the unexamined beliefs and ideas of other people. Reasoning involves thinking for oneself to determine if one's conclusions are based on good or logical foundations. More specifically, **moral reasoning** pertains to reasoning focused on moral or ethical issues. Moral reasoning for nurses usually occurs in the context of day-to-day relationships between nurses and the recipients of their care and between nurses and their coworkers.

Moral Reasoning throughout Western History

Different values, worldviews, and ways of moral reasoning have evolved throughout history and have had different points of emphasis in varying historical periods. In regard to some approaches to reasoning about moral issues, what was old becomes new again, as in the case of the renewed popularity of virtue ethics—the concept of reasoning as would a person with good character.

Third Edition

Nursing *Ethics*

Across the Curriculum and Into Practice

Janie B. Butts, DSN, RN
The University of Southern Mississippi
School of Nursing
Hattiesburg, Mississippi

Karen L. Rich, PhD, MN, RN
The University of Southern Mississippi
School of Nursing
Long Beach, Mississippi

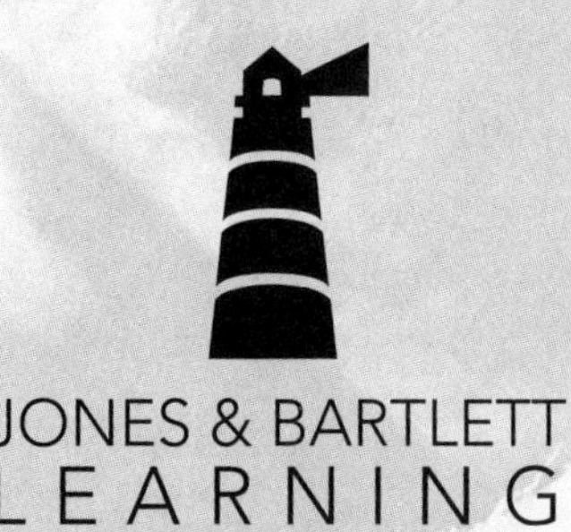

World Headquarters
Jones & Bartlett Learning
5 Wall Street
Burlington, MA 01803
978-443-5000
info@jblearning.com
www.jblearning.com

Jones & Bartlett Learning books and products are available through most bookstores and online booksellers. To contact Jones & Bartlett Learning directly, call 800-832-0034, fax 978-443-8000, or visit our website, www.jblearning.com.

Substantial discounts on bulk quantities of Jones & Bartlett Learning publications are available to corporations, professional associations, and other qualified organizations. For details and specific discount information, contact the special sales department at Jones & Bartlett Learning via the above contact information or send an email to specialsales@jblearning.com.

Production Credits
Publisher: Kevin Sullivan
Acquisitions Editor: Amanda Harvey
Editorial Assistant: Sara Bempkins
Associate Production Editor: Cindie Bryan
Marketing Manager: Elena McAnespie
Associate Marketing Manager: Katie Hennessy
V.P., Manufacturing and Inventory Control: Therese Connell
Composition: Paw Print Media
Cover Design: Kristin E. Parker
Cover & Part Opener Image: © Cleo/ShutterStock, Inc.
Chapter Opener Image: © Ints Vikmanis/ShutterStock, Inc.
Printing and Binding: Edwards Brothers Malloy
Cover Printing: Edwards Brothers Malloy

To order this product, use ISBN: 978-1-4496-4900-5

Library of Congress Cataloging-in-Publication Data
Butts, Janie B.
Nursing ethics : across the curriculum and into practice / Janie B. Butts, Karen L. Rich.—3rd ed.
p. ; cm.
Includes bibliographical references and index.
ISBN-13: 978-1-4496-2218-3 (pbk.)
ISBN-10: 1-4496-2218-6 (pbk.)
I. Rich, Karen, MN. II. Title.
[DNLM: 1. Ethics, Nursing. 2. Nurse-Patient Relations—ethics. WY 85]

174.2—dc23

2011037565

6048

Printed in the United States of America
16 15 14 13 12 10 9 8 7 6 5 4 3 2

Special Acknowledgments

We want to express our sincere appreciation to the staff at Jones & Bartlett Learning, especially Amanda, Cindie, and Sara, for their continued encouragement, assistance, and support during the writing process and publication of our book.

Contents

Preface

Rules and theories matter little without the formation of good character.

We believe that this is a very exciting time in the history of nursing. Although nurses continue to experience many difficult areas in their terrain of practice, nurses have more autonomy than ever before. With autonomy comes responsibility. Nurses face many day-to-day ethical issues that they must be prepared to handle. Nurses need to develop a firm sense of practical wisdom and to think critically about the ethics of their practice. Practical wisdom and moral ways of being do not just happen—they must deliberately be formed with education and intelligent habits of practice.

We chose a potter forming clay as the theme for the third edition of *Nursing Ethics: Across the Curriculum and Into Practice*. We believe that there are several ways that forming clay can be used as a metaphor for nursing ethics, viewing the nurse as both the potter and the clay. Clay is a malleable substance, as is a person who is a nurse. Good potters prepare their clay and take great care in forming the clay to produce an excellent piece. Like excellence in forming clay, nurses are charged with forming an excellent character, that is, a virtuous character. Knowing textbook ethics is critical, but taking care to deliberately form one's character is of significant importance for nurses.

American Association of Colleges of Nursing Recommendations in 2008

The American Association of Colleges of Nursing's (AACN) *Essentials of Baccalaureate Education for Professional Nursing Practice* (2008) recommended that nursing educators include ethics and ethical decision-making strategies in nursing curricula. The AACN (2008) stated in the rationale for Essential VIII, Professionalism and Professional Values:

> Baccalaureate education includes the development of professional values and value-based behavior. Understanding the values that patients and other health professionals bring to the therapeutic relationship is critically important to providing quality patient care. Baccalaureate graduates are prepared for the numerous dilemmas that will arise in practice and are able to make and assist others in making decisions within a professional ethical framework. Ethics is

> an integral part of nursing practice and has always involved respect and advocacy for the rights and needs of patients regardless of setting. Honesty and acting ethically are two key elements of professional behavior, which have a major impact on patient safety. (p. 27)

Some of the moral issues that nurses encounter on a daily basis leave nurses on uncertain ethical ground. Whether practicing nurses become bogged down in ethical situations about death, abortion, or saving premature infants, nurses will most likely experience moral distress when they begin to question the meaning and issues of life and death. Nurses must be prepared to attach their own meanings to life and death, and nursing students and practicing nurse clinicians need to acquire foundational knowledge about ethics, ethical reasoning, and decision-making strategies to prepare them for the ethical issues that they encounter daily. Included in this book are decision-making approaches and models, rationale for decisions, and various topics about ethical patient care.

NCLEX-RN® Test Plan for 2010

The National Council of State Boards of Nursing's 2010 *NCLEX-RN® Test Plan* has as its goal for nursing care in any setting, "preventing illness; alleviating suffering; protecting, promoting, and restoring health; and promoting dignity in dying" (p. 3). Examples of the integration of ethics into the test plan are:

NCLEX-RN® Test Plan: Safe and Effective Care Environment—Management of Care (p. 5)

- Ethical practice

NCLEX-RN® Test Plan: Psychosocial Integrity (p. 7)

- End-of-life care
- Grief and loss
- Religious and spiritual influences on health

Purposes and Readership

We have four purposes for this book. First, we wanted to provide a nursing ethics book that includes an exploration of a wide array of ethical issues in nursing. We wanted to include bioethical issues that nurses encounter every day—the ones that Fry and Veatch (2000) stated were the "flesh and blood" issues (p. 1)—but we wanted to cover the issues from a humanistic perspective. In the body of the text, we have included the most current scholarly literature, related news briefs, and research and legal findings regarding ethical issues. The content of our book is also based on theoretical foundations, clinical evidence, and case study analysis for students and nurse clinicians in practice.

Second, a prominent feature of this book is its "across the curriculum" format for undergraduate nursing students. The book can be used as a supplementary textbook in each nursing course. We strongly believe that if ethical concepts and bioethical issues are integrated in the beginning of nursing programs and throughout curricula, students will become more mindful of the myriad of ethical challenges that they will face in practice and then become habituated to resolving moral conflicts. Ultimately, we believe nurses will want to find ways to participate in the large-scale bioethical deliberations and decision making regarding their patients' and families' life and death issues.

As a third purpose, the book also is intended for RN to BSN students and their curricula, especially in ethics courses, professional development courses, or leadership courses. Even though RN to BSN students bring a wealth of real flesh-and-blood experiences with them to share in the classroom, they often return to school without substantial exposure to ethics classes or ethical content.

The last part of the book's title, "Into Practice," is related to the book's fourth purpose. Nurses' work is nursing ethics. The content of the book will stimulate the moral imagination of practicing nurses so that they can integrate ethical principles, theories, and decision-making skills into their everyday practice.

Comments and Feedback

We are dedicated to making this nursing ethics book the one that will meet your needs for the future. We are interested in your comments about the book. Please email us at Janie.Butts@usm.edu or Karen.Rich@usm.edu with feedback or questions concerning the book, questions about ethics, or any questions that you may have regarding the case studies or multiple-choice questions in the book. We appreciate your support!

References

American Association of Colleges of Nursing (AACN). (2008). *The essentials of baccalaureate education for professional nursing practice.* Retrieved from http://www.aacn.nche.edu/ccne-accreditation/standards-procedures-resources/baccalaureate-graduate/standards

Fry, S. T., & Veatch, R. M. (2000). *Case studies in nursing ethics* (2nd ed.). Sudbury, MA: Jones and Bartlett Publishers.

National Council of State Boards of Nursing. (2010). *NCLEX-RN test plan.* Retrieved from https://www.ncsbn.org/2010_NCLEX_RN_Detailed_Test_Plan_Candidate.pdf

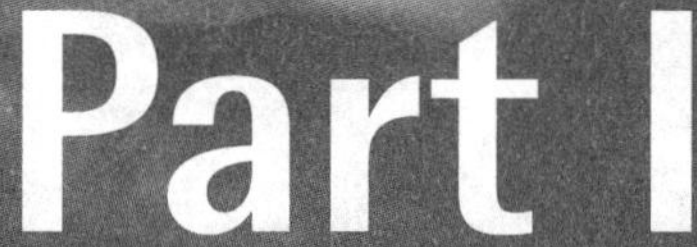

Part I

Theories and Concepts

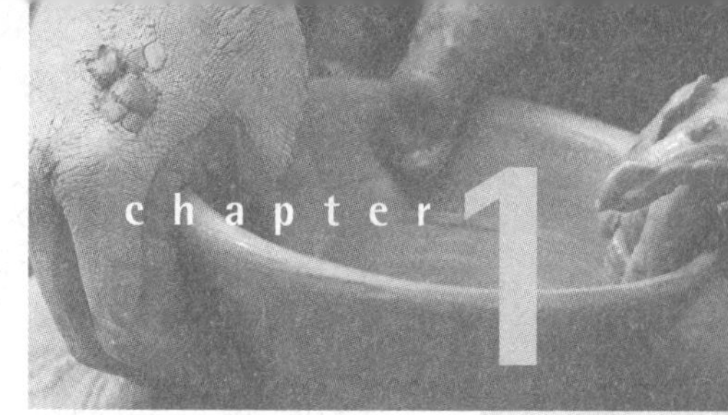

Introduction to Ethics

Karen L. Rich

A seed will only become a flower if it gets sun and water.

—Louis Gottschalk

OBJECTIVES

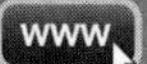

After reading this chapter, the reader should be able to:

1. Define the terms *ethics* and *morals* and discuss philosophical uses of these terms.
2. Discuss systems of moral reasoning as they have been used throughout history.
3. Evaluate a variety of ethical theories and approaches to use in personal and professional relationships.

Introduction to Ethics

In the world today, "we are in the throes of a giant ethical leap that is essentially embracing all of humankind" (Donahue, 1996, p. 484). Scientific and technological advances, economic realities, pluralistic worldviews, and global communication make it difficult for nurses to ignore the important ethical issues in the world community, their everyday lives, and their work. As controversial and sensitive ethical issues continue to challenge nurses and other healthcare professionals, many professionals have begun to develop an appreciation for traditional philosophies of ethics and the diverse viewpoints of others.

Ethical directives are not always clearly evident, and people sometimes disagree about what is right and wrong. These factors lead some people to believe that ethics can be based merely on personal opinions. However, if nurses are to enter into the global dialogue about ethics, they must do more than practice ethics based simply on their personal opinions, their intuition, or the unexamined beliefs that are proposed by other people. It is important for nurses to have a basic understanding of the concepts, principles, approaches, and theories that have been used in studying ethics throughout history so that they can identify and analyze ethical issues and dilemmas that are relevant to nurses in the 21st century. Mature ethical sensitivities are critical to ethical practice, and as Hope (2004) proposed, "we need to develop our hearts as well as our minds" (p. 6).

The Meaning of Ethics and Morals

When narrowly defined according to its original use, ethics is a branch of philosophy used to study ideal human behavior and ideal ways of being. The approaches to ethics and the meanings of related concepts have varied over time among philosophers and ethicists. For example, Aristotle believed that ideal behaviors were practices that lead to the end goal of *eudaimonia*, which is synonymous with a high level of happiness or well-being; on the other hand, Immanuel Kant, an 18th-century philosopher and ethicist, believed that ideal behavior was acting in accordance with one's duty. For Kant, well-being meant having the freedom to exercise autonomy (self-determination), not being used as a means to an end, being treated with dignity, and having the capability to think rationally.

As a philosophical discipline of study, **ethics** is a systematic approach to understanding, analyzing, and distinguishing matters of right and wrong, good and bad, and admirable and deplorable as they relate to the well-being of and the relationships among sentient beings. Ethical determinations are applied through the use of formal theories, approaches, and codes of conduct, such as codes that are developed for professions and religions. Ethics is an active process rather than a static condition, so some ethicists use the expression *doing ethics*. When people are doing ethics, they need to support their beliefs and assertions with sound reasoning; in other words, even if people believe that ethics is totally subjective, they must be able to justify their positions through logical, theoretically based arguments. Feelings and emotions are a normal part of everyday life and can play a legitimate role in doing ethics. However, people sometimes allow their emotions to overtake good reasoning, and when this happens, it does not provide a good foundation for ethics-related decisions. Evaluations generated through the practice of ethics require a balance of emotion and reason. Throughout history, people, based on their culture, have engaged in actions that they believed were justifiable only to have the light of reason later show otherwise. Following a charismatic, but egocentric, leader, such as Adolph Hitler, is an example of such a practice.

As contrasted with ethics, **morals** are specific beliefs, behaviors, and ways of being derived from doing ethics. One's morals are judged to be good or bad through systematic ethical analysis. The reverse of morality is immorality, which means that a person's behavior is in opposition to accepted societal, religious, cultural, or professional ethical standards and principles; examples of immorality include dishonesty, fraud, murder, and sexually abusive acts. *Amoral* is a term used to refer to actions that can normally be judged as moral or immoral, but are done with a lack of concern for good behavior. For example, murder is immoral, but if a person commits murder with absolutely no sense of remorse or maybe even a sense of pleasure, the person is acting in an amoral way. Acts are considered to be nonmoral if moral standards essentially do not apply to the acts; for example, choosing between cereal and toast and jam for breakfast is a nonmoral decision.

When people consider matters of ethics, they usually are considering matters about freedom in regard to personal choices, one's obligations to other sentient beings, or judgments about human character. The term *unethical* is used to describe ethics in its negative form when, for instance, a person's character or behavior is contrary to admirable traits or the code of conduct that has been endorsed by one's society, community, or profession. Because the word *ethics* is used when one may actually be referring to a situation of morals, the process-related or *doing* conception of ethics is sometimes overlooked today. People often use the word *ethics* when referring to a collection of actual beliefs and behaviors, thereby using the terms ethics and morals interchangeably. In this book, some effort has been made to distinguish the words *ethics* and *morals* based on their literal meanings; however, because of common uses, the terms have generally been used interchangeably.

Billington (2003) delineated important features regarding the concepts *morals* and *ethics*:

- Probably the most important feature about ethics and morals is that no one can avoid making moral or ethical decisions because the social connection with others necessitates that people must consider moral and ethical actions.
- Other people are always involved with one's moral and ethical decisions. Private morality does not exist.
- Moral decisions matter because every decision affects someone else's life, self-esteem, or happiness level.
- Definite conclusions or resolutions will never be reached in ethical debates.
- In the area of morals and ethics, people cannot exercise moral judgment without being given a choice; in other words, a necessity for making a sound moral judgment is being able to choose an option from among a number of choices.
- People use moral reasoning to make moral judgments or to discover right actions.

Types of Ethical Inquiry

Ethics is categorized according to three types of inquiry or study: normative ethics, meta-ethics, and descriptive ethics. The first approach, **normative ethics**, is an attempt to decide or prescribe values, behaviors, and ways of being that are right or wrong, good or bad, admirable or deplorable. When using the method of normative ethics, inquiries are made about how humans should behave, what ought to be done in certain situations, what type of character one should have, or how one should be.

Outcomes of normative ethics are the prescriptions derived from asking normative questions. These prescriptions include accepted moral standards and codes. One such accepted moral standard is the common morality. The **common morality** consists of normative beliefs and behaviors that the members of society generally agree about and that are familiar to most human beings. Because it forms what can be thought of as a universal morality, the common morality provides society with a framework of ethical stability. The belief that robbing a bank and murder are wrong is part of the common morality, whereas abortion is not a part of our common morality, because of the many varying positions about the rightness or wrongness of it.

Particular moralities adhered to by specific groups can be distinguished from the common morality (Beauchamp & Childress, 2009). Particular moralities, such as a profession's moral norms and codes, are heavily content laden and specific, rather than general, in nature. The *Code of Ethics for Nurses with Interpretive Statements* (American Nurses Association [ANA], 2001) is a specific morality for professional nurses in the United States. A normative belief posited in the *Code* is that nurses ought to be compassionate—that is, nurses should work to relieve suffering. Nurses have specific obligations toward the recipients of their care that are different from the obligations of other people. As risks and dangers for nurses become more complex, the profession's morality must evolve and be continually reexamined. Nurses might ask themselves these normative questions: Do I have an obligation to endanger my life and the life of my family members by working during a highly lethal influenza pandemic? Do I have an obligation to stay at work in a hospital during a category 5 hurricane rather than evacuating with my family? The answers to these questions may generate strong emotions, confusion, or feelings of guilt.

The focus of meta-ethics, which means "about ethics," is not an inquiry about what ought to be done or what behaviors should be prescribed. Instead, **meta-ethics** is concerned with understanding the language of morality through an analysis of the meaning of ethically related concepts and theories, such as the meaning of *good*, *happiness*, and *virtuous character*. For example, a nurse who is actively engaging in a meta-ethical analysis might try to determine the meaning of a good nurse–patient relationship.

Descriptive ethics is often referred to as a scientific rather than a philosophical ethical inquiry. It is an approach used when researchers or ethicists want to describe what people think about morality or when they want to describe how people actually behave—that is, their morals. Professional moral values and behaviors can be described through nursing research. An example of descriptive ethics is research that identifies nurses' attitudes regarding telling patients the truth about their terminal illnesses.

Ethical Perspectives

Ethical thinking, valuing, and reasoning fall somewhere along a continuum between two opposing views: ethical relativism and ethical objectivism.

Ethical Relativism

Ethical relativism is the belief that it is acceptable for ethics and morality to differ among persons or societies. There are two types of ethical relativism: ethical subjectivism and cultural relativism (Brannigan & Boss, 2001). People who subscribe to a belief in **ethical subjectivism** believe "that individuals create their own morality [and that] there are no objective moral truths—only individual opinions" (p. 7). People's beliefs about actions being right or wrong, or good or bad, depend on how people feel about actions rather than on reason or systematic ethical analysis. What is believed by one person to be wrong might not be viewed as wrong by one's neighbor depending on variations in opinions and feelings. These differences are acceptable to ethical subjectivists.

Ethical subjectivism has been distinguished from cultural relativism. Pence (2000) defined **cultural relativism** as "the ethical theory that moral evaluation is rooted in and cannot be separated from the experience, beliefs, and behaviors of a particular culture, and hence, that what is wrong in one culture may not be so in another" (p. 12). People opposed to cultural relativism argue that when it is practiced according to its extreme or literal meaning, this type of thinking can be dangerous because it theoretically may support relativists' exploitative or hurtful actions (Brannigan & Boss, 2001). An example of cultural relativism is the belief that the act of female circumcision, which is sometimes called female genital mutilation, is a moral practice. Though not considered to be a religious ritual, this act is considered ethically acceptable by some groups in countries that have a Muslim or an Egyptian Pharaonic heritage. In most countries and cultures, however, it is considered to be a grave violation in accordance with the United Nations' Declaration of Human Rights.

Ethical Objectivism

Ethical objectivism is the belief that universal or objective moral principles exist. Many philosophers and healthcare ethicists hold this view, at least to some degree,

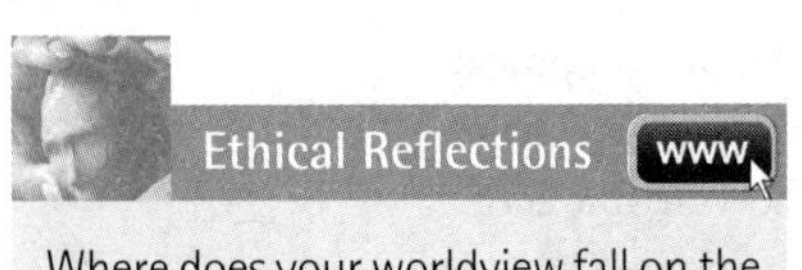

Where does your worldview fall on the continuum between ethical relativism and ethical objectivism? Explain.

because they strictly or loosely adhere to a specific approach in determining what is good. Examples of objectivist ethical theories and approaches are deontology, utilitarianism, and natural law theory, which are discussed later in this chapter. Though some ethicists believe that these different theories or approaches are mutually exclusive, theories and approaches often overlap when used in practice. "Moral judgment is a whole into which we must fit principles, character and intentions, cultural values, circumstances, and consequences" (Brannigan & Boss, 2001, p. 23).

Values and Moral Reasoning

Because ethics falls within the abstract discipline of philosophy, ethics involves many different perspectives of what people value as meaningful and good in their lives. A **value** is something of worth or something that is highly regarded. Values refer to one's evaluative judgments about what one believes is good or what makes something desirable. The things that people esteem as "good" influence how personal character develops and how people think and subsequently behave. Professional values are outlined in professional codes. A fundamental position in the ANA's (2001) *Code of Ethics for Nurses with Interpretive Statements* is that professional values and personal values must be integrated. Values and moral reasoning in nursing fall under the domain of normative ethics; that is, professional values contained in the *Code of Ethics for Nurses* guide nurses in how they ought to be and behave.

Reasoning is the use of abstract thought processes to think creatively, to answer questions, to solve problems, and to formulate strategies for one's actions and desired ways of being. When people participate in reasoning, they do not merely accept the unexamined beliefs and ideas of other people. Reasoning involves thinking for oneself to determine if one's conclusions are based on good or logical foundations. More specifically, **moral reasoning** pertains to reasoning focused on moral or ethical issues. Moral reasoning for nurses usually occurs in the context of day-to-day relationships between nurses and the recipients of their care and between nurses and their coworkers.

Moral Reasoning throughout Western History

Different values, worldviews, and ways of moral reasoning have evolved throughout history and have had different points of emphasis in varying historical periods. In regard to some approaches to reasoning about moral issues, what was old becomes new again, as in the case of the renewed popularity of virtue ethics—the concept of reasoning as would a person with good character.

Ancient Greece

In Western history, much of what is known about formal moral reasoning generally began with the ancient Greeks, especially with the philosophers Socrates (c. 469–399 B.C.E.), Plato (c. 429–347 B.C.E.), and Aristotle (384–322 B.C.E.). Though there are no primary texts of the teachings of Socrates (what we have of his teachings were recorded by Plato), it is known that Socrates was an avid promoter of moral reasoning and critical thinking among the citizens of Athens. Socrates is credited with the statement that "the unexamined life is not worth living," and he developed a method of reasoning called the Socratic method, which is still used today (see Box 1.1).

Socrates had many friends and allies who believed in his philosophy and teachings. In fact, Socrates was such a successful and well-known teacher of philosophy and moral reasoning in Athens that he was put to death for upsetting the sociopolitical *status quo*. Socrates was accused of corrupting the youth of Athens who, under his tutelage, had begun to question their parents' wisdom and religious beliefs. These accusations of corruption were based on Socrates's encouraging people to think independently and to question dogma generated by the ruling class. Though he was sentenced to death by the powerful, elite men within his society, Socrates refused to apologize for his beliefs and teachings. He ultimately chose to die by drinking poisonous hemlock rather than to deny his values.

Socrates's student, Plato, is believed by some people to have been the most outstanding philosopher to have ever lived. Plato's reasoning was based on his belief that there are two realms of reality. The first is the realm of Forms, which transcends time and space. According to Plato, an eternal, perfect, and unchanging ideal copy (Form)

BOX 1.1 ETHICAL FORMATIONS: THE SOCRATIC METHOD

Socrates posited challenging questions, and he would then ask another question about the answers that he received. An example of his method of questioning might be as follows:

Socrates: Why should nurses study ethics?
Nurse: To be good nurses.
Socrates: What is a good nurse?
Nurse: It means that my patients are well taken care of.
Socrates: How do you know that your patients are well taken care of?

This line of questioning continues on until the concepts stemming from the original question are thoroughly explored. Socratic questioning does not mean that one ends up with a final answer; however, this form of discussion leads people to think critically and reflectively.

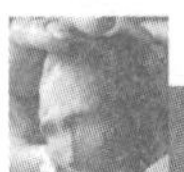

Ethical Reflections WWW

- Begin a Socratic dialogue with classmates or colleagues. Develop your own questions or use one of the following examples:
  - What does lying to a patient mean?
  - What does caring mean in nursing?
  - How are competence and ethics related in nursing?

of all phenomena exists in the realm of Forms, which is beyond everyday human access. Plato believed that the realm of Forms contains the essence of concepts and objects, and even the essence of objects' properties. Essences that exist in the realm of Forms included, for example, a perfect Form of good, redness (the color red), and a horse. In the realm of Forms, the essence of good exists as ideal Truth and redness (a particular property of some objects, such as an apple) exists as the color red in its most perfect state. A horse in the realm of Forms is the perfect specimen of the animal that is a horse, and this perfect horse contains all the "horseness" factors that, for example, distinguish a horse from a cow. Plato considered the world of Forms to be the real world, though humans do not live in that world.

The second realm is the world of Appearances, which is the everyday world of imperfect, decaying, and changing phenomena; this is the world in which humans live. The underlying purpose or goal of imperfect phenomena in the world of Appearances is to emulate their associated essences and perfect Forms. For example, a horse's purpose in life is to strive toward becoming identical to the perfect specimen of a horse that exists in the world of Forms.

Plato also proposed that humans have a tripartite soul. The three parts of the soul consist of the Faculty of Reason, associated with thought and Truth, which is located in one's head; the Faculty of Spirit that expresses love, beauty, and the desire for eternal life, which is located in one's chest; and the Faculty of Appetite that is an expression of human desires and emotions, which is located in one's gut. Plato believed that the influences of these three parts of the soul exist in greater to lesser degrees in each person. Therefore, one person may be more disposed to intellectual pursuits as compared to another person, who is more interested in physical pleasures. Plato based other associations, such as one's best-suited occupation, on the degree of influence of the three parts of the soul. The founder of modern nursing, Florence Nightingale, was a passionate student of ancient Greek philosophy. It is believed that Nightingale may have aligned the function of nurses with the Faculty of Spirit (see Box 1.2).

One of Plato's most famous stories about reasoning is his allegory of the cave. In this story, a group of people lived their lives chained to the floor of a cave. Behind them burned a fire that cast shadows of people moving on the wall in front of the people who are chained. The chained prisoners believe that the shadows are actually real people. When one of the prisoners is freed from his chains, he leaves the cave. First, he is blinded by the brightness of the sun. After his sight adjusts to the light, he sees objects that he realizes are more real than the shadows within the cave. The freed person returns to the cave to encourage the other prisoners to break their chains and to enter the more expansive world of reality. The meaning of this story has been interpreted in many different ways. Whatever Plato's intended meaning,

BOX 1.2 ETHICAL FORMATIONS: NURSES AS GUARDIANS

Plato associated the tripartite soul with three classes of Greek society. Persons were believed to have an individual aptitude that particularly suited them to their purpose in society:

1. Philosopher Kings were associated with the Faculty of Reason and wisdom.
2. Societal guardians were associated with the Faculty of Spirit and protecting others.
3. Artisans and craftsmen were associated with the Faculty of Appetite and technical work.

Because of her education in classical Greek literature and culture and her views about nursing, it has been proposed that Florence Nightingale might have compared her purpose as a nurse with the role of a societal guardian. In contrast, early physicians, whose profession developed through apprenticeship guilds that emphasized technical practices, might best be compared to the artisan class.

Source: LeVasseur, J. (1998). Plato, Nightingale, and contemporary nursing. *Image: Journal of Nursing Scholarship, 30*(3), 281–285.

the story does prompt people to think about the problems that result when they remain chained by their closed minds and flawed reasoning.

Plato's student, Aristotle, developed science, logic, and ethics to world-altering proportions. Though he was influenced by his teacher, Plato, Aristotle took a more practical approach to reasoning than believing in an other-worldly realm of ideal Forms. He was guided in his reasoning by his belief in the importance of empirical inquiry. He also believed that all things have a purpose or end goal (*telos*), similar to Plato's proposition that the goal of all things is to strive to be like their perfect Form. In *Nichomachean Ethics*, Aristotle (trans. 2002) discussed practical wisdom (*phronesis*) as being necessary for deliberation about what is good and advantageous if people want to move toward their human purpose or desired end goal of happiness or well-being (*eudaimonia*). Aristotle believed that a person needed education to cultivate *phronesis* to achieve intellectual excellence.

Aristotle's conception of *phronesis* is similar to Plato's conception of the virtue of prudence. Wisdom is focused on the good achieved from being wise, which means that one knows how to act in a particular situation, deliberates well, and has a disposition that embodies excellence of character. Therefore, in ancient Greece, prudence was more than simply having good intentions or meaning well—it was knowing what to do and how to be, but it also involved transforming that knowledge into well-reasoned actions. Aristotle believed that people

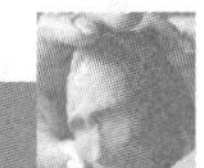

Ethical Reflections

- Discuss how and when nurses are and are not the guardians of their patients.
- How are nurses and physicians different in their roles as guardians? How are they similar?

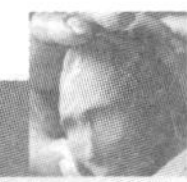

Ethical Reflections

- Compare Plato's allegory of the cave to critical thinking in nursing.
- Think of a few personal examples of when you have been "chained in the cave." What were the circumstances? What were the outcomes? What made a difference in your thinking?

are social beings whose reasoning should lead them to be good citizens, good friends, and to act in moderate ways.

The Middle Ages

After the Roman Empire was divided by barbarians (c. 476 C.E.), the golden age of intellectualism and cultural progress in Western Europe ended. The next historical period was the Middle or Dark Ages, which lasted until about 1500 C.E. In the gap left by the failed political system of Rome, Christianity became the dominant religion in Western Europe as the Catholic Church took on the powerful role of educating the European people. Christianity is a monotheistic (one God), revelatory religion, whereas ancient Greek philosophy was based on the use of reason and polytheism (many gods). Because Greek philosophy was believed to be heretical, its examination was discouraged during the Church-dominated Middle Ages. However, it is interesting that two Catholic saints, Augustine and Aquinas, who provided the major ethical influence during the Middle Ages, were both influenced by the ancient Greeks.

St. Augustine (354–430 C.E.) is often considered to be the Plato of the Middle Ages. Though Augustine was a Christian and Plato was a non-Christian, Augustine's belief in a heavenly place of unchanging moral truths is similar to Plato's belief in the realm of ideal Forms. Augustine believed that these Truths are imprinted by God on the soul of each human being. According to Augustine, one has a duty to love God, and moral reasoning should direct one's senses in accordance with that duty; being subject to this obligation is what leads to moral perfection. Generally, St. Augustine believed only in the existence of good, similar to how the essence of good would exist if it was an ideal Form. Therefore, evil is present only when good is missing or has in some way been perverted from its existence as an ideal Truth.

Augustine was 56 years old when the Roman Empire fell. In one of his most famous writings, *The City of God*, Augustine used the fall of the Roman Empire to explain a philosophy that is sometimes compared to Plato's conception of the worlds of Forms and Appearances. People who live according to the spirit live in the City of God (world of perfection/Forms), while people who live according to the flesh live in the City of Man (world of imperfection/Appearances). To move away from evil, one must have the grace of God. Humans were viewed as finite beings that must have the divine aid of grace in order to bridge the gap required to have a relationship with the infinite being of God.

The Crusades influenced Europe's exodus from the Dark Ages. When Christians entered Islamic lands, such as Spain, Portugal, and North Africa, they were reintroduced to intellectualism, including texts of the ancient Greeks, especially Aristotle. The moral teachings of St. Thomas Aquinas (1224–1274) are sometimes viewed as a Christianized version of Aristotle's ethical teachings. Aquinas tried to reconcile Aristotle's teachings with the teachings of the Catholic Church.

Like Aristotle, Aquinas believed that people have a desirable end goal or purpose and that developing excellences of character (virtues) leads to human happiness and good moral reasoning. Aristotle's non-Christian moral philosophy was based on humans moving toward an end goal or dynamic state of *eudaimonia* (happiness or well-being) through the cultivation of excellent intellect and excellent moral character.

Aquinas expanded Aristotle's conception of the end goal of perfect happiness and grounded the requirements for happiness in the knowledge and love of God and Christian virtues. Aquinas replaced Aristotle's emphasis on the virtue of pride with an emphasis on the virtue of humility. Aristotle believed that pride is an important characteristic of independent, strong men, while Aquinas valued the characteristic of humility because it represented to him one's need to depend on the benevolence of God. In addition to virtue ethics, Aquinas is associated with a belief in reasoning according to the natural law theory of ethics. Both of these ethical approaches are covered later in this chapter.

Modern Philosophy and the Age of Enlightenment

The period of modern philosophy began when the major intellectual force during the Middle Ages, the Catholic Church, began to have a diminishing influence within society, while the influence of science began to increase. The scientific revolution began in 1543 with the Copernican theory but did not rapidly advance until the 17th century, when Kepler and Galileo moved scientific debates to the forefront of society.

With these changes came a new freedom in human moral reasoning, which was based on people being autonomous, rational-thinking creatures rather than primarily being influenced and controlled by Church dogma and rules. During the 18th-century Enlightenment era, humans believed that they were coming out of the darkness of the Middle (Dark) Ages into the light of true knowledge.

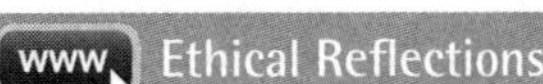

Ethical Reflections

- Identify examples of mechanistic practices in health care.
- Are all mechanistic healthcare practices bad? Why or why not?

Some scientists and philosophers were bold enough to believe that humans could ultimately be perfected and that all knowledge would be discovered. As the belief in empirical science grew, a new way of thinking was ushered in that compared both the universe and people to machines. Many scientists and philosophers believed that the world, along with its inhabitants, could be reduced through analyses into their component parts. These reductionists hoped that after most or all knowledge was discovered, the universe and human behavior could be predicted and controlled. People still demonstrate evidence of this way of thinking in health care today when *cure* is highly valued over *care*, and uncertainty is considered to be something that can be, or needs to be, eliminated in regard to health and illness. A **mechanistic approach** is one that focuses on fixing problems as if one is fixing a machine, as contrasted to a humanistic or holistic approach, in which one readily acknowledges that well-being and health occur along a complex continuum and that some situations and health problems cannot be predicted, fixed, or cured.

During the 18th century, David Hume (1711–1776) proposed an important idea about moral reasoning. Hume argued that there is a distinction between facts and values when moral reasoning is practiced. This *fact/value distinction* also has been called the *is/ought gap*. A skeptic, Hume suggested that a person should not acknowledge a fact and then make a value judgment based on that fact, as one logically cannot take a fact of what *is* and then determine an ethical judgment of what *ought to be*. If Hume's position is accepted as valid, people should not make assumptions such as: (a) if all dogs have fleas (assuming that this is a known fact), and (b) Sara is a dog (a fact), therefore, (c) Sara ought not be allowed to sleep on the sofa because having fleas on the sofa is a bad thing (a value statement). According to people who believe in the truth of the fact/value distinction, the chance of Sara spreading her fleas to the sofa might be a fact if she sleeps on it, but determining that having fleas on the sofa is a bad thing is based only on one's feelings.

Postmodern Era

After the scientific hegemony of the Enlightenment era, people began to question whether a single-minded allegiance to science was creating problems for human societies. Postmodernism often is considered to have begun around 1950, after the end of World War II. However, some people trace its beginnings back to the German philosopher Friedrich Nietzsche in the late 1800s. Pence (2000) defined **postmodernism** as "a modern movement in philosophy and the humanities that rejects the optimistic view that science and reason will improve humanity; it rejects the notion of sustained progress through reason and the scientific method" (p. 43). The postmodern mind is one that is formed by a pluralistic view, or a diversity of intellectual and cultural influences. People who live according to a postmodern philosophy acknowledge that reality is constantly changing and that scientific investigations cannot provide one grand theory or correct view of an absolute Truth that can guide human behavior, relationships, and life. Human knowledge is thought instead to be shaped by multiple factors, with storytelling and narrative analysis being viewed as core components of knowledge development.

Care-Based Versus Justice-Based Reasoning

A care approach to moral reasoning often is associated with a feminine way of thinking, and a cure approach is usually associated with a masculine, Enlightenment-era way of thinking. In 1981, Lawrence Kohlberg, a psychologist, reported his landmark research about moral reasoning based on 84 boys that he had studied for over 20 years. Based on the work of Jean Piaget, Kohlberg defined 6 stages of moral development ranging from childhood to adulthood. Interestingly, Kohlberg did not include any women in his research, but he expected that his 6-stage scale could be used to measure moral development in both males and females.

When the scale was applied to women, they seemed to score only at the third stage of the sequence, a stage in which Kohlberg described morality in terms of interpersonal relationships and helping others. Kohlberg viewed this third stage of development as somewhat deficient in regard to mature moral reasoning. Because of Kohlberg's exclusion of females in his research and his negative view of this third stage, one of Kohlberg's associates, Carol Gilligan, raised the concern of gender bias. Gilligan, in turn, published an influential book in 1982, *In a Different Voice*, in which she argued that women's moral reasoning is different, but it is not deficient. The distinction that is usually made between moral reasoning as it is suggested by Kohlberg and Gilligan is that Kohlberg's is a male-oriented ethic of justice and Gilligan's is a more feminine ethic of care (covered later in this chapter).

Learning from History

Often, it is only in hindsight that people are able to analyze a historical era in which there is a converging of norms and beliefs that are held in high esteem or valued by large groups within a society. Like the overlapping approaches used by some ethical objectivists, the influences of historical eras also build upon each other and often are hard to separate. Christians still base much of their ethical reasoning on the philosophy generated during the Middle Ages. At the same time, it is evident that individualistic ways of thinking that were popular during the Enlightenment era remain popular today in Western societies because autonomy (self-direction) is so highly valued. The varied historical influences that have affected moral reasoning, consequently, have formed a pattern of rich and interesting values, perspectives, and practices that are evident in the globally connected world that people live in today.

Ethical Theories and Approaches

Normative ethical theories and approaches function as moral guides to answer the questions, "What ought I do or not do?" and "How should I be?" A theory can provide individuals with guidance in moral thinking and reasoning, as well as provide justification for moral actions. The following theories and approaches are not all-inclusive, nor do they necessarily include all variations of the theories and approaches that are discussed.

Western Ethics

Virtue Ethics

Watch your thoughts; they become words.
Watch your words; they become actions.
Watch your actions; they become habits.
Watch your habits; they become character.
Watch your character; it becomes your destiny.

—*Frank Outlaw*

Rather than centering on what is right or wrong in terms of one's duties or the consequences of one's actions, the excellence of one's character and considerations of what sort of person one wants to be is emphasized in **virtue ethics**. Since the time of Plato and Aristotle, virtues, called *arête* in Greek, have referred to excellences in regard to persons or objects being the best that they can be in accordance with their purpose. As the ancient Greeks originally conceived the concept, even an inanimate object can have virtue. For example, the purpose of a knife is to cut, so *arête* in regard to a knife means that the knife has a sharp edge that cuts very well. If one needs the services of a knife, it is probably safe to assume that a knife that exhibits excellence in cutting would be the type of knife that one wants to use; most people want to use a knife that accomplishes its purpose in the best way possible.

For humans, virtue ethics addresses the question, "What sort of person must I be to be an excellent person?" rather than "What is my duty?" **Virtues** for humans are habitual, excellent traits that are intentionally developed throughout one's life. A person of virtue, consistent with Aristotle's way of thinking, is a person who is an excellent friend to other people, an excellent thinker, and an excellent citizen of a community.

Aristotle's (trans. 2002) approach to virtue ethics is grounded in two categories of excellence: intellectual virtues and character or moral virtues. According to Aristotle, "the intellectual sort [of virtue] mostly . . . comes into existence and increases as a result of teaching (which is why it requires experience and time), whereas excellence of character results from habituation" (p. 111). The habituation that Aristotle had in mind is an intelligent, mindful attention to excellent habits, rather than a thoughtless routinization of behaviors.

Though Aristotle divided virtues into two sorts—those of the intellect and those of character—the two categories of virtues cannot be distinctly separated. Aristotle made this point by proposing that "it is not possible to possess excellence in the primary sense [that is, having excellence of character] without wisdom, nor to be wise without excellence of character" (p. 189).

Aristotle realized that good things taken to an extreme could become bad. He therefore proposed that there is a "Golden Mean" in ways of being. Most virtues are considered to exist as a moderate way of being between two kinds of vices or faults: the extremes of excess at one end and deficiency on the other. For instance, Aristotle named courage as a virtue, but the extremes of rashness at one end of a continuum and cowardice at the other end of the same continuum are its related vices. Another example is the virtue of truthfulness, which is the mean between boastfulness and self-deprecation. The mean for each virtue is unique for each type of virtue and situation; in other words, the mean is not a mathematical average that is consistent for all virtues.

Other examples of virtues include benevolence, compassion, fidelity, generosity, and patience. Plato designated the four virtues of prudence (wisdom), fortitude (courage), temperance (moderation), and justice as cardinal virtues, meaning that all other virtues hinge on these primary four. Prudence corresponds to Plato's idea of the Faculty of Reason, fortitude corresponds to the Faculty of Spirit, and temperance corresponds to the Faculty of Appetite; the virtue of justice is an umbrella virtue that encompasses and ties together the other three.

The ancient Greeks most frequently are associated with virtue ethics, but other philosophers and ethicists also have proposed views about virtues. The Scottish philosopher David Hume (1711–1776) and the German philosopher Frederick Nietzsche (1844–1900) each proposed an interesting philosophy of virtue ethics that differs from the philosophies of the Greeks, though Hume's and Nietzsche's are not the only other approaches to virtue ethics.

Hume, whose approach is used by some feminist philosophers, believed that virtues flow from a natural human tendency to be sympathetic or benevolent toward other people. Virtues are human character traits that are admired by most people and are judged to be generally pleasing, as well as being useful to other people, useful to oneself, or useful to both other people and to oneself. Because of Hume's focus on the usefulness of virtues, his approach to ethics also is associated with utilitarianism, which is discussed later in this chapter. Hume's philosophy of ethics is based on emotion as the primary human motivator for admirable behavior, rather than motivation by reason. However, Hume did not propose that ethics is based merely on personal opinion. Virtuous behavior is validated by the consensus of members of communities according to what is useful for a whole community's well-being.

A different and more radical view of virtue ethics is based on the philosophy of Nietzsche. Rather than viewing people as caring, sympathetic beings, Nietzsche proposed that the best character for people to cultivate is based on a "will to power." Nietzsche believed that the "will to power" rightly should motivate people to achieve dominance in the world. Strength was praised as virtuous whereas "feminine" virtues, such as caring and kindness, were considered by Nietzsche to be signs of weakness. This means that, according to Nietzsche, virtue is consistent with hierarchical power or power over other people, which makes the Christian virtue

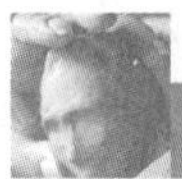

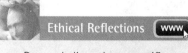

Ethical Reflections www

- Do you believe that a specific set of virtues can be identified as being essential for the nursing profession?
- If so, what are the virtues contained in the set? Why did you select them? Why are other virtues excluded?
- If you do not believe that a specific set of virtues is identifiable, defend your position.
- Partner with a colleague and list several real-life examples that are related to each line of Frank Outlaw's quotation at the beginning of the *Virtue Ethics* section.
- What do you believe might be legitimate criticisms of virtue ethics?

of humility a vice. It is believed that another German, Adolph Hitler, adopted the philosophy of Nietzsche as his worldview. Though Nietzsche is a well-known and important person in the history of philosophy, Nietzsche's approach to virtue ethics has little place in nursing ethics.

Although virtue ethics is again popular today, over the years, interest in this ethical approach experienced a significant decline among Western philosophers and nurses (MacIntyre, 1984; Tschudin, 2003). Many Western philosophers lost interest in the virtues when they became entrenched in the schools of thought popularized during the Enlightenment era that emphasize individualism and autonomy (MacIntyre, 1984).

Over time, nurses concluded that it was unfashionable to follow the tradition of Florence Nightingale because Nightingale's view of virtues in nursing included a virtue of obedience (Sellman, 1997). However, Nightingale's valuing of obedience needs to be viewed within the context of the time in which she lived. Also, Nightingale's liberal education in Greek philosophy may have influenced her use of the virtue of obedience to reflect her belief in the value of practical wisdom as conceived by Aristotle (LeVasseur, 1998; Sellman, 1997). In connecting obedience to practical wisdom, some nurses now understand that Nightingale's conception was one that approached something akin to intelligent obedience, rather than a subservient allegiance of nurses to physicians.

Natural Law Theory

> *There is in fact a true law—namely, right reason—which is in accordance with nature, applies to all men, and is unchangeable and eternal. By its commands this law summons men to the performance of their duties; by its prohibitions it restrains them from doing wrong . . .*
>
> —*Marcus Tullius Cicero,* The Republic *(51 B.C.E.)*

Natural law theory has a long and varied history, dating back to the work of Plato and Aristotle. In fact, attempting to present its essence would be to oversimplify the theory (Buckle, 1993). Even the terms *nature* and *natural* are ambiguous. Most modern versions of natural law theory have their basis in the religious philosophy of St. Thomas Aquinas. People who use natural law theory believe that the rightness of actions is self-evident because morality is inherently determined by nature, not by customs and preferences. According to this theory, the law of reason is implanted in the order of nature, and this law provides the rules or commands for human actions.

Though natural law theory and divine command theory sometimes are confused, they have a fundamental difference. According to divine command theory, an action is good because a divine being, such as God, commands it, whereas with natural law theory, a divine being commands an action because it is moral irrespective of said divine being. However, natural law theory is often associated with rule-based Judeo-Christian ethics, and it is the basis for religious prohibitions against acts that some people consider *unnatural*, such as homosexuality and the use of birth control.

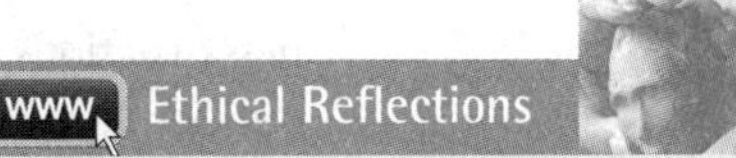

- What do you believe might be legitimate criticisms of a natural law approach to ethics?

Deontology

Deontology, literally the "study of duty," is an approach to ethics that is focused on duties and rules. The most influential philosopher associated with the deontological way of thinking was Immanuel Kant (1724–1804). Kant defined a person as a rational, autonomous (self-directed) being with the ability to know universal, objective moral laws and the freedom to decide to act morally. **Kantian deontology** prescribes that each rational being is ethically bound to act only from a sense of duty; when deciding how to act, the consequences of one's actions are considered to be irrelevant.

According to Kant, it is only through dutiful actions that people can be moral. Even when individuals do not want to act from duty, Kant believed that they are ethically bound to do so. In fact, Kant asserted that having one's actions motivated by duty is superior to acting from a motivation of love. Because rational choice is within one's control, as compared to one's tenuous control over personal emotions, Kant was convinced that only reason, and not emotion, is sufficient to lead a person to moral actions.

Kant believed that people are ends in themselves and should be treated accordingly. Each autonomous, self-directed person has dignity and is due respect, and one should never act in ways that involve using other people as a means to one's personal ends. In fact, when people use others as a means to an end, even if they believe that they are attempting to reach ethical goals, Kant believed that people could be harmed. An example of this today is the failure to obtain informed consent from a research participant even when the researcher steadfastly believes that the research will be beneficial to the participant.

Kant identified rules to guide people in thinking about their obligations. He drew a distinction between two types of duties or obligations: the hypothetical imperative and the categorical imperative. Hypothetical imperatives are optional duties or rules that people ought to observe or follow if certain ends are to be achieved. Hypothetical imperatives are sometimes called *if–then imperatives*, which means that they involve conditional or optional actions; for instance, "If I want to become a nurse, then I have to graduate from nursing school."

However, where moral actions are concerned, Kant believed that duties and laws are absolute and unconditional. Kant proposed that people ought to follow a universal, unconditional framework of maxims, or rules, as a guide to know the rightness of actions and one's moral duties. He called these absolute and unconditional duties *categorical imperatives*. When deciding about matters of ethics, one should act according to a categorical imperative and ask the question: "If I perform this action, could I will that it should become a universal law for everyone to act in the same way?" No action can ever be judged as right, according to Kant, if it is not reasonable that the action could be used as a binding, ethical law for all people. For example, Kant's ethics imposes the categorical imperative that one should never tell a lie, because a person cannot rationally wish that all people should be able to pick and choose when they have permission not to be truthful. Another example of a categorical imperative is that suicide is never acceptable. A person, when committing suicide, should not rationally wish that all people should feel free to commit suicide, or the world would become chaotic.

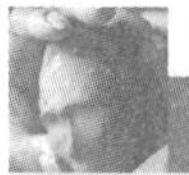

Ethical Reflections 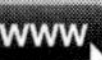

- Are there categorical imperatives (absolute duties) that nurses must follow to be ethical professionals? If so, identify examples. If not, defend your answer.
- Answer the following question and provide philosophical support for your answer: Is it more important for a nurse to have a virtuous character or to be dutiful?
- Review the ANA's (2001) *Code of Ethics* in the appendix. Is the code based on a deontological approach to nursing? Is it based on a virtue ethics approach? Discuss specific examples in the code that support your answers.
- What do you believe might be legitimate criticisms of deontological ethics?

Consequentialism

Consequentialists, as distinguished from deontologists, do consider consequences to be an important indication of the moral value of one's actions. Utilitarianism is the most well-known consequentialist theory of ethics. Utilitarianism means that actions are judged by their utility; that is, they are evaluated according to the usefulness of their consequences. When people use the theory of **utilitarianism** as the basis for ethical behavior, they attempt to promote the greatest good (happiness or pleasure) and to produce the least amount of harm (unhappiness, suffering, or pain) that is possible in a situation. In other words, utilitarians believe that it is useful to society to achieve "the greatest good for the greatest number" of people who may be affected by an action.

The British philosopher Jeremy Bentham (1748–1832), a contemporary and associate of Florence Nightingale's father, was an early promoter of the principle of utilitarianism. During Bentham's life, British society functioned according to aristocratic privilege. Poor people were mistreated by people in the upper classes and were given no choice other than to work long hours in deplorable conditions. Bentham tried to develop a theory that could be used to achieve a fair distribution of pleasure among all British citizens. He went as far as to develop a systematic decision-making method using mathematical calculations. Bentham's method was designed to determine ways to allocate pleasure and to diminish pain by using the measures of intensity and duration, though his approach to utilitarianism has been criticized because he equated all types of pleasure as being equal.

Another Englishman, John Stuart Mill (1806–1873), challenged Bentham's views when he clearly pointed out that particular experiences of pleasure and happiness do have different qualities, and that different situations do not necessarily produce equal consequences. For example, Mill stated that the higher intellectual pleasures may be differentiated from lower physical pleasures. The higher pleasures, such as enjoying a work of art or a scholarly book, are considered to be better because only human beings, not other animals, possess the mental faculties to enjoy this higher level of happiness.

According to Mill, happiness and pleasure are measured by quality and not quantity (duration or intensity). In making these distinctions between higher and lower levels of happiness and pleasure, Mill's philosophy is focused more on ethics than politics and social utility: each person's happiness is equally important.

Mill believed that communities usually agree about what is good and about the things that best promote the well-being of the most people. An example of an application of Mill's utilitarianism is the use of mandatory vaccination laws—individual liberties are limited so that the larger society is protected from diseases, and the consequence is that people generally are happier because they are free of diseases. People using Mill's form of utilitarian theory often can use widely supported traditions to guide them in deciding about rules and behaviors that probably will produce the best consequences for the most people, such as the maxim that stealing is wrong. Through experience, humans have generally identified many behaviors that will produce the most happiness or unhappiness for society as a whole.

Over time, people subscribing to a theory of utilitarianism generally have divided themselves into subgroups. Two types of utilitarianism that have developed over the years are rule utilitarianism and act utilitarianism. **Rule utilitarians** believe that there are certain rules—such as do not kill, do not break promises, and do not lie—that, when followed, generally create the best consequences for the most people. Based on this definition, someone might ask, "What is the difference between rule utilitarianism and deontology?" The answer is that all utilitarian theories of ethics, whether based on rules or individual actions, are predicated on achieving good consequences for the most people. Deontologists, on the other hand, make decisions based on right duty rather than on right consequences.

Act utilitarians believe that each action in a particular circumstance should be chosen based on its likely good consequences rather than on following an inherently moral, universal rule. The utility of each action in achieving the most happiness is the aim of act utilitarians, while rule utilitarians are willing to accept causing more suffering than happiness in a particular situation to avoid violating a generalized rule. For example, promise-breaking is permitted according to act utilitarianism if

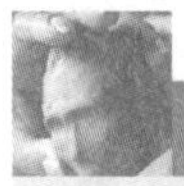

Ethical Reflections www

- Achieving the greatest good for the greatest number of people is an essential principle of public health nursing. Can you identify examples of utilitarian ethics in the ANA's (2001) *Code of Ethics for Nurses* in the appendix? If so, list examples.
- Identify specific situations in which nurses need to use a utilitarian approach to nursing care.
- What do you believe might be legitimate criticisms of utilitarian or consequentialist ethics?

the consequences of the action (breaking a promise) cause more happiness than suffering in a particular situation. In the same situation, a rule utilitarian would say that a promise should be upheld because, in most cases, promise-keeping causes more happiness than suffering.

Prima Facie Rights

The term *prima facie* means that on one's first impression ("on the face of things"), something is accepted as correct until or unless it is shown to be otherwise. For example, promise-keeping is considered to be an accepted ethical rule. However, if a nurse had promised her spouse that she would be on time for dinner, but as she was about to leave the hospital she was told that the nurse replacing her will be late for work, it is expected that the nurse would break her promise to be on time for dinner so that she could attend to her patients until the other nurse arrives.

Prima facie ethics is associated with the philosopher Sir William David Ross (1877–1971) and his 1930 book, *The Right and the Good.* Ross is called an ethical intuitionist because he believed that certain things are intrinsically good and self-evidently true. Ross understood ethics to suggest that certain acts are *prima facie* good: keeping promises, repaying kindnesses, helping others, and preventing distress. However, when these *prima facie* good actions conflict, one has to decide where one's actual duty lies. Ross conceded that human knowledge is imperfect and that the best that people can expect to do is to use their imperfect knowledge to assess the context of each situation and to make an informed judgment, although they are uncertain about the correctness of their choices.

Ross's approach to ethics has quite a bit of relevance for nurses, who frequently must make quick determinations of how to prioritize important actions that can cause distress for one person while helping another. See Box 1.3 for a case example.

Principlism

Principles are rule-based criteria for conduct that naturally flow from the identification of obligations and duties. Consequently, the theory of deontology, discussed earlier in this chapter, is a forerunner of the approach of principlism. Principles usually are reducible to concepts or statements, such as the principle of beneficence or the respect for a person's autonomy. Principles often are used as the basis for ethically related documents, such as documents that reflect positions about human rights. Examples of principle-based documents include the American Hospital Association's (2003) "The Patient Care Partnership" and the Universal Declaration

BOX 1.3 ETHICAL FORMATIONS: PRIMA FACIE RIGHTS

Suzie has been Mrs. G.'s nurse for several years because Mrs. G. frequently is admitted to the hospital where Suzie works. Suzie and Mrs. G. have developed a close relationship based on trust and respect. During this admission, Mrs. G.'s condition has been deteriorating, and she has elected to initiate a Do Not Attempt Resuscitation (DNAR) order. Today, she is experiencing agonal breathing and is nearing death. On a number of occasions, Mrs. G. stated that she is scared of dying and asked Suzie to promise to be with her when she dies, if she is working at the time. Mrs. G.'s daughter is scared and alone with Mrs. G. in her hospital room. While Mrs. G. progresses toward an imminent death, Suzie's newly post-operative patient suddenly and unexpectedly has a seizure and experiences a respiratory arrest and circulatory collapse. Suzie just met this patient when he returned from surgery earlier in the morning. The patient's wife is hysterical. As the patient's primary nurse, Suzie begins to go into action caring for the post-op patient and coordinating the Code Blue. A nursing assistant comes to Suzie and tells her that Mrs. G. is about to die.

- What should Suzie do?
- Explain the rationale for your decision.

of Human Rights, formulated in 1948 by the United Nations. Because principlism is so popular in the field of bioethics, this approach is discussed in Chapter 2.

Casuistry

Casuistry is an approach to ethics that is based in Judeo-Christian history. When people use **casuistry**, they make decisions inductively based on individual cases. The analysis and evaluation of strongly similar or outstanding cases (i.e., paradigm cases) provides guidance in ethical decision making. When people use casuistry, their ethical decision making begins as a bottom-up approach considering the details of specific cases, rather than beginning from the top down and applying absolute rules and principles. Long ago, Jewish people often tried to sort out the relevance of sacred laws in specific situations in ways that were practical and case based rather than absolute and inflexibly rule based. In Catholic history, the practice of persons individually confessing their sins to priests to receive absolution reflects the use of casuistry. Based on the confessor's specific case (i.e., the circumstances surrounding the occasion of sinning) a person receives a personal penance from the priest that is required for absolution.

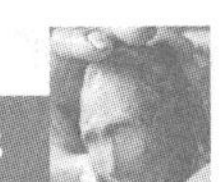

WWW Ethical Reflections

- Conduct an Internet search for landmark cases in healthcare ethics.
- Summarize two important cases.
- How have these two cases affected subsequent healthcare ethics decisions and debates?
- What do you believe might be legitimate criticisms of casuistry as an approach to ethics?

Today, casuistry is often the method used by healthcare ethics committees to analyze the ethical issues surrounding specific patient cases. The Four Topics

Method of ethical decision making that is discussed in Chapter 2 is based on a casuistry approach.

Narrative Ethics

> *There are stories and stories. There are the songs, also, that are taught. Some are whimsical. Some are very intense. Some are documentary. Everything I have known is through teachings, by word of mouth, either by song or by legends.*
>
> —*Terrance Honvantewa, Hopi (as cited in Cleary, 1996, p. 40)*

Because it is a story-based approach, narrative ethics has similarities to casuistry. Also, according to one of the foremost modern-day virtue ethicists, Alasdair MacIntyre (1984), narrative thinking and virtue ethics are closely connected. Both narrative ethics and virtue ethics are firmly embedded in human relationships. MacIntyre proposed that a human is "essentially a story-telling animal"; a person is "a teller of stories that aspire to truth" (p. 216). Narratives, such as novels and literary stories, change us in remarkable ways (Murray, 1997). Most people from childhood obtain moral education about character development from stories such as fairy tales and fables. When using a **narrative** approach to ethics, nurses are open to learning from a storied, nuanced view of life; that is, they are sensitive to how personal and community stories evolve, are constructed, and can be changed. Narratives are stories that are being lived, read, watched, heard, discussed, analyzed, or compared.

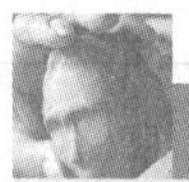

Ethical Reflections www

Discuss several specific stories in books and movies that have affected your moral views.

Obtain a copy of one or all of the following children's books:

- "The Three Questions" by Jon J. Muth
- "Stone Soup" by Jon J. Muth
- An original edition of "The Little Engine that Could" by Watty Piper
- "Old Turtle" by Douglas Wood

Identify themes and symbolism in the story.

Apply the themes and symbolism to nursing, including the nursing meta-paradigm of person, health, environment, and nursing.

As much as possible, apply the information in Chapter 1 to these stories.

- What do you believe might be legitimate criticisms of a narrative approach to ethics?

Narratives are very context or situation bound. For people to decide what they should do in particular circumstances, they may first identify how their moral character and actions fit within the greater stories of their culture. People are situated within their personal life narratives and their stories intersect with and are interwoven into the narratives of other people with whom they interact. Nurses who use narrative ethics are aware that there is much more to a patient's story than is usually known or discussed among healthcare providers. People are not solitary creatures, and as they interact with other people and their environment, they must make choices about what they believe and how they will act. They create their own stories.

When using a narrative approach to ethics, nurses realize that individual human stories are being constantly constructed in relation to the stories of a greater community of people. In nursing, a good example of narrative ethics involves nurses encountering each patient's unfolding life story in everyday practice with sensitive awareness. These nurses know that their actions while caring for patients influence the unfolding stories of those patients in both large and small ways. A "narrative approach to bioethics focuses on the patients themselves: these are the moral agents who enact choices" (Charon & Montello, 2002, p. xi). In narrative ethics, patients' and nurses' stories matter; however, no one story should be accepted without critical reflection.

Critical Theory

Critical theory, sometimes referred to as critical social theory, is a broad term that identifies theories and worldviews that address the domination perpetrated by specific powerful groups of people and the resulting oppression of other specific groups of people. There are a number of different critical theories that are included under the one broad heading. In citing the group of German philosophers who originated the concept of critical theory, Bohman (2005) stated that critical theories can be distinguished from traditional theories because the purpose of critical theories is to promote human emancipation. Specifically, the purpose of using critical theories is "to liberate human beings from the circumstances that enslave them" (Horkheimer, 1982, p. 244, as cited in Bohman, 2005, para. 1). According to Brookfield (2005), there are three core assumptions in critical theory that explain how the world is organized. Critical theory purports:

1. That apparently open, Western democracies are actually highly unequal societies in which economic inequity, racism, and class discrimination are empirical realities.
2. That the way this state of affairs is reproduced and seems to be normal, natural, and inevitable (thereby heading off potential challenges to the system) is through the dissemination of dominant ideology.
3. That critical theory attempts to understand this state of affairs as a necessary prelude to changing it. (p. viii)

One critical theory that is widely used by nurses is a feminist approach to ethics. Under this broad feminist approach is the ethic of care that originated from the Gilligan–Kohlberg debate that was discussed earlier in this chapter.

WWW Ethical Reflections

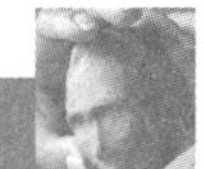

- In what areas of nursing can critical theory be applied? To which populations?
- What do you believe might be legitimate criticisms of using a critical theory approach to ethics?
- Do you believe that *caring* is a virtue? Support your answer.

Feminist Ethics

According to Tong (1997), "to a greater or lesser degree, all feminist approaches to ethics are filtered through the lens of gender" (p. 37). This means that **feminist ethics** is specifically focused on evaluating ethically related situations in terms of how these situations affect women. The concept of feminist ethics tends to have a political connotation and addresses the patterns of women's oppression as this oppression is perpetrated by dominant social groups, especially socially powerful men.

An ethic of care is grounded in the moral experiences of women and feminist ethics. It evolved into an approach to ethics that gained popularity because of the Gilligan–Kohlberg debate about the differences in women's and men's approaches to moral reasoning. Rather than being based on duty, fairness, impartiality, or objective principles (ethic of justice) similar to the values that were popularized during the Enlightenment era, an **ethic of care** emphasizes the importance of traditionally feminine traits such as love, compassion, sympathy, and concern about the well-being of other people. The natural partiality in how people care more about some people as compared to others is acknowledged as being acceptable in an ethic of care. Also, the role of emotions in moral reasoning and behavior is accepted as being a necessary and natural complement to rational thinking. This position distinguishes an ethic of care from an ethic of justice and duty-based ethics that emphasize the preeminence of reason and minimize the importance of emotion in guiding moral reasoning and the moral nature of one's relationships.

Eastern Ethics

Ethics in Asian societies has similarities to and important differences from Western ethics. In both cultures, ethics often is intertwined with spiritual or religious thinking, but ethics in Eastern societies is usually indistinguishable from general Eastern philosophies. Both Eastern and Western philosophies of ethics examine human nature and what is needed for people to move toward well-being. However, some of the differences in the two cultural systems are quite interesting and distinct.

Whereas the goal of Western ethics is generally for people to achieve self-direction and to understand themselves personally, the goal of Eastern ethics often is to understand universal interconnections (see Box 1.4), to be liberated from the self, or to understand that people really do not consist of a self at all (Zeuschner, 2001). Ethics viewed from Christian or other theological perspectives tends to be based on a belief in human flaws that require an intermediary (God) to transcend these imperfections. Eastern ethical systems usually are focused on individuals' innate but unrecognized perfection and the ability to transcend earthly suffering and dissatisfaction through one's own abilities. Therefore, Eastern ethics is not imposed from outside of a person, but instead is imposed from within oneself. Eastern ethics tends to be a discipline of training the mind, and unethical behavior leads to karmic results (i.e., the quality of one's actions results in fair consequences according to the universal law of cause and effect). The four largest Eastern ethical systems, which contain myriad variations and now exist in a number of different countries, are Indian ethics (Hinduism and Buddhism) and Chinese ethics (Taoism and Confucianism).

Indian Ethics

Hinduism

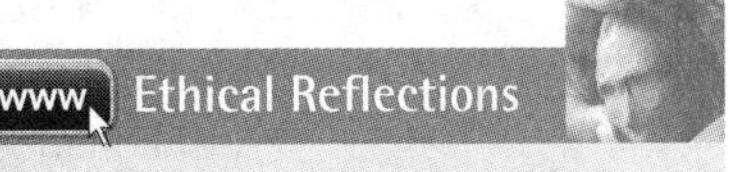

- How is the story about the Net of Indra in Box 1.4 related to ethics?

Hinduism is an ancient ethical system. It originated with writings called the Vedas (c. 2000 to 1000 B.C.E.), which include magical, religious, and philosophical teachings, that existed long before the well-known ethical philosophy of the ancient Greeks. The main emphasis in Hindu ethics is cosmic unity. Because of reincarnation, people are stuck in *maya*, an illusory, everyday, impermanent experience. The quality of one's past actions, *karma*, influences one's present existence and future incarnations or rebirths. Therefore, people need to improve the goodness of their actions, which will subsequently improve their karma. Liberation, *moksha*, means that the soul of each person is no longer reincarnated but becomes one with the desirable cosmic or universal self, *atman*, and the absolute reality of *Brahman*.

Buddhism

The historical Buddha, Siddhartha Gautama (6th century B.C.E.) was a Hindu prince. Because Siddhartha's father wanted to prevent the fulfillment of a prophecy that Siddhartha might become a spiritual teacher, he tried to shield his son from the world outside of his palace. However, Siddhartha left the confinement of his palace and saw in his fellow human beings the suffering associated with sickness, old age, and death. He decided to devote his life to understanding and ending suffering.

The Buddha's core teachings, the teachings that all Buddhist sects profess, are called the Four Noble Truths. The First Noble Truth is that unsatisfactoriness or suffering (*dukkha*) exists as a part of all forms of existence. This suffering is different from the common Western notion of physical or mental misery; suffering in a Buddhist sense, for example, arises when people are ego-centered and cling to their impermanent existence and impermanent things. Suffering is emphasized in Buddhism, not to suggest a negative outlook toward life but instead as a realistic assessment of the human condition. The Second and Third Noble Truths suggest

BOX 1.4 ETHICAL FORMATIONS: THE NET OF INDRA

The Buddhist Avatamsaka Sutra contains a story about how all perceiving, thinking beings are connected in a way that is similar to a universal community. The story is about the heavenly net of the god Indra. "In the heaven of Indra, there is said to be a network of pearls, so arranged that if you look at one you see all the others reflected in it. In the same way each object in the world is not merely itself but involves every other object and in fact is everything else. In every particle of dust there is present Buddhas without number."

—Sir Charles Eliot, as cited in Capra, 1999

that the cause of suffering is attachment (clinging or craving) to impermanent things and that suffering can be transcended (enlightenment). The Fourth Noble Truth contains the path for transforming suffering into enlightenment or liberation. This path is called the Eightfold Path, and it is composed of eight right practices: Right View, Right Thinking, Right Mindfulness, Right Speech, Right Action, Right Diligence, Right Concentration, and Right Livelihood.

Because of the central place of virtues in Buddhist philosophy, one interpretation of Buddhist ethics is to identify Buddhism as an ethic of virtue. There are four virtues that are singled out by Buddhists as being immeasurable because, when these virtues are cultivated, it is believed that they will grow in a way that can encompass and transform the whole world. The Four Immeasurable Virtues are compassion (*karuna*), loving-kindness (*metta*), sympathetic joy (*mudita*), and equanimity (*upekkha*).

Chinese Ethics

The two most influential Chinese ethical systems were developed between 600 and 200 B.C.E. during a time of social chaos in China. The two systems are Taoism and Confucianism.

Taoism

The beginning of Taoism is attributed to Lao-tzu (c. 571 B.C.E.), who wrote the Taoist guide to life, the *Tao Te Ching*. The word *Tao* is translated in English as *way* or *path*, meaning the natural order or harmony of all things. Like Buddhists, Taoists do not believe in a creator God. Instead, Taoists have a very simple perspective toward reality—the underlying purpose of humans and the underlying purpose of nature cannot be separated. Based on the cyclic nature of life observed by ancient Chinese farmers, Taoist philosophy underscores the flux and balance of nature through *yin* (dark) and *yang* (light) elements. Living well or living ethically is living authentically, simply, and unselfishly in harmony and oneness with nature.

Confucianism

K'ung Fu-tzu (551–479 B.C.E.), who was later called Confucius by Christians visiting China, originated the Confucian ethical system. The teachings of Confucian ethics are generally contained in the moral maxims and sayings attributed to K'ung Fu-tzu, along with the later writings of his followers. Confucian ethics is described through the concepts of *li* and *yi* (Zeuschner, 2001). *Li* provides guidance in regard to social order and how humans should relate to one another, including rules of etiquette, such as proper greetings and social rituals. *Yi* emphasizes the importance of one's motivations toward achieving rightness rather than emphasizing consequences. Sincerity, teamwork, and balance are critically important to ethical behavior. The primary virtue of Confucian ethics is *jen*, which is translated in English as benevolence or human goodness. Overall, Confucianism is a communitarian ethical system in which social goals, the good of society, and the importance of human relationships are valued.

KEY POINTS

- Ethics refers to the analysis of matters of right and wrong, whereas morals refer to actual beliefs and behaviors. However, the terms often are used interchangeably.
- Values refer to judgments about what one believes is good or what makes something desirable. Values influence how a person's character is developed and how people think and subsequently behave.
- Normative ethics is an attempt to decide or prescribe values, behaviors, and ways of being that are right or wrong, good or bad, admirable or deplorable. When doing normative ethics, people ask questions such as: How ought humans behave? What should I do? and What sort of person should I be?
- Ethical thinking, valuing, and reasoning generally fall along a continuum between ethical relativism and ethical objectivism.
- The study of values and ways of moral reasoning throughout history can be useful for people living in the 21st century. Specific values and ways of moral reasoning tend to overlap and converge over time.
- Virtue ethics emphasizes the excellence of one's character.
- Deontological ethics emphasizes one's duty rather than the consequences of one's actions.
- Utilitarian ethics emphasizes the consequences of one's actions in regard to achieving the most good for the most people that may be affected by a rule or action.
- Eastern philosophies and systems of ethics often are inseparable.

References

American Nurses Association. (2001). *Code of ethics for nurses with interpretive statements.* Silver Spring, MD: Author.

Beauchamp, T. L., & Childress, J. F. (2009). *Principles of biomedical ethics* (6th ed.). New York, NY: Oxford University Press.

Billington, R. (2003). *Living philosophy: An introduction to moral thought* (3rd ed.). London, UK: Routledge—Taylor & Francis Group.

Bohman, J. (2005). Critical theory. In E. N. Zalta (Ed.), *The Stanford encyclopedia of philosophy.* Retrieved from http://plato.stanford.edu/archives/spr2005/entries/critical-theory/

Brannigan, M. C., & Boss, J. A. (2001). *Healthcare ethics in a diverse society.* Mountain View, CA: Mayfield.

Brookfield, S. D. (2005). *The power of critical theory: Liberating adult learning and teaching.* San Francisco, CA: Jossey-Bass.

Buckle, S. (1993). Natural law. In P. Singer (Ed.), *A companion to ethics* (pp. 161–174). Malden, MA: Blackwell.

Capra, F. (1999). *The Tao of physics* (4th ed.). Boston, MA: Shambhala.

Charon, R., & Montello, M. (2002). Introduction: The practice of narrative ethics. In R. Charon & M. Montello (Eds.), *Stories matter* (pp. ix–xii). New York, NY: Routledge.

Cleary, K. M. (1996). *Native American wisdom.* New York, NY: Barnes & Noble Books.

Donahue, M. P. (1996). *Nursing the finest art: An illustrated history* (2nd ed.). St. Louis, MO: Mosby.

Gilligan, C. (1982). *In a different voice: Psychological theory and women's development.* Cambridge, MA: Harvard University Press.

Hope, T. (2004). *Medical ethics: A very short introduction.* New York, NY: Oxford University Press.

LeVasseur, J. (1998). Plato, Nightingale, and contemporary nursing. *Image: Journal of Nursing Scholarship, 30*(3), 281–285.

MacIntyre, A. (1984). *After virtue: A study of moral theory* (2nd ed.). Notre Dame, IN: University of Notre Dame Press.

Murray, T. H. (1997). What do we mean by "narrative ethics"? *Medical Humanities Review, 11*(2), 44–57.

Pence, G. (2000). *A dictionary of common philosophical terms.* New York, NY: McGraw-Hill.

Ross, W. D. (1930/2002). *The right and the good.* Oxford, UK: Oxford University Press. (Original work published 1930)

Sellman, D. (1997). The virtues in the moral education of nurses: Florence Nightingale revisited. *Nursing Ethics, 4*(1), 3–11.

Tong, R. (1997). *Feminist approaches to bioethics: Theoretical reflections and practical applications.* Boulder, CO: Westview Press.

Tschudin, V. (Ed.). (2003). *Approaches to ethics: Nursing beyond boundaries.* Edinburgh, UK: Butterworth-Heinemann.

Zeuschner, R. B. (2001). *Classical ethics East and West: Ethics from a comparative perspective.* Boston, MA: McGraw-Hill.

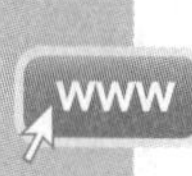

For a full suite of assignments and additional learning activities, use the access code located in the front of your book to visit this exclusive website: http://go.jblearning.com/butts. If you do not have an access code, you can obtain one at the site.

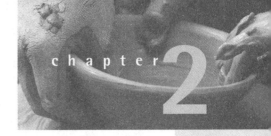

chapter 2

Introduction to Bioethics and Ethical Decision Making

Karen L. Rich

The tiniest hair casts a shadow.

—*Johann Wolfgang von Goethe, German poet and dramatist (1749–1832)*

OBJECTIVES

www

After reading this chapter, the reader should be able to:

1. Discuss the history of bioethics.
2. Use the approach of ethical principlism in nursing practice.
3. Analyze bioethical issues in practice and from news media.
4. Identify the criteria that define an ethical dilemma.
5. Consider how critical thinking is used in ethical nursing practice.
6. Use selected models of reflection and decision making in ethical nursing practice.

Introduction to Bioethics

The terms bioethics and healthcare ethics sometimes are used interchangeably. **Bioethics**, born out of the rapidly expanding technical environment of the 1900s, is a specific domain of ethics that is focused on moral issues in the field of health care. During World War II, President Franklin D. Roosevelt assembled a committee to improve medical scientists' coordination in addressing the medical needs of the military (Jonsen, 2000). As often happens with wartime research and advancements, the work aimed at addressing military needs also affected civilian sectors, such as the field of medicine.

> Between 1945 and 1965, antibiotic, antihypertensive, antipsychotic, and cancer drugs came into common medical use; surgery entered the heart and the brain; organ transplantation was initiated; and life-sustaining mechanical devices, the dialysis machine, the pacemaker, and the ventilator were invented. (Jonsen, 2000, p. 99)

However, with these advances also came increased responsibility and distress among healthcare professionals. Patients who would have died in the past began to have a lingering, suffering existence. Healthcare professionals were faced with trying to decide how to allocate newly developed, scarce medical resources. During the 1950s, scientists and medical professionals began meeting to discuss these confusing problems. Eventually, healthcare policies and laws were enacted to address questions of "Who lives, Who dies, and Who decides?" A new field of study was developed that was called *bioethics*, a term that first appeared in the literature in 1969 (Jonsen, 1998, 2000, 2005). Key events in the early days of bioethics are listed in Box 2.1.

Ethical Principles

Because shocking information surfaced about serious ethical lapses, such as the heinous World War II Nazi medical experiments in Europe and the unethical Tuskegee research in the United States (see Box 2.2), societies around the world

BOX 2.1 ETHICAL FORMATIONS: EARLY EVENTS IN BIOETHICS

August 19, 1947: The Nuremberg trials of Nazi doctors who conducted heinous medical experiments during WWII begin.
April 25, 1953: Watson and Crick publish a one-page paper about DNA.
December 23, 1954: First renal transplant.
March 9, 1960: First use of chronic hemodialysis.
December 3, 1967: First heart transplant by Dr. Christiaan Barnard.
August 5, 1968: Definition of brain death developed by an ad hoc committee at Harvard Medical School.
July 26, 1972: Revelations appear about the unethical Tuskegee syphilis research.
January 22, 1973: Roe v. Wade.
April 14, 1975: A comatose Karen Ann Quinlan was brought to Newton Memorial Hospital; she becomes the basis of a landmark legal case about the removal of life support.
July 25, 1978: Baby Louise Brown was born, the first "test-tube baby."
Spring 1982: Baby Doe becomes the basis of a landmark case that resulted in legal and ethical directives about the treatment of impaired neonates.
December 1982: The first artificial heart was implanted into the body of Barney Clark who, thereafter, lived 112 days.
April 11, 1983: *Newsweek* publishes a story that a mysterious disease called AIDS is at epidemic levels.

Source: Jonsen, A. R. (2000). *A short history of medical ethics.* New York, NY: Oxford University Press, pp. 99–114.

BOX 2.2 ETHICAL FORMATIONS: RESEARCH ETHICS

During the late 1920s in the United States, syphilis rates were extremely high in some areas. The private Rosenwald Foundation teamed with the United States Public Health Service (USPHS) to begin efforts to control the disease using the drug Neosalvarsan, an arsenic compound. Macon County, Alabama, particularly the town of Tuskegee, was targeted because of its high rate of syphilis, as identified through a survey. However, the Great Depression derailed the plans and the private foundation withdrew from the work. The USPHS repeated the Rosenwald survey in Macon County and identified a syphilis rate of 22% among African American men in the county and a 62% rate of congenital syphilis cases. The natural history (progression) of syphilis had not been studied yet in the United States, and the Surgeon General suggested that 399 African American men with syphilis in Tuskegee should be observed, rather than treated, and compared with a group of 200 African American men who were uninfected. The men were not told about the particular details of their disease. They underwent painful, nontherapeutic spinal taps to provide data about the natural history of syphilis and were told that these procedures were treatments for "bad blood." The men were given free meals, medical treatment for diseases other than their syphilis, and free burials. Even after penicillin was discovered in the 1940s, the men were not offered treatment. In fact, the USPHS researchers arranged to keep the uninformed study participants out of WWII, because the men would have been tested for syphilis, treated with penicillin, and lost from the study. The unethical research continued for 40 years, from 1932 to 1972. During the 40 years of research, an astonishing number of articles about the study were published in medical journals and no attempt was made to hide the surreptitious terms of the research. Yet no one intervened to stop the travesty. Finally, a medical reporter learned of the study and the ethical issues were exposed.

After reading Chapter 2 and researching more information on the Internet about the Tuskegee research, answer the following questions:

1. What were the main social issues with ethical implications that were involved with this study? For example, was racism an issue?
2. Which bioethical principles were violated by the Tuskegee study? Explain.
3. How does Kantian ethics relate to the Tuskegee study? See Chapter 1.
4. What procedures are in place today to prevent this type of unethical research?

became very conscious of the ethical pitfalls in conducting biomedical and behavioral research. In the United States, the National Research Act became law in 1974, and a commission was created to outline the underlying principles that must be supported during research involving human subjects (National Institutes of Health, 1979). In 1976, to carry out their charge, the commission held an intensive four-day meeting at the Belmont Conference Center at the Smithsonian Institute. Thereafter, discussions continued until 1978, when the commission released its report, called the Belmont Report.

The report outlined three basic principles for all human subjects research: respect for persons, beneficence, and justice (National Institutes of Health, 1979).

The principle of beneficence, as set forth in the Belmont Report, is the rule to do good. However, the description of beneficence also included the rule that is now commonly known as the principle of nonmaleficence—that is, to do no harm. The report contained guidelines regarding how to apply the principles in research through informed consent, the assessment of risks and benefits to research participants, and the selection of research participants.

In 1979, as an outgrowth of the Belmont Report, Beauchamp and Childress published the first edition of their book, *Principles of Biomedical Ethics*, which featured four bioethical principles: autonomy, nonmaleficence, beneficence, and justice. Currently, the book is in its sixth edition, and the principle of autonomy is described as respect for autonomy.

Doing ethics based on the use of principles—that is, ethical principlism—does not involve the use of a theory or a formal decision-making model; rather, ethical principles provide guidelines that can be used to make justified moral decisions and to evaluate the morality of actions. Ideally, when using the approach of principlism, no one principle should automatically be assumed to be superior to the other principles. Each principle is considered to be *prima facie* binding; see Chapter 1 for a discussion and examples of the term *prima facie.*

Some people have criticized the use of ethical principlism because they believe that it is a top-down approach that does not include allowances for the context of individual cases and stories. Critics contend that simply applying principles when making ethical determinations results in what might be described as a linear way of doing ethics—that is, the fine nuances present in relationship-based situations are not considered adequately. Nevertheless, the approach of ethical principlism using the four principles outlined by Beauchamp and Childress (2009) has become one of the most popular tools used today for analyzing and resolving bioethical problems.

Autonomy

Autonomy is the freedom and ability to act in a self-determined manner. It represents the right of a rational person to express personal decisions independent of outside interference and to have these decisions honored. It can be argued that autonomy occupies a central place in Western healthcare ethics because of the popularity of the Enlightenment-era philosophy of Immanuel Kant. However, it is noteworthy that autonomy is not emphasized in an ethic of care and virtue ethics, and these also are popular approaches to ethics today (see Chapter 1).

The principle of autonomy sometimes is described as respect for autonomy (Beauchamp & Childress, 2009). In the domain of health care, respecting a patient's autonomy includes obtaining informed consent for treatment; facilitating and supporting patients' choices regarding treatment options; allowing patients to refuse treatments; disclosing comprehensive and truthful information, diagnoses, and treatment options to patients; and maintaining privacy and confidentiality.

Respecting autonomy also is important in less obvious situations, such as allowing home care patients to choose a tub bath versus a shower when it is safe to do so and allowing an elderly long-term care resident to choose her favorite foods when they are medically prescribed. In fact, if the elder is competent and has been properly informed about the risks, she has the right to choose to eat foods that are not medically prescribed. Restrictions on an individual's autonomy may occur in cases where a person presents a potential threat for harming others, such as exposing other people to communicable diseases or committing acts of violence; people generally lose the right to exercise autonomy or self-determination in such instances.

Respecting patients' autonomy is important, but it also is important for nurses to receive respect for their professional autonomy. In considering how the language that nurses choose defines the profession's place in health care, Munhall (2007) used the word autonomy (*auto-no-my*) as an example. She reflected on how infants and children first begin to express themselves through nonverbal signs, such as laughing, crying, and pouting, but by the time children reach the age of two, they usually "have learned to treasure the word *no*" (p. 40). Munhall calls the word *no* "one of the most important words in any language" (p. 40). Being willing and able to say *no* is part of exercising one's autonomy.

Informed Consent

Informed consent in regard to a patient's treatment is a legal, as well as an ethical, issue of autonomy. At the heart of **informed consent** is respecting a person's autonomy to make personal choices based on the appropriate appraisal of information about the actual and/or potential circumstances of a situation. Though all conceptions of informed consent must contain the same basic elements, the description of these elements is presented differently by different people. Beauchamp and Childress (2009) have outlined informed consent according to seven elements (see Box 2.3). Dempski (2009) presented three basic elements necessary for informed consent to occur:

1. Receipt of information: Includes receiving a description of the procedure, information about the risks and benefits of having or not having the treatment, reasonable alternatives to the treatment, probabilities about outcomes, and "the credentials of the person who will perform the treatment" (p. 78). Because it is too demanding to inform a patient of every possible risk or benefit involved with every treatment or procedure, the obligation is to inform the person about the information that a reasonable person would want and need to know. Information should be tailored specifically to a person's personal circumstances, including providing information in the person's spoken language.
2. Consent for the treatment must be voluntary: A person should not be under any influence or be coerced to provide consent. This means that patients should not be asked to sign a consent form when they are under

the influence of mind-altering medications, such as narcotics. Depending on the circumstances, consent may be verbalized, written, or implied by behavior. Silence does not convey consent when a reasonable person would normally offer another sign of agreement.

3. Persons must be competent: Persons must be able to communicate consent and to understand the information provided to them. If a person's condition warrants transferring decision-making authority to a surrogate, informed consent obligations must be met with the surrogate.

It is neither ethical nor legal for a nurse to be responsible for obtaining informed consent for procedures that are performed by a physician (Dempski, 2009). Nurses may need to display the virtue of courage if physicians attempt to delegate this responsibility to them. Though both nurses and physicians in some circumstances may believe that nurses are well versed in assuring that the elements of informed consent are met for medical or surgical invasive treatments or procedures performed by a physician, nurses must refrain from accepting this responsibility. On the other hand, it is certainly within a nurse's domain of responsibility to help identify a suitable person to provide informed consent if a patient is not competent; to verify that a patient understands the information communicated, including helping to secure interpreters and/or appropriate information for the patient in the patient's spoken language (see Box 2.4); and to notify appropriate parties if the nurse knows that a patient has not given an informed consent for a procedure or treatment. In fact, it is ethically incumbent upon nurses to facilitate patients' opportunities to give informed consent. Nurses also may be legally liable if they know or should have known that informed consent was not obtained, and if nurses do not appropriately notify physicians or supervisors about this deficiency.

BOX 2.3 ETHICAL FORMATIONS: ELEMENTS OF INFORMED CONSENT

I. Threshold elements (preconditions)
  1. Competence (to understand and decide)
  2. Voluntariness (in deciding)

II. Information elements
  3. Disclosure (of material information)
  4. Recommendation (of a plan)
  5. Understanding (of 3 and 4)

III. Consent elements
  6. Decision (in favor of a plan)
  7. Authorization (of the chosen plan)

Source: Beauchamp, T. L., & Childress, J. F. (2009). *Principles of biomedical ethics* (6th ed.). New York, NY: Oxford University Press, pp. 120–121.

BOX 2.4 ETHICAL FORMATIONS: CULTURAL CONSIDERATIONS WITH INFORMED CONSENT

Mrs. Mendoza, a Hispanic woman, needed a medically necessary hysterectomy to remove a tumor. The patient's bilingual son agreed to serve as the interpreter to convey information to his mother to obtain an informed consent. It seemed that the consent process was progressing smoothly, and the patient's son even appeared to be pointing to the appropriate anatomical area when translating information for his mother. The patient willingly signed the consent form. The morning after the surgery, the patient became very upset when she realized that her uterus had been removed. The hospital staff wondered what went wrong.

The staff learned that among some Hispanic people, it is inappropriate for a male family member to discuss his mother's private parts or anything remotely related to her sexuality. In deference to the authority of the healthcare professionals, the son did not divulge his dilemma. Instead of mentioning his mother's uterus, he told her that the surgery would be performed on her abdomen. The patient threatened to sue the hospital when she realized that she could no longer have children.

- What lessons can be learned from this case?

Source: Galanti, G-A. (2008). *Caring for patients from different cultures* (4th ed.). Philadelphia, PA: University of Pennsylvania Press.

Advanced-practice nurses are legally and ethically obligated to obtain informed consent before performing risky or invasive treatments or procedures within their scope of practice. All nurses are required to explain nursing treatments and procedures to patients before performing them. If a patient understands the treatment or procedure and allows the nurse to begin the nursing care, consent has been implied. Nursing procedures do not need to meet all of the requirements of informed consent if the procedures are not risky or invasive (Dempski, 2009).

Intentional Nondisclosure

In the past, medical and nursing patient-care errors were something to be "swept under the rug" and care was taken to avoid patient discovery of these errors. When healthcare leaders realized that huge numbers of patients, as many as 98,000 per year, were dying from medical errors, the Institute of Medicine (IOM) began a project to analyze medical errors and try to reduce them. One outcome of the project is the book, *To Err Is Human: Building a Safer Health Care System* (Institute of Medicine [IOM], 2000). The IOM project committee determined that to err really is human, and that good people working within unsafe systems make the most errors.

It is now expected that errors involving serious, preventable adverse events be reported to patients, as well as to other organizational reporting systems, on a mandatory basis (IOM, 2000). Reporting "near misses" (i.e., errors that cause no harm to patients) are more controversial (Lo, 2009). Some professionals tend to avoid telling patients about "near miss" errors since no harm was done to the patient, but ethicists recommend disclosure of these events. Being honest and forthright with patients promotes trust, and secrecy is unethical (Jonsen, Siegler, & Winslade, 2010).

BOX 2.5 ETHICAL FORMATIONS: WAIVING ONE'S RIGHT TO INFORMATION

Suken Hashimoto, a 78-year-old Japanese woman, was hospitalized with a diagnosis of cancer. Mrs. Hashimoto's physician initially spoke with her son about his mother's diagnosis and discussed a detailed plan of care for her. Chemotherapy was ordered. Her son told the physician and nurses not to tell his mother her diagnosis. The oncology nurses' normal procedure is to explain the chemotherapy treatment to the patient, including why she will receive it. The medical and nursing staff were perplexed about how to handle the son's request.

- Before reading below about how Mrs. Hashimoto's case was managed, discuss how you think that the physicians and nurses should resolve the situation and provide your rationale. See information below about actions taken by the hospital staff in this case.

1. Mrs. Hashimoto was asked how much detail that she wanted to know about her diagnosis and treatment. She said that she did not want details and told the staff members to allow her son to make decisions for her.
2. The staff consulted the hospital ethics committee to help ensure that they would make an ethical decision.
3. Ultimately, Mrs. Hashimoto's and her son's wishes were respected. The hospital staff asked Mrs. Hashimoto to sign a durable power of attorney that granted her son authority to make her healthcare decisions. She was happy to do this.

Source: Galanti, G-A. (2008). *Caring for patients from different cultures* (4th ed.). Philadelphia, PA: University of Pennsylvania Press.

Intentionally not disclosing information to a patient is legal in situations of emergency, incompetence, or when patients waive their right to be informed. Respecting a patient's right *not* to be informed is especially important in culturally sensitive care (see Box 2.5). Other more legally and ethically controversial circumstances of intentionally not disclosing relevant information to a patient involve three healthcare circumstances (Beauchamp & Childress, 2009). The first circumstance falls under therapeutic privilege. The second relates to therapeutically using placebos. The third involves withholding information from research subjects in order to protect the integrity of the research.

Invoking **therapeutic privilege** allows physicians to withhold information from patients if physicians, based on sound medical judgment, believe that "divulging the information would potentially harm a depressed, emotionally drained, or unstable patient" (Beauchamp & Childress, 2009, p. 124). There are varying standards about what constitutes therapeutic privilege in different legal jurisdictions. Standards range from withholding information if the physician believes that the information would have *any* negative effect on the patient's health condition to withholding information only if divulging it is likely to have a *serious* effect.

Placebos, when used therapeutically, are inactive substances given to patients in an attempt to induce a positive health outcome through the patients' belief that the inert substance really carries some beneficial power. It is interesting that at least one study has shown that placebos can have a positive effect in a majority of patients even when the patients know that they are receiving an inert pill (Scuderi, 2011). Proponents of using placebos say that the action is covered under a patient's general consent to treatment, though the consent is not entirely informed. However, there is a general consensus that the therapeutic use of placebos is unethical (Jonsen et al., 2010), in that it violates a patient's autonomy and can seriously damage trust between patients and healthcare professionals. The use of placebos is ethical when used properly during experimental research. Participants in a research control group often are given a placebo so that they can be compared to an experimental group that receives the treatment being studied. Research participants are fully informed that they may receive a placebo rather than the actual treatment. See Box 2.6 for a case involving the use of a placebo.

Strict rules apply to research studies requiring that research subjects be protected from manipulation and personal risks. Thus, informed consent in research has stringent requirements. Withholding information from research subjects should never be undertaken lightly. Intentional nondisclosure sometimes is allowed only if the research is relatively risk-free to the participants and when the nature of the research is behavioral or psychological and disclosure might seriously skew the outcomes of the research.

Patient Self-Determination Act

The Patient Self-Determination Act (PSDA) passed by the U.S. Congress in 1990 is the first federal statute designed to facilitate a patient's autonomy through the knowledge and use of advance directives. Healthcare providers and organizations must provide written information to adult patients regarding state laws covering the right to make healthcare decisions, to refuse or withdraw treatments, and to write advance directives. One of the underlying aims of the PSDA is to increase meaningful dialogue about patients' rights to make autonomous choices about

BOX 2.6 ETHICAL FORMATIONS: WOULD IT BE ETHICAL TO GIVE THIS PATIENT A PLACEBO?

Callie is a nurse who just began a new job in an emergency department (ED). Mrs. J. arrived at the ED complaining of left-leg pain and is assigned to Callie. Mrs. J. is known to the ED physicians and other nurses because of her frequent visits for back pain. Mrs. J. is assessed by Callie and is seen briefly by the ED physician. The physician walks out of Mrs. J.'s room and tells Callie to give the patient saline IV push as a placebo.

- What questions should Callie ask?
- What should Callie do?
- Where might she seek guidance about the physician's request?

receiving or not receiving health care. See Appendix D for an example of one state's patient self-determination document.

It is important that dialogue about end-of-life decisions and options not be lost in organizational admission processes, paperwork, and other ways. Nurses provide the vital communication link between the patient's wishes, the paperwork, and the provider. When the opportunity arises, nurses need to take an active role in increasing their dialogue with patients in regard to patients' rights and end-of-life decisions. In addition to responding to the direct questions that patients and families ask about advance directives and end-of-life options, nurses would do well to listen and observe patients' subtle cues that signal their anxiety and uncertainty about end-of-life care. A good example of compassionate care is when nurses actively listen to patients and try to alleviate patients' uncertainty and fears in regard to end-of-life decision making.

The Health Insurance Portability and Accountability Act of 1996 (HIPAA) Privacy and Security Rules

"Within [Health and Human Services] HHS, the Office for Civil Rights (OCR) has responsibility for enforcing the [HIPAA] Privacy and Security Rules with voluntary compliance activities and civil money penalties" (United States Department of Health and Human Services [USDHHS], n.d.b., para. 2). The HIPAA Privacy Rule is a federal regulation designed to protect people from disclosure of their personal health information other than for the provision of health care and for other "need-to-know" purposes on a "minimum necessary" basis (USDHHS, n.d.c.; USDHHS, 2003). The intent of the Rule is to ensure privacy while facilitating the flow of information necessary to meet the needs of patients.

> The Privacy Rule protects all "individually identifiable health information" held or transmitted by a covered entity or its business associate, in any form or media, whether electronic, paper, or oral. The Privacy Rule calls this information "protected health information (PHI)." (45 C.F.R. § 160.103 as cited in USDHHS, 2003, p. 3)

The Security Rules of the Act operationalize the Privacy Rules. These rules contain standards that address privacy safeguards for electronic protected health information (USDHHS, n.d.b.) The Rule is designed to "assure the confidentiality, integrity, and availability of electronic protected health information" (USDHHS, n.d.b., para. 2).

All patient-identifiable protected health information is to be kept private unless it is being used for patient care, a patient agrees to a release, or it is released according to legitimate, limited situations covered by the act. It is incumbent on all healthcare professionals to be familiar with the content of the act. Other special health information privacy issues that are addressed by the USDHHS (n.d.a.) include:

- Public health: There is sometimes a legitimate need to release medical information for the protection of public health.

- Research: Private information is protected, but processes are used to allow researchers to conduct well-designed studies.
- Emergency preparedness: As with other public health issues, access to protected information sometimes is allowed to facilitate emergency preparedness.
- Health information technology: The confidential maintenance and exchange of information via electronic formats is supported by the act.
- Genetic information: The Genetic Information Nondiscrimination Act (GINA) of 2008 identifies genetic information as health information and requires Privacy Rule modifications to ensure that no one is discriminated against in employment or for insurance coverage based on genetic information.

Nonmaleficence

Nonmaleficence is the principle used to communicate the obligation to "do no harm." Emphasizing the importance of this principle is as old as organized medical practice. Healthcare professionals have historically been encouraged to do good (beneficence), but if for some reason they cannot do good, they generally are required to at least do no harm. Because of the "two sides of the same coin" connotation between these two principles, some people consider them to be essentially one and the same. However, Beauchamp and Childress (2009) do make a distinction between the two of them.

Nonmaleficence is the maxim or norm that "one ought not to inflict evil or harm" (Beauchamp & Childress, 2009, p. 151), whereas beneficence includes the following three norms: "one ought to prevent evil or harm, one ought to remove evil or harm, [and] one ought to do or promote good" (p. 151). As evidenced by these maxims, beneficence involves action to help someone and nonmaleficence requires "*intentionally refraining* from actions that cause harm" (p. 151). In addition to violating the maxim not to intentionally harm another person, some of the issues and concepts listed by Beauchamp and Childress as frequently involving or requiring the obligation of nonmaleficence are included in Box 2.7.

Best practice and due-care standards are adopted by professional organizations and regulatory agencies to minimize harm to patients. Regulatory agencies develop oversight procedures to ensure that healthcare providers maintain the competency and skills needed to properly care for patients. Nonmaleficence has a wide scope of implications in health care that includes the need to avoid negligent care, the need to avoid harm when deciding whether to provide treatment or to withhold or withdraw it, and considerations about rendering extraordinary or heroic treatment.

The distinctions included in Box 2.7 often are associated with end-of-life care. Violating the principle of nonmaleficence, particularly in the first three distinctions, may involve issues of medical futility. Though it sometimes is difficult to accurately predict the outcomes of all interventions, **futile treatments** are treatments that a

BOX 2.7 ETHICAL FORMATIONS: ISSUES AND CONCEPTS ASSOCIATED WITH THE PRINCIPLE OF NONMALEFICENCE

1. Upholding standards of due care: the standards specific to one's profession, the acceptable and expected care that a reasonable person in a profession would render
2. Negligence: "the absence of due care" (Beauchamp & Childress, 2009, p. 153) and imposing a *risk* of harm—imposing an unintended careless risk of harm or imposing an intentional reckless risk of harm
3. Distinctions of and rules governing nontreatment and end-of-life decisions (Beauchamp & Childress, 2009, p. 155):
   a. Withholding and withdrawing life-sustaining treatment
   b. Extraordinary (or heroic) and ordinary treatment
   c. Sustenance technologies and medical treatments
   d. Intended effects and merely foreseen effects
   e. Killing and letting die

Source: Beauchamp, T. L., & Childress, J. F. (2009). *Principles of biomedical ethics* (6th ed.). New York, NY: Oxford University Press.

healthcare provider, when using good clinical judgment, does not believe will provide a beneficial outcome for a patient. Consequently, these treatments may instead cause harm to a patient, such as a patient having to endure a slow and painful death that may have otherwise occurred in a quicker and more natural or humane manner. Clinical judgments usually are made in the face of uncertainty (Jonsen et al., 2010), even though medical probabilities often are fairly clear.

The **rule of double effect** is described in Box 2.7. Performing some actions may have two potential outcomes. One is the intended good outcome, but in order to achieve the good outcome, a second, less acceptable outcome also might be foreseen to occur. In these situations, one has to gauge and balance actions according to their good, intended effects as compared to their possible harmful, adverse effects. For example, although research has shown that giving morphine in regular, increasing increments for pain and/or respiratory distress at the end of life rarely causes complete cessation of respirations, it is possible for respiratory arrest to occur in this type of situation. It is legal and ethical for healthcare professionals to treat pain and respiratory distress, particularly at the end-of-life, with increasing increments of morphine even though it is foreseen that cessation of respirations *may* occur. A nurse never should intend to end a person's life, but it is ethical for nurses to try to relieve suffering (American Nurses Association [ANA], 2001; see Appendix A). Considering the terms *killing* and *letting die* raises issues of legality, ethics, homicide, suicide, euthanasia, acts of commission and omission, and active–passive distinctions, which are beyond the scope of this chapter.

Slippery Slope Arguments

Often, a slippery slope argument is a metaphor that is used as a "beware the Ides of March" warning with no justification or formal, logical evidence to back it up (Ryan, 1998, p. 341). A **slippery slope** situation is one that may be morally acceptable when the current, primary event is being discussed or practiced, but one that later could hypothetically slip toward a morally unacceptable situation. A slippery slope situation is somewhat like a runaway horse that cannot be stopped once the barn door is left open. People using a slippery slope argument tend to believe the old saying that when people are given an inch, they eventually may take a mile. Because it is argued that harm may be inflicted if the restraints on a particular practice are removed, the concept of the slippery slope sometimes is considered to fall under the principle of nonmaleficence.

Slippery slope arguments may move toward illogical extremes. Therefore, people who are afraid of a dangerous slide to the bottom of the slope on certain issues need to find evidence that justifies their arguments rather than trying to form public opinions and policies based only on alarmist comparisons. One example of a slippery slope debate occurred with the legalization of physician-assisted suicide (PAS), such as the acts legalized by the Oregon Death with Dignity Act. Proponents of the slippery slope argument say that allowing PAS, which involves a patient's voluntary decision and self-administration of lethal drugs in well-defined circumstances, may or may not in itself be morally wrong. However, slippery slope proponents argue that the widespread legalization of PAS may lead to the eventual legalization of nonvoluntary practices of euthanasia (see Chapter 9 for more explanation on euthanasia). The Oregon Death with Dignity Act was passed in October 1997, and as of 2011, no slide toward the legalization of nonvoluntary euthanasia has occurred in the United States. Opponents of slippery slope arguments believe that people proposing this type of argument mistrust people's abilities to make definitive distinctions between moral/legal and immoral/illegal issues and to exercise appropriate societal controls.

www Ethical Reflections

- Another common slippery slope argument surrounds the issues of stem-cell research and cloning. What, specifically, are the slippery slope arguments that surround issues of stem-cell research and cloning? What are your positions? Support your answer.
- Do you believe that most people can be trusted to make ethical decisions based on the overall well-being of human beings? Explain.

Beneficence

The principle of beneficence consists of performing deeds of "mercy, kindness, and charity" (Beauchamp & Childress, 2009, p. 197). **Beneficence** means that people take actions to benefit and promote the welfare of other people. Examples of moral rules and obligations underlying the principle of beneficence are listed in Box 2.8.

Whereas people are obligated to act in a nonmaleficent manner toward all people—that is, not to harm anyone—

BOX 2.8 ETHICAL FORMATIONS: RULES OF BENEFICENCE

1. Protect and defend the rights of others.
2. Prevent harm from occurring to others.
3. Remove conditions that will cause harm to others.
4. Help persons with disabilities.
5. Rescue persons in danger.

Source: Beauchamp, T. L., & Childress, J. F. (2009). *Principles of biomedical ethics* (6th ed.). New York, NY: Oxford University Press, p. 199.

there are limits to beneficence or to the benefits that people are expected to bestow on other people. Generally, people act more beneficently toward people whom they personally know or love rather than toward people not personally known to them, though this certainly is not always the case.

Because of professional standards and social contracts, physicians and nurses have a responsibility to be beneficent in their work. Nurses are directed in the *Code of Ethics for Nurses with Interpretive Statements* (ANA, 2001; see Appendix A) to have their patients' interests and well-being as their primary concern. Therefore, though there sometimes are limits to the good that nurses can do, nurses have a more stringent obligation to act according to the principle of beneficence than does the general public. Doing good toward and facilitating the well-being of one's patients is an integral part of being a moral nurse.

Paternalism

Occasionally, healthcare professionals may experience ethical conflicts when confronted with having to make a choice between respecting a patient's right to self-determination (autonomy) and doing what is good for a patient's well-being (beneficence). Sometimes healthcare professionals believe that they, not their patients, know what is in a patient's best interest. In these situations, healthcare professionals may be tempted to act in ways that they believe promote a patient's well-being (beneficence) when the actions actually are a violation of a patient's right to exercise self-determination (autonomy). The deliberate overriding of a patient's opportunity to exercise autonomy because of a perceived obligation of beneficence is called **paternalism**. The word itself reflects its roots in fatherly or male (paternal) hierarchical relationships, governance, and care.

If a nurse avoids telling a patient that her blood pressure is elevated because the nurse believes that this information will upset the patient and consequently further elevate her blood pressure, this is an example of paternalism. A more ethical approach to the patient's care is to unexcitedly give the patient truthful information while helping her to remain calm and educating her about successful ways to manage her blood pressure.

BOX 2.9 ETHICAL FORMATIONS: JUSTIFYING PATERNALISM

1. Soft paternalism: A term used to describe the use of paternalism to protect persons from their own nonvoluntary conduct. People justify its acceptance when a person may be unable to make reasonable, autonomous decisions. Examples of when soft paternalism is used include situations involving depression, substance abuse, and addiction.
2. Justified hard paternalism: A term used to describe "actions that prevent major harms or provide major benefits while only trivially disrespecting autonomy [and that] have a plausible paternalistic rationale" (Beauchamp & Childress, 2009, p. 214).

According to Beauchamp and Childress (2009), the following is a summary of justifiable reasons to practice hard paternalism (Beauchamp & Childress, 2009, p. 216):

1. A patient is at risk of a significant, preventable harm.
2. The paternalistic action will probably prevent the harm.
3. The projected benefits to the patient of the paternalistic action outweigh its risks to the patient.
4. There is no reasonable alternative to the limitation of autonomy.
5. The least autonomy-restrictive alternative that will secure the benefits and reduce the risks is adopted.

Source: Beauchamp, T. L., & Childress, J. F. (2009). *Principles of biomedical ethics* (6th ed.). New York, NY: Oxford University Press.

Two positions used to justify paternalism are listed in Box 2.9. Generally, however, the practice of paternalism is discouraged today, although it once was a common practice among healthcare professionals. Paternalism is still a common practice among people of some cultures who, for example, believe that people with authority, such as physicians or male family members, should be allowed to make decisions in the best interests of patients and that patients should not be given bad news, such as a terminal diagnosis.

Justice

Justice, as a principle in healthcare ethics, refers to fairness, treating people equally and without prejudice, and the equitable distribution of benefits and burdens, including assuring fairness in biomedical research. Most of the time, difficult healthcare resource allocation decisions are based on attempts to answer questions regarding who has a right to health care, how much health care a person is entitled to, and who will pay for healthcare costs. Remember, however, that justice, as it was discussed in Chapter 1, is one of Plato's cardinal virtues. This means that justice is a broad concept in the field of ethics and is considered to be both a principle and a virtue.

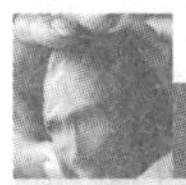

Ethical Reflections

- Read the Tarasoff case in Box 10.10, Chapter 10. Discuss how the principles of autonomy, nonmaleficence, and beneficence do or do not relate to this case.
- Discuss the following issues as they relate to obligations of beneficence. What specific circumstances might be relevant to decision making in these cases?
  - Rescuing a person who is drowning.
  - Alleviating global poverty.
  - Working as a nurse during a highly lethal influenza pandemic.
  - Defending the rights of immigrants.
- Refer to Mrs. Hashimoto's case, presented in Box 2.5. Consider the ethical implications if Mrs. Hashimoto had not been given the option to waive her right to information. As the patient's nurse, what would you do?
- Have you practiced paternalism with any of your patients? If so, discuss the circumstances and your rationale for this practice. Evaluate the ethics of this action using the approach of principlism.
- Do you believe that paternalism is ever justified? If not, defend your position. If so, suggest an example of when it is acceptable.

Social Justice

Distributive justice refers to the fair allocation of resources, while **social justice** represents the position that benefits and burdens should be distributed fairly among members of a society, or ideally, that all people in a society should have the same rights, benefits, and opportunities. The mission to define and attain some measure of social justice is an ongoing and difficult activity for the world community. One only needs to think about the obligations of beneficence to identify how these two principles are related. For example, what are the limits of the obligation that people have to "do good" in distributing their assets to help others?

An analysis of social justice mostly has been used to evaluate the powers of competing social systems and the application of regulatory principles on an impartial basis. Theories of social justice differ to some extent, but most of the theories are based on the notion that justice is related to fair treatment and that similar cases should be treated in similar ways. People who take a communitarian approach to social justice will seek the common good of the community rather than individual benefits and freedoms. If people think beyond borders in promoting social justice, they consider how basic health care for all people can be provided and what can be done to prevent social injustice worldwide, such as trying to alleviate poverty and hunger.

In his book, *A Theory of Justice*, John Rawls (1971) proposed that fairness and equality be evaluated under a **veil of ignorance**. This concept means that if people had a veil to shield themselves from their own or others' economic, social, and class standing, each person would be likely to make justice-based decisions from a position that is free from biases. Consequently, each person would view the distribution of resources in impartial ways. Under the veil, people would view social conditions neutrally because they would not know what their own position might be at the time the veil is lifted. This "not knowing" or ignorance of persons about their own social position means that they would not gain any type of advantage for themselves by their choices. Rawls advocated two principles of equality and justice: (1) everyone should be given equal liberty regardless of their adversities, and (2) differences among people should be recognized by making sure that the least-advantaged people are given opportunities for improvement.

In 1974, Robert Nozick presented the idea of an entitlement system in his book, *Anarchy, State, and Utopia*. He proposed that individuals should be entitled to health care and the benefits of insurance only if they are able to pay for these benefits. Nozick emphasized a system of **libertarianism,** meaning that justice and fairness are based on rewarding only those people who contribute to the system. People who cannot afford health insurance are disadvantaged if Nozick's entitlement theory is used as a philosophy of social justice.

In his book, *Just Health Care*, Norman Daniels (1985) used the basis of Rawls's concept of justice and suggested a liberty principle. Daniels advocated national healthcare reform and proposed that every person should have equal access to health care and reasonable access to healthcare services. Daniels suggested that there should be critical standards for a fair and equitable healthcare system, and he provided points of reference, or benchmarks, for this application of fairness in the implementation and development of national health reform.

Distributing and allocating healthcare resources continues to be a major problem in the United States. As of 2009, 50.7 million people did not have health insurance (U.S. Census Bureau, 2010). This number reflects an increase of 4.4 million uninsured people from 2008. No matter what theory is applied, there needs to be a standard by which health care and other resources are distributed. Brannigan and Boss (2001) stated that some version of the following standards can be applied or considered when distributions are made:

- Distribute according to market—that is, to those who can afford to pay
- Distribute according to social merit
- Distribute according to medical need
- Distribute according to age
- Distribute according to queuing, or first-come, first-served
- Distribute according to random selection (p. 619)

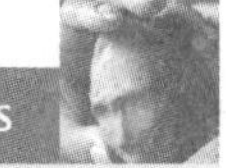

WWW Ethical Reflections

- Discuss personal experiences with justice in your work with patients.
- Do you believe that health care is a basic human right? Defend your answer.
- Of the standards for distributing resources listed in the social justice section, which one(s) best fit(s) your beliefs and value system? Justify your choice(s).
- Do you believe that it is ethical to ration health care? Explain.
- Do we ration health care in the United States? Explain.
- Discuss your views about the limits of social justice. What do you believe people "owe" one another? Defend your answers.

Professional–Patient Relationships

To a disciple who was constantly complaining about others the Master said, "If it is peace you want, seek to change yourself, not other people. It is easier to protect your feet with slippers than to carpet the whole earth."

—*Anthony De Mello,* One Minute Wisdom, *1985, p. 38*

The quality of patient care rendered by healthcare professionals and patients' satisfaction with health care often depends on the existence of harmonious relationships between professionals and patients and between the members of professions themselves. Good professional–patient relationships are built using much of the information that has been covered in Chapters 1 and 2. If healthcare professionals view life as a web of interrelationships, all of their relationships potentially can affect the well-being of patients. After reading the *Professional–Patient Relationships* section of this chapter, go to Box 2.10 and read Anne Sexton's poem, "The Operation" and answer the questions that follow.

Unavoidable Trust

When patients enter the healthcare system, they usually are entering a foreign and frightening environment (Chambliss, 1996; Zaner, 1991). Intimate conversations and activities, such as being touched and probed, that normally do not occur between strangers are commonplace between healthcare professionals and patients. Patients frequently are stripped of their clothes, subjected to sitting alone in cold and barren rooms, and made to wait anxiously for frightening news regarding the continuation of their very being. When patients are in need of help from healthcare professionals, they frequently feel a sense of vulnerability and uncertainty. The tension that patients feel when accessing health care is heightened by the need for what Zaner called **unavoidable trust**. In most cases, when they are in need of care, patients have no option but to trust nurses and other healthcare professionals.

This unavoidable trust creates an asymmetrical, or uneven, power structure in professional–patient and family relationships (Zaner, 1991). Nurses' responsiveness to this trust needs to include the promise to be the most excellent nurses that they can be. According to Zaner, healthcare professionals must promise "not only to take care of, but to care for the patient and family—to be candid, sensitive, attentive, and never to abandon them" (p. 54). It is paradoxical that trust is necessary *before* health care is rendered, but it can be evaluated in terms of whether the trust was warranted only *after* care is rendered. To practice ethically, nurses must never take for granted the fragility of patients' trust.

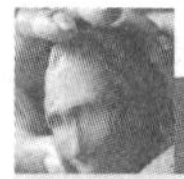

Ethical Reflections

- Explain how a nurse might assess if a patient is feeling vulnerable and experiencing uncomfortable feelings associated with unavoidable trust.
- Suggest nursing actions that may help decrease patients' uncomfortable feelings when they are experiencing unavoidable trust.
- Why is unavoidable trust an ethical issue?

Human Dignity

In the first provision of the *Code of Ethics for Nurses with Interpretive Statements*, the ANA (2001) included the standard that a nurse must have "respect for human dignity" (p. 7). Typically, people refer to maintaining dignity in regard to the circumstances of how people look, behave, and express themselves when they are being watched by others or when they are ill, aging, or dying; in circumstances of how people respect themselves and are respected by others; and in the honor accorded to the privacy of one's body, emotions, and personhood. Nurses are charged with protecting a person's dignity during all nursing care, and often, a patient's nurse is the primary person who guards a patient's dignity during medical procedures. Healthcare settings can be scenes of professionals rushing through treatments so that they can efficiently move on to the next patient and job to be done. Nurses have many opportunities to stop and be mindful of the person who is the patient: a person who wants to be respected.

Shotton and Seedhouse (1998) said that the term *dignity* has been used in vague ways. They characterized dignity as persons being in a position to use their capabilities and proposed that a person has dignity "if he or she is in a situation where his or her capabilities can be effectively applied" (p. 249). For example, a nurse can enhance dignity when caring for an elderly person by assessing the elder's priorities and determining what the elder has been capable of doing in the past and what the person is capable of doing and wants to do in the present.

A lack of or loss of capability is frequently an issue for consideration when caring for patients such as children, elders, and the physically and mentally disabled. Having absent or diminished capabilities is consistent with what MacIntyre (1999) was referring to in his discussion of human vulnerability. According to MacIntyre, people generally progress from a point of vulnerability in infancy to achieving varying levels of independent, practical reasoning as they mature. However, all people, including nurses, would do well to realize that all persons have been or will be vulnerable at some point in their lives. Taking a "there but for the grace of God go I" stance may prompt nurses to develop what MacIntyre called the virtues of acknowledged dependence. These virtues include *just generosity*, *misericordia*, and *truthfulness* and are exercised in communities of giving and receiving. Just generosity is a form of giving generously without "keeping score" of who gives or receives the most, *misericordia* is a Latin word that signifies giving based on urgent need without prejudice, and truthfulness involves not being deceptive. Nurses who cultivate these three virtues, or excellences of character, can move toward preserving patients' dignity and toward working for the common good of a community.

Patient Advocacy

> *The virtue of the candle lies not in the wax that leaves its trace, but in its light.*
>
> —*Antoine de Saint-Exupéry*, The Wisdom of the Sands

Nurses acting from a point of patient advocacy try to identify unmet patient needs and then follow up to address the needs appropriately (Jameton, 1984). Advocacy, as opposed to advice, involves the nurse's moving from the patient to the healthcare system rather than moving from the nurse's values to the patient. The concept of advocacy has been a part of the ethics codes of the International Council of Nurses' (ICN) and the ANA since the 1970s (Winslow, 1988). In the *Code of Ethics for Nurses with Interpretive Statements*, the ANA (2001) continues to support patient advocacy by elaborating on the "primacy of the patient's interest" (p. 9) and requiring nurses to work collaboratively with others to attain the goal of addressing the healthcare needs of patients and the public. Nurses are called upon to ensure that all appropriate parties are involved in patient-care decisions, that patients are provided with the information needed to make informed decisions, and that collaboration is used to increase the accessibility and availability of health care to all patients who need it. The ICN (2006), in *The ICN Code of Ethics for Nurses*, affirms that the nurse must share "with society the responsibility for initiating and supporting action to meet the health and social needs of the public, in particular those of vulnerable populations" (p. 2).

Moral Suffering

Many times, healthcare professionals experience a disquieting feeling of anguish, uneasiness, or angst that can be called **moral suffering**. Suffering in a moral sense has similarities to the Buddhist concept of *dukkha*, a Sanskrit word that is translated as suffering. *Dukkha* "includes the idea that life is impermanent and is experienced as unsatisfactory and imperfect" (Sheng-yen, 1999, p. 37). The concept of *dukkha* evolved from the historical Buddha's beliefs that the human conditions of birth, sickness, old age, and death involve suffering and *are* suffering. Nurses confront these human conditions every day. Not recognizing, and in turn struggling against, the reality that impermanence, or the changing and passing away of all things, is inherent to human life, the world, and all objects is a cause of suffering.

Moral suffering can be experienced when nurses attempt to sort out their emotions if they find themselves in imperfect situations that are morally unsatisfactory or when forces beyond their control prevent them from positively influencing or changing unsatisfactory moral situations. Suffering occurs because nurses believe that situations must be changed or fixed in order to bring well-being to themselves and others or to alleviate the suffering of themselves and others.

Moral suffering may arise, for example, from disagreements with imperfect institutional policies, such as an on-call policy or work schedule that the nurse believes does not allow relaxation time for the nurse's psychological well-being. Nurses also may disagree with physicians' orders that the nurses believe are not in patients' best interests, or they may disagree with the way a family treats a patient or makes patient-care decisions. Moral suffering can result when a nurse is with a patient when she receives a terminal diagnosis, or when a nurse's compassion is aroused when caring for a severely impaired neonate or an elder who is suffering and life-sustaining care is either prolonged or withdrawn. These are but a few examples of the many types of encounters that nurses may have with moral suffering.

Another important, but often unacknowledged, source of moral suffering may occur when nurses freely choose to act in ways that they, themselves, would not defend as being morally commendable if the actions were honestly analyzed. For example, a difficult situation that may cause moral suffering for a nurse would be "covering up" a patient-care error made by a valued nurse friend. On the other hand, nurses may experience moral suffering when they act virtuously and courageously by doing what they believe is morally right despite anticipated disturbing consequences. Sometimes, doing the right thing or acting as a virtuous person would act is hard, and it is incumbent upon nurses to habitually act in virtuous ways, that is, to exhibit habits of excellent character.

The Dalai Lama (1999) proposed that how people are affected by suffering is often a matter of choice or personal perspective. Some people view suffering as something to accept and to transform, if possible. Causes may lead toward certain effects, and nurses often are able to change the circumstances or conditions of events so that positive effects occur. Nurses can choose and cultivate their perspectives, attitudes, and emotions in ways that lead toward happiness and well-being even in the face of suffering.

> www Ethical Reflections
>
> - Have you experienced moral suffering during your work as a nurse or student nurse? Explain.

The Buddha was reported to have stated, "Because the world is sick, I am sick. Because people suffer, I have to suffer" (Hanh, 1998, p. 3). However, in the Four Noble Truths, the Buddha postulated that the cessation of suffering can be a reality through the Eightfold Path of eight right ways of thinking, acting, and being, sometimes grouped under the three general categories of wisdom, morality, and meditation. In other words, suffering can be transformed. When nurses or other healthcare professionals react to situations with fear, bitterness, and anxiety, it is important to remember that wisdom and inner strength often are increased most during times of the greatest difficulty. Thich Nhat Hanh (1998) wisely stated, "without suffering, you cannot grow" (p. 5). Therefore, nurses can learn to take their disquieting experiences of moral anguish and uneasiness—that is, moral suffering—and transform them into experiences that lead to well-being.

Ethical Dilemmas

An **ethical dilemma** is a situation in which an individual is compelled to choose between two actions that will affect the welfare of a sentient being, and both actions are reasonably justified as being good, neither action is readily justified as being good, or the goodness of the actions is uncertain. One action must be chosen, thereby generating a quandary for the person or group who is burdened with the choice.

Kidder (1995) focused on one characteristic of an ethical dilemma when he described the heart of an ethical dilemma as "the ethics of right versus right" (p. 13). Though the best choice about two right actions is not always self-evident, according

BOX 2.10 ETHICAL FORMATIONS: "THE OPERATION" BY ANNE SEXTON

1.
After the sweet promise,
the summer's mild retreat
from mother's cancer, the winter months of
her death,
I come to this white office, its sterile sheet,
its hard tablet, its stirrups, to hold my breath
while I, who must, allow the glove its oily rape,
to hear the almost mighty doctor over me
equate
my ills with hers
and decide to operate.

It grew in her
as simply as a child would grow,
as simply as she housed me once, fat and
female.
Always my most gentle house before that embryo
of evil spread in her shelter and she grew frail.
Frail, we say, remembering fear, that face we
wear
in the room of the special smells of dying, fear
where the snoring mouth gapes
and is not dear.

There was snow everywhere.
Each day I grueled through
its sloppy peak, its blue-struck days, my boots
slapping into the hospital halls, past the retinue
of nurses at the desk, to murmur in cahoots
with hers outside her door, to enter with the
outside
air stuck on my skin, to enter smelling her pride,
her upkeep, and to lie
as all who love have lied.

No reason to be afraid,
my almost mighty doctor reasons.
I nod, thinking that woman's dying
must come in seasons,
thinking that living is worth buying.
I walk out, scuffing a raw leaf,
kicking the clumps of dead straw
that were this summer's lawn.
Automatically I get in my car,
knowing the historic thief
is loose in my house
and must be set upon.

2.
Clean of the body's hair,
I lie smooth from breast to leg.
All that was special, all that was rare
is common here. Fact: death too is in the egg.
Fact: the body is dumb, the body is meat.
And tomorrow the O.R. Only the summer was
sweet.

The rooms down the hall are calling
all night long, while the night outside
sucks at the trees. I hear limbs falling
and see yellow eyes flick in the rain. Wide eyed
and still whole I turn in my bin like a shorn
lamb.
A nurse's flashlight blinds me to see who I am.

The walls color in a wash
of daylight until the room takes its objects
into itself again. I smoke furtively and squash
the butt and hide it with my watch and other
effects.
The halls bustle with legs. I smile at the nurse
who smiles for the morning shift. Day is worse.

Scheduled late, I cannot drink
or eat, except for yellow pills
and a jigger of water. I wait and think
until she brings two mysterious needles: the skills
she knows she knows, promising, soon you'll be out.
But nothing is sure. No one. I wait in doubt.

BOX 2.10 (continued)

I wait like a kennel of dogs
jumping against their fence. At ten
she returns, laughs and catalogues
my resistance to drugs. On the stretcher, citizen
and boss of my own body still, I glide down the halls
and rise in the iron cage toward science and
pitfalls.

The great green people stand
over me; I roll on the table
under a terrible sun, following their command
to curl, head touching knee if I am able.
Next, I am hung up like a saddle and they begin.
Pale as an angel I float out over my own skin.

I soar in hostile air
over the pure women in labor,
over the crowning heads of babies being born.
I plunge down the backstair
calling *mother* at the dying door,
to rush back to my own skin, tied where it was
torn.
Its nerves pull like wires
snapping from the leg to the rib.
Strangers, their faces rolling lilke hoops, require
my arm. I am lifted into my aluminum crib.

3.
Skull flat, here in my harness,
thick with shock, I call mother
to help myself, call toe to frog,
that woolly bat, that tongue of dog;
call God help and all the rest.
The soul that swam the furious water
sinks now in flies and the brain
flops like a docked fish and the eyes
are flat boat decks riding out the pain.

My nurses, those starchy ghosts,
hover over me for my lame hours
and my lame days. The mechanics
of the body pump for their tricks.
I rest on their needles, am dosed
and snoring amid the orange flowers
and the eyes of visitors. I wear,
like some senile woman, a scarlet
candy package ribbon in my hair.

Four days from home I lurk on my
mechanical parapet with two pillows
at my elbows, as soft as praying cushions.
My knees work with the bed that runs
on power. I grumble to forget the lie
I ought to hear, but don't. God knows
I thought I'd die—but here I am,
recalling mother, the sound of her
good morning, the odor of orange and jam.

All's well, they say. They say I'm better.
I lounge in frills or, picturesque,
I wear bunny pink slippers in the hall.
I read a new book and shuffle past the desk
to mail the author my first fan letter.
Time now to pack this humpty-dumpty
back the frightened way she came
and run along, Anne, and run along now,
my stomach laced like a football
for the game.

1. Analyze the story and feelings conveyed in the poem.
2. Discuss your perception of the quality of the patient–provider relationships reflected in this poem.
3. Apply to the poem concepts, theories, and approaches that you have read about in Chapters 1 and 2.

Source: Anne Sexton, "The Operation" from *The Complete Poems of Anne Sexton*, published by Houghton Mifflin Harcourt.

to Kidder, "right versus right" choices clearly can be distinguished from "right versus wrong" choices. Right versus right choices bring us nearer to common societal and personal values, whereas the closer one analyzes right versus wrong choices, "the more they begin to smell" (p. 17). He proposed that people generally can judge wrong choices according to three criteria: violation of the law, departure from the truth, and deviation from moral rectitude. Of course, the selection and meaning of these three criteria can be a matter of debate among people.

It needs to be noted, however, that when a person is facing a real ethical dilemma, often none of the options available feel right. Both choices actually may feel wrong. For a daughter trying to decide whether to withdraw life support from her 88-year-old mother, it may feel wrong not to try to save her mother's life, but allowing her mother to suffer in a futile medical condition probably also will feel wrong. On the other hand, for a healthcare professional considering this same case, there may be no real dilemma involved—the healthcare professional may see clearly that the right choice is to withhold or withdraw life support.

Considering the explanations given above, it is important to note that the words *ethical dilemma* often are used loosely and inappropriately. Weston (2011) stated "today you can hardly even mention the word 'moral' without 'dilemma' coming up in the next sentence, if it waits that long" (p. 99). He called an ethical dilemma "a very special thing" (p. 99), contending that often when people believe that they face a dilemma, they are facing a "false dilemma"; the person only needs to work on identifying "new possibilities or reframing the problem itself" (p. 99) to solve the problem. As an example, he presented the classic case of the "Heinz dilemma" used by Lawrence Kohlberg in his research. The story is about Heinz, whose wife is dying of cancer. She needs a particular drug to save her life. The pharmacist who makes the drug charges much more than it costs him to make it. The cost is way beyond what Heinz can afford to pay. Heinz tries to borrow the money needed but is not successful. He asks the pharmacist to sell him the drug at a lower cost, but the pharmacist refuses his request. Finally, Heinz robs the pharmacy to obtain the drug. The question is whether or not Heinz should have done this. Did Heinz face a dilemma? Weston discussed the Heinz dilemma with his students and found that they generated some very creative ways of approaching the problem that did not involve robbing the pharmacy. A case similar to the Heinz dilemma is presented in Box 2.11.

Introduction to Critical Thinking and Ethical Decision Making

In health care and nursing practice, moral matters are so ever-present that nurses often do not even realize that they are faced with minute-to-minute opportunities to make ethical decisions (Chambliss, 1996; Kelly, 2000). It is vitally important that nurses have the analytical thinking ability and skills to respond to many of the everyday decisions that must be made. Listening attentively to other people,

BOX 2.11 ETHICAL FORMATIONS: MAN ROBS BANK FOR $1 TO RECEIVE HEALTH CARE

The following story was published by NBC News on June 21, 2011:

A North Carolina man robbed a bank, but it wasn't money he was after.

James Verone, 59, walked into the RBC Bank in Gastonia and handed the teller a note. "This is a bank robbery. Please give me one dollar," the note read.

Then Verone made the opposite of a getaway.

"I started to walk away from the teller, then I went back and said, 'I'll be sitting right over there in the chair waiting for the police,'" Verone told WCNC.

Verone said he does not have medical insurance, but has an assortment of health problems. He said he is hoping for a three-year sentence, which would give him health care until he qualifies for Medicare. A jail doctor told him he was manipulating the system.

"If it is called manipulation, then out of necessity because I need medical care then I guess I am manipulating the courts to get medical care," Verone said.

One potential kink in Verone's plan: His $1 demand only netted a larceny charge, according to WCNC. He may be looking at less jail time than he thought.

1. Try to generate new possibilities to solve Mr. Verone's problem.
2. Can you reframe the problem itself? If so, how? If not, why?
3. Did Mr. Verone face an ethical dilemma? Why or why not?

Source: Wilson, G. (2011, June 21). Man robs bank for $1 to go to jail, get health care. *NBC News*. Retrieved from http://www.nbcnewyork.com/news/weird/Man-Robs-Banks-for-1-to-Go-to-Jail-Get-Health-Care-124287474.html

including patients, and not developing hasty conclusions are essential skills for nurses to conduct reasoned, ethical analyses. Personal values, professional values and competencies, ethical principles, and ethical theories and approaches are variables that must be considered when a moral decision is made. Pondering the questions: "What is the right thing to do?" and "What ought I do in this circumstance?" are ever-present normative considerations in nursing.

Critical Thinking

The concept of critical thinking is used quite liberally today in nursing. Many nurses probably have a general idea about the meaning of the concept, but they may not be able to clearly articulate answers to questions about its meaning. Examples of such questions include: Specifically, what is critical thinking? Are critical thinking and problem solving interchangeable concepts? If not, what distinguishes them? Can critical thinking skills be learned or does critical thinking either occur naturally or not at all? If the skill can be learned, how does one become a critical thinker? Is there a difference between doing critical thinking and reasoning?

Socrates's method of teaching and questioning (see Chapter 1) is one of the oldest systems of critical thinking. In modern times, the American philosopher

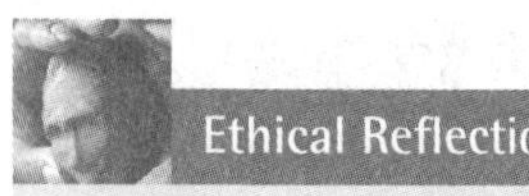

- Read about the Terri Schiavo case in Chapter 9 and on the Internet. Was the decision to remove Terri's feeding tube a real ethical dilemma? Why or why not? Consider, was there good ethical and legal support for removing the tube or leaving the tube in place? Legal precedence? Ethical support based on theory and landmark cases?
- What criteria do you use to identify unethical or wrong choices in your life? Were your criteria developed subjectively or objectively? Explain.
- Describe an ethical dilemma that you have encountered during your personal life or during your work as a nurse or student nurse.
- Explain why your example fits the criteria of an ethical dilemma.
- What were your thoughts and feelings during the experience?
- Describe the process that you used to make a decision in the situation.
- What was the outcome of the situation?

John Dewey (1859–1952) is considered to be one of the early proponents of critical thinking. In his book, *How We Think*, Dewey (1910/1997) summarized reflective thought as

> active, persistent, and careful consideration of any belief or supposed form of knowledge in light of the grounds that support it, and the further conclusions to which it tends. . . . [O]nce begun it is a conscious and voluntary effort to establish belief upon a firm basis of reasons. (p. 6)

Paul and Elder (2006), directors of the Foundation for Critical Thinking, defined critical thinking as "the art of analyzing and evaluating thinking with a view to improving it" (p. 4). They proposed that critical thinkers have certain characteristics. Critical thinkers:

- ask clear, pertinent questions and identify key problems;
- analyze and interpret relevant information by using abstract thinking;
- are able to generate reasonable conclusions and solutions that are tested according to sensible criteria and standards;
- remain open-minded—they consider alternative thought systems; and
- solve complex problems by effectively communicating with other people.

The process of **critical thinking** is summarized by Paul and Elder (2006) as "self-directed, self-disciplined, self-monitored, and self-corrective thinking [that] requires rigorous standards of excellence and mindful command of their use" (p. 4). Fisher (2001) described the basic way to develop critical thinking skills as simply "thinking about one's thinking" (p. 5).

Moral Imagination

> *[Persons], to be greatly good, must imagine intensely and comprehensively; [they] must put [themselves] in the place of another and of many others. . . . The great instrument of moral good is the imagination.*
>
> —*Percy Bysshe Shelley*, Defense of Poetry

The foundation underlying the concept of moral imagination, an artistic or aesthetic approach to ethics, is based on the philosophy of the American philosopher John Dewey. Imagination, as Dewey proposed it, is "the capacity to concretely perceive what is before us in light of what could be" (Fesmire, 2003, p. 65). Dewey (1934) stated that imagination "is a way of seeing and feeling things as they compose an integral whole" (p. 267). **Moral imagination** is moral decision making through reflection that involves "empathetic projection" and "creatively tapping a situation's possibilities" (Fesmire, 2003, p. 65). It involves moral awareness and decision making that goes beyond the mere application of standardized ethical meanings, decision-making models, and bioethical principles to real-life situations.

The use of empathetic projection helps nurses be responsive to patients' feelings, attitudes, and values. To creatively reflect on a situation's possibilities helps prevent nurses from becoming stuck in their daily routines and instead encourages them to look for new and different possibilities in problem solving and decision making that go beyond mere habitual behaviors. Although Aristotle taught that habit is the way that people cultivate moral virtues, Dewey (1922/1988) cautioned that mindless habits can be "blinders that confine the eyes of mind to the road ahead" (p. 121). Dewey proposed that habit should be combined with intellectual impulse. He stated:

> Habits by themselves are too organized, too insistent and determinate to need to indulge in inquiry or imagination. And impulses are too chaotic, tumultuous and confused to be able to know even if they wanted to. . . . A certain delicate combination of habit and impulse is requisite for observation, memory and judgment. (p. 124)

Dewey (1910/1997) provided an example of a physician trying to identify a patient's diagnosis without proper reflection:

> Imagine a doctor being called in to prescribe for a patient. The patient tells him some things that are wrong; his experienced eye, at a glance, takes in other signs of a certain disease. But if he permits the suggestion of this special disease to take possession prematurely of his mind, to become an accepted conclusion, his scientific thinking is by that much cut short. A large part of his technique, as a skilled practitioner, is to prevent the acceptance of the first suggestions that arise; even, indeed, to postpone the occurrence of any very definite suggestions till the trouble—the nature of the problem—has been thoroughly explored. In the case of a physician this proceeding is known as a diagnosis, but a similar inspection is required in every novel and complicated situation to prevent rushing to a conclusion. (p. 74)

Although Dewey's example is about an individual physician–patient clinical relationship, the example also is applicable for illustrating the dangers of rushing to conclusions in the moral practice of the art and science of nursing with individuals, families, communities, and populations. The following story provides an

www Ethical Reflections

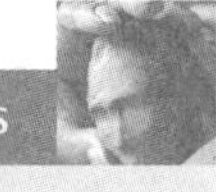

- Perform a written self-analysis of your critical thinking skills. What are your strengths? In what ways do you need to improve? Be specific with your analysis.
- Explain why asking intelligent questions is essential to good nursing practice. What type of questions do you routinely ask of yourself during your work? What type of questions do you routinely ask of other people during your work?
- Provide a personal example of a good question that you asked about an important issue that arose during your clinical work. Provide a personal example of a time when you should have asked a question but did not do so. Analyze the different circumstances of these situations.
- From what you have learned about ethics and critical thinking, discuss why critical thinking is an important element of doing ethics.

example of a nurse not using moral imagination. A young public health nurse moves from a large city to a rural town and begins working as the occupational health nurse at a local factory. The nurse noticed that a large number of workers at the factory have developed lung cancer. He immediately assumes that the workers have been exposed to some type of environmental pollution at the factory and that the factory owners are morally irresponsible people. The nurse discusses his assessment with his immediate supervisor and an official at the district health department. Upon further assessment, the nurse finds data showing that the factory's environmental pollution is unusually low. However, the nurse does learn that radon levels are particularly high in homes in the area and that a large percentage of the factory workers smoke cigarettes.

In the following example, a home health nurse uses moral imagination. The nurse visits Mrs. S., a homebound patient diagnosed with congestive heart failure. The patient tells the nurse that she has difficulty affording her medications and that she does not buy the low-sodium foods that the nurse recommends because the fresh foods are too expensive. However, the patient's television set broke, and she bought a new television that she usually is watching when the nurse visits. The home health aide that visits the patient tells the nurse, "No wonder Mrs. S. can't afford her medications—she spent her money on a television." Rather than judging the patient, the nurse uses her moral imagination to try to empathetically envision what it must be like to be Mrs. S.—homebound, consistently short of breath, and usually alone. The nurse decides that Mrs. S.'s television may have been money well spent in terms of the patient's quality of life. With Mrs. S.'s physician and social worker, the nurse explores ways to help the patient obtain her medications. The nurse also works patiently with Mrs. S. to try to develop a healthy meal plan that is affordable for her.

Dewey (1910/1997) seemed to be trying to make the point that critical thinking and moral imagination require suspended judgment until problems and situations are fully explored and reflected upon. Moral imagination includes engaging in frequent considerations of "What if?" with regard to day-to-day life events as well as novel situations. In a public interview on July 22, 2004, immediately after the U.S. Congress released its 9/11 Commission Report, former New Jersey Governor and the September 11 Commission's chairman, Thomas Kean, made a statement with regard to the findings about the probable causes of the failure to prevent the terrorist attacks on September 11, 2001 (Mondics, 2004). The commission concluded that, above all, there was a "failure of imagination" (p. A4).

An important role for nurses is to provide leadership and to help create healthy communities through individual-, family-, and population-based assessments; program planning; program implementation; and evaluation. When assuming this key leadership role, nurses continually must make choices and decisions that may affect the well-being of both individuals and populations. Opinions should not be formed hastily, nor should actions be taken without nurses cultivating and using their moral imaginations.

The High, Hard Ground and Swampy Low Ground

It generally is agreed that nursing is based on the dual elements of art and science. Schön (1987) postulated that professional decision points sometime arise when there is tension between how to attend to knowledge based on technical, scientific foundations and indeterminate issues that lie beyond scientific laws. Schön described this tension as follows:

> In the varied topography of professional practice, there is a high, hard ground overlooking a swamp. On the high ground, manageable problems lend themselves to solution though the application of research-based theory and technique. In the swampy lowland, messy, confusing problems defy technical solutions. The irony of this situation is that the problems of the high ground tend to be relatively unimportant to individuals or society at large, however great their technical interest may be, while in the swamp lie the problems of greatest human concern. The practitioner must choose. (p. 3)

Gordon and Nelson (2006) argued that nursing has suffered by not emphasizing the profession's scientific basis and the specialized skills that are required for nursing practice. These authors proposed that the professional advancement of nursing has been hurt by nurses and others (including the general members of society) focusing too much on the virtues of nurses and the caring nature of the profession, essentially the art of nursing. According to Gordon and Nelson,

> Although much has changed for professional women in the twentieth century, nurses continue to rely on religious, moral, and sentimental symbols and rhetoric—images of hearts, angels, touching hands, and appeals based on diffuse references to closeness, intimacy, and making a difference. . . . When repeated in recruitment brochures and campaigns, appeals to virtue are unlikely to help people understand what nurses really do and how much knowledge and skill they need to do it. (pp. 26–27)

www Ethical Reflections

- Nurses might ask: Should we firmly try to stay primarily on the high, hard ground founded on rigid scientific standards or is it equally and sometimes more important to descend into the swampy low ground full of important problems that are relatively unnoticed by people who are not directly affected? Discuss.
- Are nurses really faced with choosing "either/or" in terms of nursing science and art? Explain.
- Discuss your views about the state of the profession of nursing. Does a focus on the virtues and caring ways of nurses help or hinder the advancement of nursing as a profession?
- Can there be a good balance between describing nursing as a caring profession and a profession that requires specialized knowledge and skills? If so, how would you describe the balance point?

Reflective Practice

Schön (1987) distinguished reflection-*on*-action from reflection-*in*-action. Reflecting on action involves looking back on one's actions, whereas reflection in action involves stopping to think about what one is choosing and doing before and during one's actions. In considering the value of reflection-in-action, Schön stated, "in an

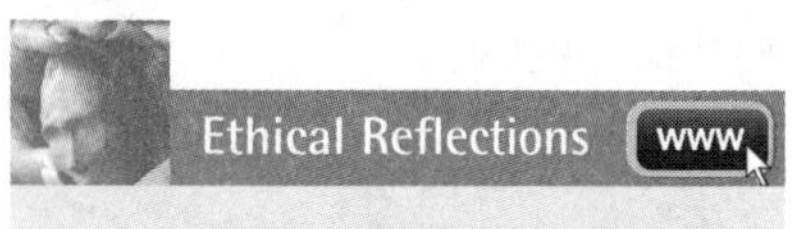

- Use Gibbs's Reflective Cycle to reflect on a challenging, personal, ethical situation that occurred during your nursing practice.

action present—a period of time, variable with the context, during which we can still make a difference to the situation at hand—our thinking serves to reshape what we are doing while we are doing it" (p. 26). Mindful reflection while we are still able to make choices about our behaviors is preferable to looking backward. However, as the saying goes, hindsight is 20/20, so there is certainly learning that can occur from hindsight.

Since ethics is an active process of doing, reflection in any form is crucial to the practice of ethics. Making justified ethical decisions requires healthcare professionals to know themselves and their motives, to ask good questions, to challenge the status quo, and to be continual learners (see Box 2.12). There is no one model of reflection and decision making that can provide healthcare professionals with a cookie cutter approach to ethical practice. However, there are a number of models that professionals can use to improve their skills of reflection and decision making during their practice. Figure 2.1 includes an example of a model that is helpful for reflection-on-action. The Four Topics Method, discussed later in this chapter, is an example of reflection-in-action.

The Four Topics Approach to Ethical Decision Making

Jonsen, Siegler, and Winslade's (2010) Four Topics Method for ethical analysis is a practical approach for nurses and other healthcare professionals. The nurse or

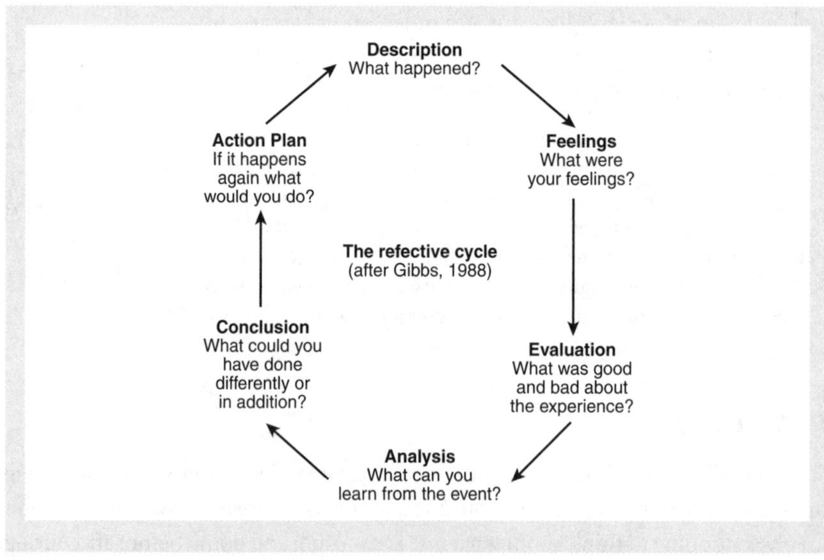

Figure 2.1
Gibbs's Reflective Cycle

Source: Retrieved from http://www.nursesnetwork.co.uk/images/reflectivecycle.gif

Original out of print publication: Gibbs, G. (1988). *Learning by doing: A guide to teaching and learning methods.* Oxford, UK: Oxford Polytechnic.

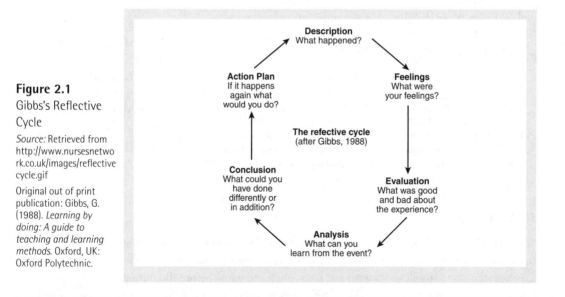

BOX 2.12 ETHICAL FORMATIONS: THE FIVE R'S APPROACH TO ETHICAL NURSING PRACTICE

1. Read
   Read and learn about ethical philosophies, approaches, and the ANA's *Code of Ethics for Nurses*. Insight and practical wisdom are best developed through effort and concentration.
2. Reflect
   Reflect mindfully on one's egocentric attachments—values, intentions, motivations, and attitudes. Members of moral communities are socially engaged and focus on the common good. This includes having good insight regarding life events, cultivating and using practical wisdom, and being generous and socially just.
3. Recognize
   Recognize ethical bifurcation points, whether they are obvious or indistinct. Because of indifference or avoidance, nurses may miss both small and substantial opportunities to help alleviate human suffering in its different forms.
4. Resolve
   Resolve to develop and practice intellectual and moral virtues. Knowing ethical codes, rules, duties, and principles means little without being combined with a nurse's good character.
5. Respond
   Respond to persons and situations deliberately and habitually with intellectual and moral virtues. Nurses have a choice about their character development and actions.

Intellectual Virtues	**Moral Virtues**
Insight	Compassion
Practical wisdom	Loving-kindness
Equanimity	
Sympathetic joy	

Insight: awareness and knowledge about universal truths that affect the moral nature of nurses' day-to-day life and work

Practical wisdom: deliberating about and choosing the right things to do and the right ways to be that lead to good ends

Equanimity: an evenness and calmness in one's way of being; balance

Sympathetic joy: rejoicing in other persons' happiness

Compassion: the desire to separate other beings from suffering

Loving-kindness: the desire to bring happiness and well-being to oneself and other beings

Considerations for Practice

- Trying to apply generic algorithms or principles when navigating substantial ethical situations does not adequately allow for variations in life narratives and contexts.
- Living according to a philosophy of ethics already must be a way of being for nurses before they encounter critical situations.

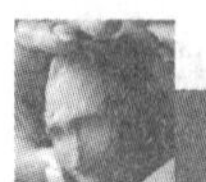

Ethical Reflections www

- Gather information about the case of Terri Schiavo from Chapter 9, other literature, and the Internet. Use the information about her case to complete the following:
  - Summarize key information and events in the case. Think about the information that would be needed by an ethics committee reviewing this case.
  - Clearly identify (list) the specific ethical issues involved in her case.
  - Imagine that you are a member of an ethics committee that has been consulted for a decision about whether Terri's feeding tube should be removed. As a member of the ethics committee, complete the questions of the Four Topics Method shown in Table 2.1. Some of the questions will require more discussion than other questions because of the direct relationship to the Schiavo case. Do your best to answer the questions comprehensively.
  - Summarize "the committee's" specific determination(s) based on the answers to the Four Topics questions and your research of the case.
  - Speak for the committee to recommend removal of the feeding tube or not to remove the feeding tube and provide your rationale.

team begins with relevant facts about a particular case and moves toward a resolution through a structured analysis. In healthcare settings, ethics committees often resolve ethical problems and answer ethical questions by using a case-based, or bottom-up, inductive, casuistry approach. (See Chapter 1 for a discussion of casuistry.) The Four Topics Method, sometimes called the Four Box Approach (see Table 2.1) was first published in 1982 in the book, *Clinical Ethics: A Practical Approach to Ethical Decisions in Clinical Medicine.* The book is now in its seventh edition.

This case-based approach allows healthcare professionals to construct the facts of a case in a structured format that facilitates critical thinking about ethical problems. Cases are analyzed according to four topics: "medical indications, patient preferences, quality of life, and contextual features" (Jonsen et al., 2010, p. 8). Nurses and other healthcare professionals on the team gather information in an attempt to answer the questions in each of the four boxes. The Four Topics Method facilitates dialogue between the patient–family/surrogate dyad and members of the healthcare ethics team or committee. By following the outline of the questions, healthcare providers are able to inspect and evaluate the full scope of the patient's situation, as well as the central ethical conflict. Once the ethics team has gathered the facts of a case, an analysis is conducted. Each case is unique and should be considered as such, but the subject matter of particular situations often involves common threads with other ethically and legally accepted precedents, such as landmark cases that involved withdrawing or withholding treatment. Though each case analysis begins with facts, the four fundamental principles—autonomy, beneficence, nonmaleficence, and justice—along with the Four Topics Method are considered together as the process and resolution take place (Jonsen et al., 2010). In Table 2.1, each box includes principles appropriate for each of the four topics. Fairness and loyalty are included in the contextual features box. To see an analysis of a specific case, go to http://depts.washington.edu/bioethx/tools/cecase.html.

Frustration, anger, and other intense emotional conflicts may occur among healthcare professionals or between healthcare professionals and the patient or the patient's surrogates. Unpleasant verbal exchanges and hurt feelings can result. Openness and sensitivity toward other healthcare professionals, patients, and family members are essential behaviors

TABLE 2.1 FOUR TOPICS METHOD FOR ANALYSIS OF CLINICAL ETHICS CASES

Medical Indications

The Principles of Beneficence and Nonmaleficence

1. What is the patient's medical problem? history? diagnosis? prognosis?
2. Is the problem acute? chronic? critical? emergent? reversible?
3. What are the goals of treatment?
4. What are the probabilities of success?
5. What are the plans in case of therapeutic failure?
6. In sum, how can this patient be benefited by medical and nursing care, and how can harm be avoided?

Patient Preferences

The Principle of Respect for Autonomy

1. Is the patient mentally capable and legally competent? Is there evidence of incapacity?
2. If competent, what is the patient stating about preferences for treatment?
3. Has the patient been informed of benefits and risks, understood this information, and given consent?
4. If incapacitated, who is the appropriate surrogate? Is the surrogate using appropriate standards for decision making?
5. Has the patient expressed prior preferences, e.g., Advance Directives?
6. Is the patient unwilling or unable to cooperate with the medical treatment? If so, why?
7. In sum, is the patient's right to choose being respected to the extent of possible in ethics and law?

Quality of Life

The Principles of Beneficence and Non-maleficence and Respect for Autonomy

1. What are the prospects, with or without treatment, for a return to normal life?
2. What physical, mental, and social deficits is the patient likely to experience if treatment succeeds?
3. Are there biases that might prejudice the provider's evaluation of the patient's quality of life?
4. Is the patient's present or future condition such that his or her continued life might be judged undesirable?
5. Is there any plan and rationale to forgo treatment?
6. Are there plans for comfort and palliative care?

Contextual Features

The Principles of Loyalty and Fairness

1. Are there family issues that might influence treatment decisions?
2. Are there provider (physicians and nurses) issues that might influence treatment decisions?
3. Are there financial and economic factors?
4. Are there religious and cultural factors?
5. Are there limits on confidentiality?
6. Are there problems of allocation of resources?
7. How does the law affect treatment decisions?
8. Is clinical research or teaching involved?
9. Is there any conflict of interest on the part of the providers or the institution?

Source: Jonsen, A. R., Siegler, M., & Winslade, W. J. (2006). *Clinical ethics: A practical approach to ethical decisions in clinical medicine* (6th ed.). New York, NY: McGraw-Hill.

for nurses during these times. As information is exchanged and conversations take place, nurses need to maintain an attitude of respect as a top priority. If respect and sensitivity are maintained, lines of communication more likely will remain open.

The Healthcare Team

When patients and families are experiencing distress and suffering, it often is during times when decisions need to be made about risky procedures or end-of-life care. Family members may want medical treatment for their loved one while physicians and nurses may be explaining to the family that to continue treatment most likely would be nonbeneficial or futile for the patient. When patients are weakened by disease and illness and family members are reacting to their loved one's suffering, decisions regarding care and treatment become challenging for everyone concerned.

In caring for particular patients and interacting with their families, nurses sometimes find themselves caught in the middle of conflicts. Though nurses frequently make ethical decisions independently, they also act as an integral part of the larger team of decision makers. Many problematic bioethical decisions will not be made unilaterally—not by physicians, nurses, or any other single person. By participating in reflective dialogues with other professionals and healthcare personnel, nurses are often part of a larger team approach to ethical analysis. When a team is formally assembled and is composed of preselected members that come together regularly to discuss ethical issues within an organization, the team is called an ethics committee. An organization's ethics committee usually consists of physicians, nurses, an on-staff chaplain, a social worker, a representative of the organization's administrative staff, possibly a legal representative, local community representatives, and others drafted by the team. Also, the involved patient, the patient's family, or a surrogate decision maker may meet with one or more committee members. See Box 2.13 for examples of the goals of an ethics committee.

Members of the heathcare team may question the decision-making capacity of the patient or family, and the patient's or family's decisions may conflict with the physician's or healthcare team's recommendations regarding treatment. Sometimes, a genuine ethical dilemma arises in a patient's care, difficult decisions must be made, difficult and unpleasant situations must be navigated, or no surrogate can be located to help make decisions for an incompetent patient. When these situations emerge, a team approach to decision making is helpful and is in accordance with the Institute of Medicine's (2003) call for healthcare professionals to work in interdisciplinary teams by cooperating, collaborating, communicating, and integrating care "to ensure that care is continuous and reliable" (p. 4). See Box 2.14 for an example of a case that probably should be referred to an ethics committee.

At times, nurses do not agree with physicians', family members', or surrogates' decisions regarding treatment and subsequently may experience moral uncertainty

BOX 2.13 ETHICAL FORMATIONS: GOALS OF AN ETHICS COMMITTEE

- Support, by providing guidance to patients, families, and decision makers
- Review of cases, as requested, when there are conflicts in basic values
- Provide assistance in clarifying situations that are ethical, legal, or religious in nature that extend beyond the scope of daily practice
- Help in clarifying issues, discussing alternatives, and suggesting compromises
- Promote the rights of patients
- Assist the patient and family, as appropriate, in coming to consensus with the options that best meet the patient's care needs
- Promote fair policies and procedures that maximize the likelihood of achieving good, patient-centered outcomes
- Enhance the ethical tenor of both healthcare organizations and professionals

Source: Pozgar, G. D. (2010). *Legal and ethical issues for health professionals* (2nd ed.). Sudbury, MA: Jones and Bartlett, pp. 142–143.

BOX 2.14 ETHICAL FORMATIONS: PATIENT REFUSES BLOOD

Mrs. Jones has gangrene of her left leg. Her hemoglobin slipped to 6.4. She has a major infection and is diabetic. There is no spouse and no living will. The patient has decided that she does not want to be resuscitated if she should go into cardiopulmonary arrest. She needs surgery. She has agreed to surgery but refuses a blood transfusion, even though she is not a Jehovah's Witness. The surgeon will not perform the surgery, which is urgent, without Mrs. Jones agreeing to a blood transfusion, if it becomes necessary. The attending physician questions the patient's capacity to make decisions. Her children have donated blood. She says she is not afraid to die.

1. What ethical issues and principles are involved with this case?
2. Generate questions that need to be answered to reach an ethical solution in this case.
3. Is an ethical dilemma involved in this case? Explain.
4. Should the physician refuse to treat this patient? Explain your answer.
5. Should the family have a right to override the patient's decision to refuse blood? Explain your answer.
6. What is the role of nurses in this case?

Source: Pozgar, G. D. (2010). *Legal and ethical issues for health professionals* (2nd ed.). Sudbury, MA: Jones and Bartlett, p. 152.

and anxiety. When passionate ethical disputes arise between nurses and physicians or when nurses seriously are concerned about the action of patients' decision-making representatives, nurses are the ones who often seek an ethics consultation. It is within the rights and duties of nurses to seek help and advice from other professionals when nurses experience moral uncertainty or witness unethical conduct in their work setting. This action is a part of the nurse's role as a patient advocate.

KEY POINTS

- Bioethics was born out of the rapidly expanding technical environment of the 1900s.
- The four most well-known and frequently used bioethical principles are (1) autonomy, (2) beneficence, (3) nonmaleficence, and (4) justice.
- Paternalism involves an overriding of autonomy in favor of the principle of beneficence.
- Social justice emphasizes the fairness of how the benefits and burdens of society are distributed among people.
- Ethical dilemmas involve unclear choices, not clear matters of right versus wrong.
- Nurses often experience a disquieting feeling of anguish, uneasiness, or angst in their work that is consistent with what might be called moral suffering.
- It is paradoxical that patients often must trust healthcare providers to care for them before the providers show evidence that the trust is warranted.
- When acting as patient advocates, nurses try to identify patients' unmet needs and help to address these needs.
- Nurses may develop good critical thinking skills by "thinking about their thinking."

References

American Nurses Association. (2001). *Code of ethics for nurses with interpretive statements.* Silver Spring, MD: Author.

American Nurses Association. (2004). *Nursing: Scope and standards of practice.* Silver Spring, MD: Author.

Beauchamp, T. L., & Childress, J. F. (2009). *Principles of biomedical ethics* (6th ed.). New York, NY: Oxford University Press.

Brannigan, M. C., & Boss, J. A. (2001). *Healthcare ethics in a diverse society.* Mountain View, CA: Mayfield.

Chambliss, D. F. (1996). *Beyond caring: Hospitals, nurses, and the social organization of ethics.* Chicago, IL: The University of Chicago Press.

Dalai Lama. (1999). *Ethics for the new millennium.* New York, NY: Riverhead Books.

Daniels, N. (1985). *Just health care.* New York, NY: Cambridge University Press.

Dempski, K. M. (2009). Informed consent. In S.J. Westrick & K. Dempski.*Nursing law and ethics* (pp. 77–83). Sudbury, MA: Jones and Bartlett.

Dewey, J. (1934). *Art as experience.* New York, NY: Perigee Books.

Dewey, J. (1988). *Human nature and conduct: The middle works, 1899–1924* (Vol. 14) (J. A. Boydston & P. Baysinger, Eds.). Carbondale, IL: Southern Illinois University Press. (Original work published 1922)

Dewey, J. (1997). *How we think.* Mineola, NY: Dover Publications. (Original work published 1910)

Fesmire, S. (2003). *John Dewey and moral imagination: Pragmatics in ethics.* Bloomington, IN: Indiana University Press.

Fisher, A. (2001). *Critical thinking: An introduction.* Cambridge, UK: Cambridge University Press.

Gibbs, G. (1988). *Learning by doing: A guide to teaching and learning methods.* Oxford, UK: Oxford Polytechnic.

Gordon, S., & Nelson, S. (2006). Moving beyond the virtue script in nursing. In S. Nelson & S. Gordon (Eds.), *The complexities of care: Nursing reconsidered* (pp. 13–29). New York, NY: Cornell University Press.

Hanh, T. N. (1998). *The heart of the Buddha's teaching: Transforming suffering into peace, joy, and liberation.* New York, NY: Broadway Books.

Institute of Medicine. (2000). *To err is human: Building a safer health care system.* Washington, DC: National Academy Press.

Institute of Medicine. (2003). *Health professions education: A bridge to quality.* Washington, DC: National Academy Press.

International Council of Nurses. (2006). *The ICN code of ethics for nurses.* Geneva, Switzerland: Author. Retrieved from http://www.icn.ch/icncode.pdf

Jameton, A. (1984). *Nursing practice: The ethical issues.* Englewood Cliffs, NJ: Prentice-Hall.

Jonsen, A. R. (1998). *The birth of bioethics.* New York, NY: Oxford University Press.

Jonsen, A. R. (2000). *A short history of medical ethics.* New York, NY: Oxford University Press.

Jonsen, A. R. (2005). *Bioethics beyond the headlines: Who lives? Who dies? Who decides?* Lanham, MD: Rowman & Littlefield.

Jonsen, A. R., Siegler, M., & Winslade, W. J. (2010). *Clinical ethics: A practical approach to ethical decisions in clinical medicine* (7th ed.). New York, NY: McGraw-Hill.

Kelly, C. (2000). *Nurses' moral practice: Investing and discounting self.* Indianapolis, IN: Sigma Theta Tau International Center Nursing Press.

Kidder, R. M. (1995). *How good people make tough choices: Resolving the dilemmas of ethical living.* New York, NY: Quill.

Lo, B. (2009). *Resolving ethical dilemmas: A guide for clinicians* (4th ed.). Philadelphia, PA: Wolters Kluwer.

MacIntyre. A. (1999). *Dependent rational animals: Why human beings need the virtues.* Chicago, IL: Open Court.

Mondics, C. (2004, July 23). 9/11 report details failure. *The Sun Herald*, pp. A1, A4.

National Institutes of Health. (1979). *The Belmont report.* Retrieved from http://ohsr.od.nih.gov/guidelines/belmont.html

National Institutes of Health. (2011). *NIH stops clinical trial on combination cholesterol treatment.* Retrieved from http://www.nih.gov/news/health/may2011/nhlbi-26.htm

Nozick, R. (1974). *Anarchy, state, and utopia.* New York, NY: Basic Books.

Patient Self-Determination Act, 42 U.S.C. §§ 1395–1396 (1990).

Paul, R., & Elder, L. (2006). *The miniature guide to critical thinking concepts and tools* (4th ed.). Dillon Beach, CA: Foundation for Critical Thinking.

Pozgar, G. D. (2010). *Legal and ethical issues for health professionals* (2nd ed.). Sudbury, MA: Jones and Bartlett.

Rawls, J. (1971). *A theory of justice.* Cambridge, MA: Harvard University Press.

Ryan, C. J. (1998). Pulling up the runaway: The effect of new evidence on euthanasia's slippery slope. *Journal of Medical Ethics, 24*, 341–344.

Schön, D. A. (1987). *Educating the reflective practitioner*. San Francisco, CA: Jossey-Bass.

Scuderi, B. M. (2011, February 21). Placebos found to have positive effect. *The Harvard Crimson*. Retrieved from http://www.thecrimson.com/article/2011/2/21/study-placebos-group-medicine/

Sheng-yen, M. (1999). Subtle wisdom: Understanding suffering, cultivating compassion through Ch'an Buddhism. New York, NY: Doubleday.

Shotton, L., & Seedhouse, D. (1998). Practical dignity in caring. *Nursing Ethics, 5*(3), 246–255.

U.S. Census Bureau. (2010). *Income, poverty, and health insurance coverage in the United States: 2009*. Retrieved from http://www.census.gov/prod/2010pubs/p60-238.pdf

U.S. Department of Health and Human Services. (2003). *Summary of HIPAA Privacy Rule* (Office for Civil Rights Privacy Brief). Retrieved from http://www.hhs.gov/ocr/privacy/hipaa/understanding/summary/privacysummary.pdf

U.S. Department of Health and Human Services. (n.d.a.). Special topics in health information privacy. Retrieved from http://www.hhs.gov/ocr/privacy/hipaa/understanding/special/index.html

U.S. Department of Health and Human Services. (n.d.b.). Summary of the HIPAA Security Rule: Introduction. Retrieved from http://www.hhs.gov/ocr/privacy/hipaa/understanding/srsummary.html

U.S. Department of Health and Human Services. (n.d.c.). Understanding health information privacy. Retrieved from http://www.hhs.gov/ocr/privacy/hipaa/understanding/index.html

Weston, A. (2011). *A practical companion to ethics* (4th ed.). New York, NY: Oxford University Press.

Wilson, G. (21, June 2011). Man robs bank for $1 to go to jail, get health care. *NBC News*. Retrieved from http://www.nbcnewyork.com/news/weird/Man-Robs-Banks-for-1-to-Go-to-Jail-Get-Health-Care-124287474.html

Winslow, G. (1988). From loyalty to advocacy: A new metaphor for nursing. In J. C. Callahan (Ed.), *Ethical Issues in Professional Life* (pp. 95–105). New York, NY: Oxford University Press.

Zaner, R. M. (1991). The phenomenon of trust and the patient-physician relationship. In E. D. Pellegrino, R. M. Veatch, & J. P. Langan (Eds.), *Ethics, trust, and the professions: Philosophical and cultural aspects* (pp. 45–67). Washington, DC: Georgetown University Press.

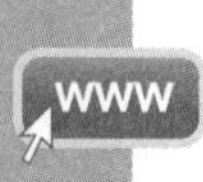

For a full suite of assignments and additional learning activities, use the access code located in the front of your book to visit this exclusive website: http://go.jblearning.com/butts. If you do not have an access code, you can obtain one at the site.

Ethics in Professional Nursing Practice

Janie B. Butts

Nursing is a profession that has its own code of conduct, its own philosophic views, and its own place in the health care team. . . .Nurses work under their own license. That means that nurses are completely responsible for their work.

—*Janet R. Katz, 2007,* A Career in Nursing: Is It Right For Me?, *p. 105*

OBJECTIVES

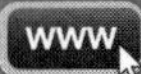

After reading this chapter, the reader should be able to:

1. Distinguish between nursing ethics, medical ethics, and bioethics.
2. Delineate key historical events that led to the development of the current American Nurses Association (ANA) and International Council of Nurses (ICN) codes of ethics for nurses.
3. Discuss examples of professional nursing boundaries and ways that boundary crossings can occur.
4. Examine the ethical nurse qualities discussed in the ANA and ICN codes (see also Appendices A and B).
5. Contrast moral distress from moral integrity.
6. Recall ways a nurse can discern whether another nurse's character fits Aristotle's description of the truthful sort.
7. Define truthtelling in terms of two ethical frameworks: deontology and a virtue ethics approach.
8. Examine the ethical implications of caring for a dying patient whose physician exercised therapeutic privilege by not disclosing the whole truth.
9. Describe examples of scenarios that would prompt a nurse to respond with moral courage.

10. Compare patient advocacy and power in relation to nurses' everyday ethical work.
11. Formulate a plan for assessing a culturally diverse patient who is a new admission to a hospital unit.
12. Characterize two types of relationships: the nurse–physician relationship and the nurse–nurse relationship.
13. Weigh nurses' use of social networking in terms of professional ethical considerations.

Introduction to Nursing Ethics

Bioethical issues are relevant to nurses' work in everyday practice, but in matters of bioethics nurses usually are not autonomous decision makers. Nursing ethics, as a unique field, continues to be debated. Fry, Veatch, and Taylor (2011) continue to support the view that both nursing ethics and medical ethics are valid subcategories of the larger field of bioethics. Additional views are that everyday ethical practice in nursing is situated within an interdisciplinary team and that nursing ethics is distinctive from other disciplines in bioethics but is not yet unique (Volker, 2003; Holm, 2006; Wright & Brajtman, 2011).

The experiences and needs of practicing nurses, along with explorations of the meaning of nursing ethics, are areas of emphasis in nursing ethics. Johnstone (2008) defined **nursing ethics** as "the examination of all kinds of ethical and bioethical issues from the perspective of nursing theory and practice, which, in turn, rest on the agreed core concepts of nursing, namely: person, culture, care, health, healing, environment and nursing itself" (p. 16).

Johnstone's definition of nursing ethics is consistent with a common view that a strong bond between nursing ethics and nursing theory distinguishes nursing ethics from other areas of healthcare ethics. Nurses' professional relationships to patient care and within the healthcare team bring about ethical issues unique to the nursing profession. To practice nursing ethically, nurses must be sensitive enough to recognize when they are facing seemingly obscure ethical issues in everyday work.

Professional Codes of Ethics in Nursing

Professional nursing can be traced to England in the 1800s, to the school that was founded by Florence Nightingale, where profession-shaping ethical precepts and values were communicated. By the end of the 1800s, modern nursing had been established, and ethics was becoming a discussion topic in nursing. The Nightingale Pledge of 1893 was written under the chairmanship of a Detroit nursing school principal, Lystra Gretter, to establish nursing as an art and a science. Six years later, in 1899, the International Council of Nurses (ICN) was established and became known as a pioneer in developing a code of ethics for nurses.

By the turn of the 20th century, the first book on nursing ethics, titled *Nursing Ethics: For Hospital and Private Use* (1900), had been written by an American nurse leader, Isabel Hampton Robb. In Robb's book, the titles of the chapters were descriptive of the times and moral milieu, such as Chapter 4: The Probationer, Chapter 7: Uniform, Chapter 8: Night-Duty, and Chapter 12: The Care of the Patient (nurse–physician, nurse–nurse, nurse–public relationships). The focus in the nursing code initially was on physicians, because, typically, male physicians trained nurses in the Nightingale era. Nurses' technical training and obedience to physicians remained at the forefront of nursing responsibilities into the 1960s. This emphasis was reflected in the ICN *Code of Ethics for Nurses* as late as 1965. However, by 1973, the ICN code reflected a shift in nursing responsibility from a focus on obedience to physicians to a focus on patient needs, where it remains to this day.

American Nurses Association's Code of Ethics for Nurses

"A Suggested Code" was published in the American Journal of Nursing (AJN) in 1926 by the American Nurses Association (ANA), but was never adopted; in 1940 "A Tentative Code" was published in AJN, but again was never adopted (Davis, Fowler, and Aroskar, 2010). The ANA adopted its first official code in 1950. Three more code revisions occurred before the creation of the interpretative statements in 1976.

The word "ethics" was not added to the title until the 1985 code was replaced with its sixth and latest revision in 2001. Within the code are nine moral provisions that are nonnegotiable with regard to nurses' work. Detailed guidelines for clinical practice, education, research, administration, and self-development are found in the accompanying interpretive statements of each provision (see Appendix A for the ANA *Code of Ethics for Nurses with Interpretive Statements*).

A clear patient focus in the 2001 code obliges nurses to remain attentive and loyal to each patient in their care, but nurses must also be cognizant of ethical issues and conflicts of interest that potentially have a negative effect on patient care and relationships with patients. Other forces to be reckoned with in today's environment are the politics in institutions and cost-cutting strategic plans (see Box 3.1).

In the code, the ANA (2001) emphasized the need for the habitual practice of virtues such as wisdom, honesty, and courage, because these virtues reflect a morally good person and promote the values of human dignity, well-being, respect, health, and independence. Values in nursing emphasize what is important for the nurse personally and for patients. The ANA emphasized the magnitude of moral respect for all human beings, including the respect of nurses for themselves. **Personal regard** involves nurses extending attention and care to their own requisite needs, as nurses who do not regard themselves as worthy of care usually cannot fully care for others. Recognizing the dignity of oneself and of each patient is essential in moral reasoning. There are other statements in the code about **wholeness of character**, which pertains to recognizing the values of the nursing profession and one's own authentic moral values, integrating these belief systems, and then expressing them appropriately.

BOX 3.1 ETHICAL FORMATIONS: *CODE OF ETHICS* APPLICATION

- In the *Code of Ethics for Nurses with Interpretive Statements*, the ANA currently emphasizes the word "patient" instead of the word "client" in referring to the recipients of nursing care. Do you agree with this change? Please explain your rationale for your answer.
- Take a few minutes to review the ANA *Code of Ethics for Nurses with Interpretive Statements* (2001) in Appendix A. In your view, should there be additional provisions of the code? Would you remove any of the nine provisions? Please explain your rationale for your answers.
- After reviewing the interpretive statements in the code, discuss random brief scenarios on how nurses can justify their actions with the following approaches or frameworks: the principles of autonomy, beneficence, nonmaleficence, and justice; Kant's categorical imperatives based on deontology; a utilitarian framework; a virtue ethics approach; and an ethic of care approach.

International Council of Nurses' Code of Ethics for Nurses

In 1953, the ICN adopted its first code of ethics for nurses. (See Appendix B for the 2006 ICN *Code of Ethics for Nurses.*) The multiple revisions illustrate a reaffirmation of the code as a universal global document for ethical practice in nursing. The four major elements contained in the code involve standards related to nurses and people, practice, the profession, and coworkers. The elements in the code form a framework that must be internalized before it can be used as a guide for nursing conduct in practice, education, research, and leadership.

Common Thread between American Nurses Association and International Council of Nurses Codes

A common theme between the ANA (2001) and ICN (2006) codes is a focus on the importance of compassionate patient care aimed at alleviating suffering. Nurses are to support patients' self-determination and are to protect the moral space where patients receive care. The interests of various nursing associations and healthcare institutions must not be placed above those of patients. Nurses are to uphold the moral agreement that they make with patients and communities when they join the nursing profession. Nursing care includes the primary responsibilities of promoting health and preventing illness, but the primacy of nursing care has always involved caring for patients who are experiencing varying degrees of physical, psychological, and spiritual suffering.

Professional Boundaries in Nursing

Professional ethical codes serve as useful, systematic, normative guidelines for providing direction and shaping behavior. The ANA and ICN codes apply to all nurses regardless of their role, although no code can provide a complete and absolute set of rules free of conflict and ambiguity—a rationale often cited in favor of the use of virtue ethics as a better approach to ethics (Beauchamp & Childress, 2009).

Some people contend that nurses who are without a virtuous character cannot be depended on to act in good or moral ways, even with a professional code as a guide. In the 30th-anniversary issue in 2006 of the *Journal of Advanced Nursing*, the editors reprinted and revisited a 1996 article by Esterhuizen titled, "Is the Professional Code Still the Cornerstone of Clinical Nursing Practice?", and solicited three responses. One respondent, Tschudin, agreed with Esterhuizen that nursing lacks opportunities for full autonomy in moral decision making. There is abundant ground for nurses to engage in moral decisions, but they still do not have enough opportunity to participate. In the current uncertain moral landscape, nurses often wonder about the benefit of codes of ethics. Tschudin's key message was that virtuous nurses with full autonomy and accountability have an internal moral compass to guide their practice and do not necessarily need a code of ethics.

However one perceives the value of the codes of ethics for nurses, they still serve as mandates for accountability in practice. Professional boundary issues occur in all settings of nursing. **Professional nursing boundaries** are commonly defined as limits that protect the space between the nurse's professional power and the patient's vulnerabilities. Boundaries facilitate a safe connection in a relationship, because they give each person in the relationship a sense of legitimate control, whether the relationships are between the nurse and patient, the nurse and physician, the nurse and administrator, or nurse and nurse. **Boundary crossings** or violations are actions that do not promote the best interest of the other person(s) in a relationship; crossings pose a potential risk, harm, or exploitation to the other(s) in the relationship. The blurring of boundaries between persons in a relationship is often subtle and unrecognizable at first. The ANA (2001) included numerous boundary issues in the code. See Box 3.2 for a few examples of these boundary topics and moral obligations.

Qualities of Ethical Nurses

Numerous qualities, or virtues, could describe the ideal ethical nurse. The foremost quality, often considered the fiber for all others, is moral integrity. Some people believe that moral integrity is necessary for the individual as a whole to flourish. A person with moral integrity usually is described as having honesty, truthfulness, trustworthiness, courage, benevolence, and wisdom. In this section, there is a discussion of (1) moral integrity—honesty, truthfulness, and moral courage; (2) concern—advocacy and power; and (3) culturally sensitive care. Other qualities, such as respect for others and confidentiality, are explored in the previous chapter.

Moral Integrity

Moral integrity represents a person's wholeness of character. T. G. Plante (2004) stated that although no one is mistake free, people with moral integrity follow a

BOX 3.2 ETHICAL FORMATIONS: PROFESSIONAL BOUNDARIES AND MORAL OBLIGATIONS FOR NURSES AS SPECIFIED BY THE ANA *CODE OF ETHICS FOR NURSES WITH INTERPRETIVE STATEMENTS* (2001)

Clinical Practice Boundaries

- Respecting patients' dignity
- Right to self-determination
- Delegating tasks appropriately
- Practicing good judgment
- Accepting accountability in practice
- Alleviating suffering
- Being attentive to patients' interests
- Working within the nurse practice acts and nursing standards of practice

Professional Practice Boundaries

- Maintaining authenticity in all relationships with others, such as nurse-to-nurse relationships, nurse–physician relationships, nurse-to-patient relationships, and multidisciplinary collaboration
- Addressing and evaluating issues of impaired practice; fraternizing inappropriately with patients or others; accepting inappropriate gifts from patients and families; confidentiality and privacy violations; and unhealthy, unsafe, illegal, or unethical environments

Self-Care and Self-Development Boundaries and Obligations

- Participating in self-care activities to maintain and promote moral self-respect, professional growth and competence, wholeness of character in nurses' actions and in relationships with others, and preservation of integrity
- Advancing knowledge and research through professionalism, practice, education, and administrative contributions
- Collaborating with other healthcare professionals and the public to promote community, national, and international efforts
- Promoting healthy practices in the community through political activism or professional organizations by addressing unsafe, unethical, or illegal health practices that have the potential to harm the community

moral compass and usually they do not vary by appeals to act immorally. Most of the time, when people speak of a person's moral integrity, they are referring to a person's quality of character.

People with moral integrity pursue a moral purpose in life, understand their moral obligations in the community, and are committed to following through without any constraints imposed on them by their moral stance. In a qualitative study on moral integrity by Laabs (2011), nurses' perceptions of the definition of **moral integrity** were, "[A] state of being, acting like, and becoming a certain kind of person. This person is honest, trustworthy, consistently doing the right thing and standing up for what is right despite the consequences" (p. 433).

Features of moral integrity include good character, intent, and performance. Nurses with moral integrity act consistently with personal and professional values. When nurses are asked or pressured to do something that conflicts with their values, such as to falsify records, deceive patients, or accept verbal abuse from others, moral distress may occur. In a healthcare system often burdened with constraints of politics, self-serving groups or interests, and organizational bureaucracy, threats to moral integrity can be a serious pitfall for nurses. When nurses with moral integrity must compromise, the compromise usually does not interfere with their personal or professional values. To have moral integrity means that a person's character is made of up several virtues; three of those virtues are honesty, truthfulness, and moral courage.

Moral Distress

Moral distress occurs when nurses or other healthcare professionals have multiple or dual expectations and cannot act according to the guidance of their moral integrity. Jameton (1984) popularized and defined the term **moral distress** as occurring "when one knows the right thing to do, but institutional constraints make it nearly impossible to pursue the right course of action" (p. 6). Nurses' work involves hard choices that sometimes result in avoidance of patients, emotional and physical suffering, painful ambiguity, contradiction, frustration, anger, and guilt. Since Jameton's initial work, authors have continued to research and develop the conception of moral distress.

Numerous scholars have linked moral distress to incompetent or poor care, unsafe or inadequate staffing, overwork, cost constraints, ineffective policy, futile care, unsuccessful advocacy, the current definition of brain death, objectification of patients, and unrealistic hope (e.g., Corley, 2002; Corley, Minick, Elswick, & Jacobs, 2005; Pendry, 2007; Schluter, Winch, Holzhauser, & Henderson, 2008; McCue, 2011). Moral distress is defined in the context of institutional constraints. Research has revealed that nurses' work environments have a strong effect on the degree of moral distress experienced (e.g., Redman & Fry, 2000).

Leaders of nursing continue to search for strategies to reduce moral distress and promote healthy work environments. The American Association of Critical-Care Nurses (AACN) published a position statement to accentuate the seriousness of moral distress in nursing:

> Moral distress is a critical, frequently ignored, problem in healthcare work environments. Unaddressed it restricts nurses' ability to provide optimal patient care and to find job satisfaction. AACN asserts that every nurse and every employer are responsible for implementing programs to address and mitigate the harmful effects of moral distress in the pursuit of creating a healthy work environment. (American Association of Critical Care Nurses [AACN], 2008, p. 1)

The AACN ethics work group developed a call-to-action plan—*The Four A's to Rise above Moral Distress*—for use by nurses to identify and analyze moral distress (AACN, 2004):

- **Ask** appropriate questions to become aware that moral distress is present.
- **Affirm** your distress and commitment to take care of yourself and address moral distress.
- **Assess** sources of your moral distress to prepare for an action plan.
- **Act** to implement strategies for changes to preserve your integrity and authenticity.

Honesty

In the 2010 Gallup poll, just as it had been over the past 11 years, nurses were rated as the most honest and ethical health professionals (Jones, 2011). Nurses continue to be ranked consistently as the most trusted voice among the healthcare professionals; nurses have earned this trust because of their commitment and loyalty to their patients. According to Laabs (2011), nurses voiced that being honest was important for three reasons: (1) honesty is a prerequisite for good care, (2) dishonesty is always exposed in the end, and (3) nurses are expected to be honest.

In a phenomenological study of nurses on honesty in palliative care, Erichsen, Danielsson, and Friedrichsen (2010) stated that nurses had some difficulty defining honesty. In an attempt to clarify their perception of honesty, nurses often defined lying or dishonesty as sharp contrasts to honesty. Nurses perceived honesty as a virtue related to facts, metaphors, ethics, and communication, while perceiving truthtelling as a palpable feature in trusting relationships.

Honesty, in simple terms, can be defined as being "real, genuine, authentic, and bona fide" (Bennett, 1993, p. 597). Honesty is more than just telling the truth: it is the substance of human relationships. It involves people having the ability to place emphasis on resolve and action to achieve a just society by exercising a willingness to dig for truth in a rational, methodical, and diligent way. A person with maturity in honesty will place bits of truths into perspective and prudently search for the missing truths before addressing the issue. In other words, honesty is well-thought out and rehearsed behavior that reflects commitment and integrity.

There are many ways that nurses can portray honesty. For example, nurses must stay committed to their promises to patients and follow through with appropriate behaviors, such as returning to patients' hospital rooms, as promised, to help them with certain tasks. If nurses do not follow through with their commitments, trust may be broken, and patients potentially will see those nurses as dishonest or untrustworthy.

Honesty is also about being honest with one's self. For example, if a nurse was in the process of administering medications and a pill fell on the hospital floor, would the nurse be justified in wiping it off and placing it back in the cup if no one was there to see the action? Nurses might be tempted to wipe off the pill and administer it just to keep from completing a required form for a replacement medication, but if nurses evaluate their problems and make decisions based on the thought "always be honest with myself," it is more likely that they will make rational, trustworthy decisions regarding the care of patients.

Truthfulness

Aristotle recognized truthfulness as the mean between imposture (excessiveness) and self-deprecation (deficiency) and as one of the 12 excellences (virtues) that he identified in his book *Nicomachean Ethics* (Aristotle, 2002, C. Row Trans.). People accomplish their ultimate goal of happiness only by exercising rational and intellectual thinking, which is known as wisdom or contemplation. Aristotle explained his view of a truthful person as being **the truthful sort** (see Box 3.3).

Based on the principle of veracity, truthfulness is what we say and how we say it. **Truthfulness**, translated to "truthtelling" in the healthcare environment, means that nurses are usually ethically obligated to tell the truth and are not intentionally to deceive or mislead patients. Because of the emphasis in the Western world on patients' right to know about their personal health care, truthtelling has become the basis for most relationships between healthcare professionals and their patients (Beauchamp & Childress, 2009). In the older, traditional approach, disclosure or truthtelling was done with more of a beneficent or paternalistic approach and involved basing actions on answers to the questions such as, "What is best for my patient to know?"

The ethical question to ask is: Are there ever circumstances when nurses should be ethically excused from telling the truth to their patients? The levels of disclosure in health care and the cultural viewpoints on truthtelling create too much fogginess for a clear line of distinction to be drawn between nurses telling or not telling the truth. The ANA *Code of Ethics for Nurses* (2001) obligates nurses to be honest in matters involving patients and themselves, and to express a moral point of view when they become aware of unethical practices.

In some Western cultures, such as the United States, autonomy is so valued that withholding information is unacceptable. Under this same autonomy principle, it is assumed that patients also have a right not to know their medical history if they so desire. Some cultures, such as those in several Eastern countries, do not prize autonomy in this way; the head of the family or the elders usually decide how much and what information needs to be disclosed to the family member as patient.

BOX 3.3 ETHICAL FORMATIONS: ARISTOTLE'S "THE TRUTHFUL SORT"

"We are not here talking about the person who tells the truth in the context of agreements, or anything of that sort . . . but about contexts in which . . . a person is truthful both in the way he talks and in the way he lives, by virtue of being such by disposition. Someone like this would seem to be a decent person. For the lover of truth, since he also tells the truth where it makes no difference, will tell the truth even more where it does make a difference; for there he will be guarding against falsehood as something shameful, when he was already guarding against it in itself. Such a person is to be praised."

Source: Quotation from Aristotle. (2002). *Nichomachean ethics.* (C. Rowe, Trans.) New York, NY: Oxford University Press.

Therapeutic Privilege

The American Medical Association (AMA, 2006) published a statement on the definition of **therapeutic privilege** and offered an explanation of its moral meaning. The following excerpt spotlights this opinion:

> [T]he practice of withholding patient medical information from patients in the belief that disclosure is medically contraindicated is known as therapeutic privilege. It creates a conflict between the physician's obligations to promote patients' welfare and respect for their autonomy by communicating truthfully. Therapeutic privilege does not refer to withholding medical information in emergency situations, or reporting medical errors.
>
> Withholding medical information from patients without their knowledge or consent is ethically unacceptable. Physicians should encourage patients to specify their preferences regarding communication of their medical information, preferably before the information becomes available [but] physicians should honor patient requests not to be informed of certain medical information or to convey the information to a designated proxy . . .
>
> All information need not be communicated to the patient immediately or all at once; physicians should assess the amount of information a patient is capable of receiving at a given time, delaying the remainder to a later, more suitable time, and should tailor disclosure to meet patients' needs. (para. 1, 2, 3)

When physicians exercise this privilege, they base their opinion on facts gathered from the patient's records and their interactions with the patient, family, and other healthcare professionals. There are several reasons nurses or physicians might avoid telling the full truth: (1) they are trying to protect patients from sad and heartbreaking news, (2) they do not know the facts, or (3) they state what they know to be untrue about the situation rather than admit everything they know to be true.

There are advantages for physicians and nurses to tell the truth, especially when patients are in advanced stages of a diagnosis (Loprinzi et al., 2010). With the full knowledge of the disease process, patients will make fully informed decisions, be prepared for the outcomes, have more meaningful dialogue with family members, and make the most of meaningful events during their remaining life. Physicians and nurses are left with a difficult decision to make, especially when a patient wants to know the full truth and physicians have decided to disclose only part of the truth—or none of it—to the patient. No matter how disappointing the news will be to patients and families, nurses must evaluate each situation carefully with wisdom and contemplation before making any decision on the degree of disclosure. A clear understanding of the communication that has transpired between the physician and patient and family members contributes to the nurse's decision on the degree of shared disclosure (see Box 3.4).

An excellent example of truthtelling is from the play *Wit* by Margaret Edson, winner of the 1998 Pulitzer Prize; the play was published as a book, then in 2001 was made into an HBO Home Movie and is available for purchase. Susie Monahan, R.N., decided to tell the truth to and be forthright with a patient despite a few physicians who chose not to do so (see Box 3.5).

BOX 3.4 ETHICAL FORMATIONS: A WOMAN WITH UTERINE CANCER

You are caring for a woman scheduled for a hysterectomy because of uterine cancer. Her surgeon is known to have a bad surgical record in general, but especially in performing hysterectomies. The woman has heard gossip to this effect and asks you about it before her surgery because she is apprehensive about using that surgeon. You know for a fact that at least one legal suit has been filed against him because you personally know the woman involved in the case—a botched hysterectomy.

Your choices are: you could be brutally honest and truthful with your preoperative patient, you could give her part of the truth by giving her information that you know to be untrue about certain gossip or not confirming the truth about certain gossip, or you could be totally untruthful by remaining silent or by telling her that you have heard nothing.

- Discuss these options and any other ideas that you may have in regard to this case. As a nurse who wants to be committed to an ethical nursing practice, what actions might you consider in this difficult circumstance? Be as objective as possible.
- Now that you have determined possible actions, please justify these actions by applying either Kant's deontological theory or a virtue ethics approach.
- Describe the major differences, or any similarities, between these two frameworks (deontology versus virtue ethics).
- Other than simply verbally telling the truth to patients and others, how else can you display honesty in ethical nursing practice? Think of how you would portray honesty in different settings and situations—bedside nursing of patients, documentation, dealing with coworkers, and administration—while taking into consideration the ANA *Code of Ethics for Nurses with Interpretive Statements.*

Moral Courage

> *Without moral courage, our brightest virtues rust from lack of use. With it, we build piece by piece a more ethical world.*
>
> —RUSHWORTH M. KIDDER, "A WHITE PAPER," INSTITUTE OF GLOBAL ETHICS

Moral courage is having the courage to be moral (Kidder, 2005). Although defined in several ways, Kidder associated five core values with moral courage: honesty, respect, responsibility, fairness, and compassion. In a hermeneutical analysis of nurses in advanced practice, Spence and Smythe (2007) found that courage is an individual and a collective phenomenon that occurs in everyday practice. From the findings, Spence and Smyth stated that **courage** "can be seen as a response to threat or challenge, real in the present, recognized in the past, and/or anticipated in the future" (p. 52).

Having moral courage means that a nurse overcomes fear by confronting an issue head on, especially when the issue is a conflict of the nurse's core values and beliefs. **Moral courage** is having the will to speak out and do the right thing even when constraints or forces to do otherwise are present. Moral courage turns principles into actions. When nurses have the courage to do what they believe is the

BOX 3.5 ETHICAL FORMATIONS: SUSIE MONAHAN, R.N.: *WIT*—TRUTHTELLING

Susie Monahan was a registered nurse who was caring for Vivian Bearing, a dying patient with cancer, at a large research hospital. Vivian was getting large doses of cancer chemotherapy without any success of remission—in fact, the cancer was progressing at an alarming rate. She was near death but the research physicians wanted to challenge her body with chemotherapy for as long as possible to observe outcome effects. Everyone on the medical staff had been cold and technically minded, and no one had shown any concern for her except for Susie. Vivian had not been informed about the chemotherapy failure, her prognosis, or that she was dying. One night, Susie found Vivian crying and in a state of panic. Susie first helped to calm her, then shared a popsicle with Vivian at the bedside while she disclosed the full truth to Vivian about her chemotherapy, her prognosis, her choices about Code Blue or DNR, and her imminent death. Susie affectionately explained:

> You can be "full code," which means that if your heart stops, they'll call a Code Blue and the code team will come and resuscitate you and take you to Intensive Care until you stabilize again. Or you can be "Do Not Resuscitate," so if your heart stops we'll . . . well, we'll just let it. You'll be "DNR." You can think about it, but I wanted to present both choices . . . " (p. 67).
>
> Susie felt an urge to be truthful and honest. By giving human respect to Vivian, Susie was showing her capacity to be human.

Source: Edson, M. (1999). *Wit.* New York, NY: Faber & Faber.

right thing in a particular situation, they make a personal sacrifice by possibly standing alone, but will feel a sense of peace in their decision. When nurses are in a potential risk of danger, they need moral courage to act according to their core values, beliefs, or their moral conscience. Nurses are susceptible to experiences of apprehension and fear because of the uncertainty in outcomes, even when they have a high degree of certitude that they are doing the right thing.

Even though physical harm could be a potential threat, it is more likely that threats will materialize in the form of "humiliation, rejection, ridicule, unemployment, and loss of social standing" (Lachman, 2007, p. 131). A few examples of having moral courage are (1) confronting or reporting a peer who is stealing and using drugs at work, (2) confronting a physician who ordered questionable treatments that are not within the reasonable standard of care, (3) confronting an administrator regarding unsafe practices or staffing patterns, (4) standing against peers who are planning an emotionally hurtful action toward another peer, and (5) reporting another nurse for exploitation of a patient or family member, such as when a nurse posts a picture or story of a patient on a social networking site.

Lachman (2007) offered two strategies to help nurses to exhibit moral courage in threatening situations. Nurses would probably regret any careless and hasty reactions, or even nonreaction or silence, on their part, so they must first try to soothe inner feelings that could trigger these behaviors. Self-talk, relaxation techniques, and moral reasoning to process information, while pushing out negative thoughts, are ways for nurses to keep calm in the face of a confrontation involving moral courage. Second, nurses must assess the whole scenario while identifying the risks and benefits involved in standing alone.

Concern

Advocacy

A general definition of **advocacy** is pleading in favor of or supporting a case, person, group, or cause, but many variations on the definition of advocacy exist. Related to professional nursing ethics, Bu and Jezewski (2006) found in their concept analysis that **patient advocacy** is defined as having three central features:

- Safeguarding patients' autonomy
- Acting on behalf of patients
- Championing social justice in the provision of health care (p. 104)

Patient advocacy, an essential element of ethical nursing practice, requires that nurses embrace the promotion of well-being and uphold the rights and interests of their patients (Vaartio, Leino-Kilpi, Salanterä, & Suominen, 2006). The ANA (2001) did not define the terms advocacy or patient advocacy in the *Code of Ethics for Nurses with Interpretive Statements*, although advocating for the patient is implied in some places in the code and is also explicit in others, such as in the interpretive statements: "Nurses are leaders and vigilant advocates for the delivery of dignified and humane care" (p. 8) and in Provision 3 of the code: "The nurse promotes, advocates for, and strives to protect the health, safety, and rights of the patient" (p. 12).

Nurses are in ideal positions for a patient advocacy role. Nurses can clarify and discuss patient rights, health goals, treatment issues, and potential outcomes with patients, but barriers to advocacy often become a nursing reality. These barriers are shadows that remain as unresolved issues. Refer to Box 3.6.

Hamric (2000) offered excellent ways for nurses to boost their patient advocacy skills: (1) nursing educators need to convert the basic ethics education to real-life action; (2) practicing nurses need to continue their education on the ethical imperatives of advocacy; and (3) institutions need to review their incentives, if any, to promote patient advocacy. Butts (2011) created an acronym labeled **PRISMS** as a reminder of strategies to promote patient advocacy (see Box 3.7).

Power

Power, by definition, means that a person or group has influence in an effective way over others—power results in action. Nurses with power have the ability to influence persons, groups, or communities. Nurses ingrained with the ideals of **socialized power** seek goals to benefit others with intent to avoid harm or negative effects—an indication of the principles of beneficience, nonmaleficence, and justice at work. Goals of social benefit to others are usually accomplished through the efforts of members of large service organizations, and individual volunteer work by

BOX 3.6 ETHICAL FORMATIONS: BARRIERS TO NURSING ADVOCACY

Barriers to nursing advocacy were identified by Hanks (2007) based on findings from existing literature.

- Conflicts of interest between the nurse's moral obligation to the patient and nurse's sense of duty to the institution
- Institutional constraints
- A lack of education and time
- Threats of punishment
- A gender-specific, historical, critical social barrier related to nurses' expectations of a subservient duty to medical doctors

Source: Adapted from Hanks, R. G. (2007). Barriers to nursing advocacy: A concept analysis. *Nursing Forum, 42*(4), 171–177.

BOX 3.7 ETHICAL FORMATIONS: PRISMS—AN ACRONYM FOR KEY ACTION VERBS FOR STRATEGIES TO PROMOTE PATIENT ADVOCACY

P Persuade
R Respect
I Intercede
S Safeguard
M Monitor
S Support

Source: Butts, J. B. (2011). PRISMS—An Acronym for key action verbs for strategies to promote patient advocacy. Personal Collection. Ellisville, MS, copyright 2011.

nurses and others at service organizations contributes to the efforts and shared goals of the larger organization and also can contribute to efforts of smaller goals for individuals, small groups, and small areas of the community. Nurses continue to take advantage of their empowerment as a profession in order to control the content of their practice, the context of their practice, and their competence in practice.

Hakesley-Brown and Malone (2007) found in their research that nurses and patients are a powerful entity evolving over time because of paradigm shifts in clinical, political, and organizational power. Nurses have facilitated patients' emancipation from a paternalistic form of care to today's autonomous decision makers seeking quality care. With nurses being directly involved in quality of care, they are in a prime position to use power to benefit patients and the professional practice of nursing.

Ponte et al. (2007) interviewed nursing leaders from six organizations to understand, from the leaders' perspectives on the concept of power, ways that nurses can acquire power and ways that these leaders demonstrate power in their practice and work. Refer to more detail on sources of leadership power in Chapter 12. According to the leaders in the study, power lies within *each nurse* who engages in patient care and in other roles, such as in organizations, with colleagues, and within the nursing profession as a whole. As nurses develop knowledge and expertise in practice from multiple domains, they integrate and use their power in a "collaborative, interdisciplinary effort focused solely on the patients and families that the nurse and care team serve and with whom they partner" (Ponte et al., 2007, Characteristics of Nursing Power section, para. 1). Ponte et al. found eight properties of a powerful professional practice, which could serve as a basis for current and future power in nursing. Refer to Boxes 3.8 and 3.9.

Culturally Sensitive Care

Culture refers to "integrated patterns of human behavior that include the language, thoughts, communications, actions, customs, beliefs, values, and/or institutions of racial, ethnic, religious, and/or social groups" (Lipson & Dibble, 2005, p. xi). Giving culturally sensitive care is a core element in closing the gap on health disparities. Spector (2004) explained that providing **culturally sensitive care** means that nurses must first have a basic knowledge of culturally diverse customs and then demonstrate constructive attitudes based on that knowledge. A culturally competent nurse or healthcare provider

BOX 3.8 ETHICAL FORMATIONS: PONTE ET AL.'S PROPERTIES OF A POWERFUL PROFESSIONAL NURSING PRACTICE

Nurses who have developed a powerful nursing practice:

- Acknowledge their unique role in the provision of patient- and family-centered care.
- Commit to continuous learning through education, skill development, and evidence-based practice.
- Demonstrate professional comportment [manner in which one conducts oneself] and recognize the critical nature of presence.
- Value collaboration and partner effectively with colleagues in nursing and other disciplines.
- Actively position themselves to influence decisions and resource allocation.
- Strive to develop an impeccable character: to be inspirational, compassionate, and have a credible, sought-after perspective (the antithesis of power as a coercive strategy).
- Recognize that the role of a nurse leader is to pave the way for nurses' voices to be heard and to help novice nurses develop into powerful professionals.
- Evaluate the power of nursing and the nursing department in organizations they enter by assessing the organization's mission and values and its commitment to enhancing the power of diverse perspectives.

Source: Quoted from Ponte, P. R., Glazer, G., Dann, E., McCollum, K., Gross, A., Tyrell, R., . . . Washington, D. (2007). The power of professional nursing practice—An essential element of patient and family centered care. *The Online Journal of Issues in Nursing, 12*(1). Retrieved from http://www.nursingworld.org/MainMenuCategories/ANAMarketplace/ANAPeriodicals/OJIN/TableofContents/Volume122007/No1Jan07/tpc32_316092.aspx

BOX 3.9 ETHICAL FORMATIONS: TWO LEVELS OF POWER

There are a variety of ways that power can be abusive, coercive, or not used at all. Nurses who do not use their power for the good of a situation are ineffective. There are two examples of power presented here, one on a smaller scale and one on a larger scale.

Power on a Smaller Scale: Ms. Gomez's diagnosis is an inoperable and incurable cancer of the liver. She is unaware of her diagnosis but realizes that she is experiencing abdominal pain that she described as 8 on a 10-point scale. Everyone in the oncology unit is involved in her care and aware of her diagnosis, except for her. The nurses had been observing Ms. Gomez's continued edginess and irritability as they interacted with her. Ms. Gomez senses something is terribly wrong and begins to panic when physicians gather in her room for clinical rounds and talk medical jargon about her "case" in front of her. Ms. Gomez experienced an acute anxiety reaction. Her outcome could have been better had her nurse beforehand discussed the situation with the physicians and tried convincing them to discuss her case somewhere else and/or asked them politely to tell her the truth about her diagnosis and prognosis. Had the nurse exerted a noncoercive power over this situation, the outcome potentially could have been averted. What specific actions could this nurse have taken on a small-scale or unit level in terms of unit policies regarding clinical rounds or disclosure to patients?

Power on a Larger Scale: Nurse Mary is a nurse at a hospice located in a coastal region and has six patients in her care. The national weather center forecasted several potential life-threatening hurricanes for her region during the next two weeks. Most of her patients are financially challenged. Mary has choices to make: (1) she could do nothing and let nature take its course; (2) she could educate her patients and families on ways to prepare for disaster; or (3) she could educate her patients and families on disaster preparedness as well as use her power to help poor, homebound patients—not just her patients—in the community to prepare for disaster. One way for Mary to exercise her power immediately on a large, community-wide scale is to have a fundraiser and supply drive, then work with agencies such as the American Red Cross to recruit community or nurse volunteers for distributing the supplies, handing out disaster preparedness information, and verbally educating the families. What are other strategies that Mary could implement?

> develops an awareness of his or her existence, sensations, thoughts, and environment without letting these factors have an undue effect on those for whom care is provided. Cultural competence is the adaptation of care in a manner that is consistent with the culture of the client and is therefore a conscious process and nonlinear. (Purnell, 2002, p. 193)

Purnell (2011) explained that the process of nurses getting to know themselves and their values, beliefs, and moral compass is fundamental to providing culturally competent care. Without some degree of cultural knowledge, nurses cannot possibly provide ethical care; one example is that relationships with others cannot develop into a trusting, respectful exchange.

Lipson and Dibble's (2005) trademark name, ASK, serves as an acronym that nurses can use when approaching patients of various cultures; it refers to awareness, sensitivity, and knowledge. There are many cultural views in the United

States, and these are based on each culture's belief system on health, illness, pain, suffering, birth, parenting, death, dying, health care, communication, and truth, among others. Lipson and Dibble (2005) emphasized that nurses need to conduct a quick assessment on cultural diversity needs. The following basic cultural assessment questions are based on ASK:

1. What is the patient's ethnic affiliation?
2. Who are the patient's major support persons and where do they live?
3. With whom should we speak about the patient's health or illness?
4. What are the patient's primary and secondary languages, and speaking and reading abilities?
5. What is the patient's economic situation? Is income adequate to meet the patient's and family's need? (Lipson & Dibble, 2005, p. xiii)

Nurses' authentic attention to cultural diversity and the diversity within each culture promotes ethically competent care, which is essential in everyday nursing practice. Nurses must be open-minded to increasing their knowledge and awareness to the needs of culturally diverse patients. The *Code of Ethics for Nurses with Interpretive Statements* (ANA, 2001) contains explicit guidelines for giving care to individuals regardless of social or economic status, personal attributes, or nature of health problems. Nursing care based on the code includes giving care with cultural sensitivity.

Refer to Boxes 3.10 and 3.11 to test your moral grounding. In this section on qualities of ethical nurses, you have read about selected qualities that make up ethical nurses—moral integrity, honesty, truthtelling, advocacy, power, and culturally sensitive care.

Nursing Professional Relationships

Nurse–Physician Relationships

Women endured many centuries of oppression from male-dominated hierarchies, such as religious institutions. Women healers, accused of being witches, were burned at the stake from the 1300s to the 1600s (Ehrenreich & English, 1973), and other events also gave rise to oppression of women during that time. By the early 20th century, Florence Nightingale's work from the 1800s had achieved some respect for the role of nurses, but nurses and other mostly female occupations "were presented as simple extensions of women's 'natural' domestic role" (Ehrenreich & English, 1973, p. 38). Nurses, to varying degrees, have been working since that time to overcome this perception.

Stein (1967), a physician, characterized a type of relationship between physicians and nurses that he called the **doctor–nurse game**. The game is based on a hierarchical relationship with doctors being in the position of the superior. The hallmark of the game is that open disagreement between the disciplines is to be avoided, and

BOX 3.10 ETHICAL FORMATIONS: TEST YOUR MORAL GROUNDING!

Thus far, you have learned about the qualities that define ethical nursing. The codes of ethics and the qualities of ethical nurses assist nurses in developing moral grounding for professional practice, education, research, and leadership.

Test your personal moral grounding! List the ethical qualities of a nurse on a piece of paper and write down how they might relate to your ethical nursing practice. Briefly summarize an ethical situation or conflict that could arise with each ethical quality and a corresponding resolution.

- Moral integrity
- Honesty
- Truthfulness
- Moral courage
- Advocacy
- Power
- Culturally sensitive care

avoidance of conflict is achieved when an experienced nurse, who is able to provide helpful suggestions to a doctor regarding patient care, cautiously offers the suggestions in such a way so that the physician does not directly perceive that consultative advice is coming from a nurse. In the past, student nurses were educated about the rules of the game while attending nursing school. Over the years, others have given credence to the historical accuracy of Stein's characterization of doctor–nurse relationships (Fry & Johnstone, 2002; Jameton, 1984; Kelly, 2000).

Stein, Watts, and Howell (1990) revisited the doctor–nurse game concept 23 years after Stein first coined the phrase. They proposed that nurses unilaterally had decided to stop playing the game; some of the reasons for this change and ways the change was accomplished have involved nurses' increased use of dialogue rather than gamesmanship, the profession's goal of equal partnership status with other healthcare professionals, the alignment of nurses with the civil rights and women's movements, the increased percentage of nurses who are receiving higher education, and collaboration between nurses and physicians on projects. In the process of the dismantling of the game, many nurses took a less than communitarian stance with physicians.

There are nurses who believe that an adversarial fight needs to continue in order to establish nursing as an autonomous profession. Nurses' reports and opinions of strained relationships between nurses and physicians have steadily appeared in the literature across many countries of the world despite efforts by some nurses to have friendlier relationships with physicians. Reported reasons for the strained relationships include: (1) the hierarchical way that ethical care decisions are made, both institutional system decisions and physician decisions; (2) competency and quality of care conflicts; and (3) the lack of communication.

BOX 3.11 ETHICAL FORMATIONS: TEST YOUR MORAL GROUNDING! SHOULD I BUY THIS PAPER?

Megan, a nursing student, found a site on the Internet advertising a company that, for a fee, would customize a nursing school paper on any topic. She needed a paper in APA format on the concept of compassion in nursing practice and realized that she was overloaded with assignments from school, so she asked herself, "Should I buy this paper?" Without further thought, however, she completed the form and ordered the paper. The company sent the paper to her within 3 days. Megan then submitted the paper electronically to the professor as her own work.

- Who is the rightful owner of the paper?
- Is buying the paper unethical, illegal, or both? Please explain your rationale.
- Is this action cheating, plagiarism, or both, by common university or college standards of academic honesty? Please explain your rationale.
- What are some ethical implications that Megan needed to consider before buying the paper?
- What was an alternative action for Megan, based on Kant's deontology framework or a virtue ethics approach?
- What is a creative strategy that Megan's professor could use instead of the paper assignment to reduce the chance of students buying a paper on the Internet?
- What are some examples of other similar Internet incidents considered illegal or unethical?

(The story continues.)

The professor required that electronic versions of the paper be submitted, and Megan did not realize that the professor opened each document to review the name appearing in the properties of the document. The property name on Megan's document was National Nursing Papers. Megan was shocked when the professor questioned her about the name in the properties. She did not realize that a property name even existed. She could not give an adequate explanation for the existing name and finally admitted to buying the paper. She failed the course. Megan was not dismissed from the program for this one academic honesty violation, but the dean and professor gave her a one-time warning notice that if she cheated or plagiarized in any form in the future, she would be dismissed from the school of nursing and the university as instructed in the university's handbook. Megan signed the warning notice. She had no other choice if she wanted to remain in the nursing program.

- Do you believe, based on your analysis of the deontology framework, that Megan deserved another opportunity to remain in the nursing program? Please explain your rationale.

One example of research of an organizational culture is a qualitative focus group study by Malloy et al. (2009). Forty-two nurses from a variety of settings in four nations (Canada, Ireland, Australia, and Korea) participated to identify ethical dilemmas and decisions in the everyday care of elders with dementia, as well as to identify how end-of-life decisions are made. The researchers extracted four themes in conjunction with the unexpected finding that nurses from all countries consistently voiced strained and powerless hierarchical relationships with some physicians. The first theme arose as a result of two different philosophies: Care (nurses) versus treatment (physicians) was a source of tension between nurses and physicians on end-of-life decisions. The second theme was a constrained obligation in terms of the nurse–physician hierarchy, established protocol, and the way that decisions were made. Third, nurses perceived that physicians, patients, families, and the system silenced the nurse's voice; they also believed themselves to be unequal participants in the care of patients, largely because of the system. The fourth theme was a lack of respect for the profession of nursing from other professionals.

Pullon's (2008) qualitative study of 18 nurses and physicians in primary care settings from New Zealand is an example of research of the features that build an interprofessional nurse–physician relationship. Pullon identified certain extrinsic and intrinsic factors of this relationship, but focused the article only on the intrinsic nature of individual interprofessional relationships. A key feature of interprofessional relationships, demonstrated professional competence, served as the foundation for respect for each other and, in turn, formed trust calculated over time with reliable and consistent behavior.

Pullon found that nurses and physicians identified their professional groups as distinct but complementary to each other. Nurses described the formation and maintenance of quality professional relationships with patients and others as the heart of their professional work and described teamwork as one means for achieving those relationships. Physicians depicted the physician–patient relationship as the crux of their practice, but only in the context of consultation. Nurses and physicians both unveiled several shared values and attitudes, such as the provision of continuity of care; the ability to cope with unpredictable and demanding care; the importance of working together and building a relationship; and the significance of professional competence, mutual respect for each other, and trust in an ongoing relationship, but with the realization that trust could be broken quickly in the early stages of a trustworthy relationship.

Other studies have reflected findings similar to these highlighted studies. Nurses' perceptions of inequality with physicians reveal that the solutions are complex and currently do not exist universally. Churchman and Doherty (2010) found that certain factors contribute to the challenge of finding answers: nurses are discouraged from confronting physicians in everyday practice, fear of conflict and aggression by physicians, and fear of having their views disregarded. The institutional hierarchy continues to be a source for unequal rewards and power between nurses and physicians.

Nurse–Nurse Relationships

In the provisions of the code, the ANA (2001) characterized various ways that nurses demonstrate their primary responsibility to their patients (families and communities). Some key indicators found in the code that reflect this responsibility include having compassion for patients, showing respect to patients and to each other, collaborating with other healthcare professionals, protecting the rights and safety of patients, advocating for the patient and family, and caring for and preserving the integrity of self and others. Patient and family relationships are important, but good relationships with other nurses and with other healthcare professionals are necessary for the successful follow-through of that responsibility to patients.

Unfortunately, nurses often treat other nurses in hurtful ways through what some people have called lateral or horizontal violence (Kelly, 2000; McKenna, Smith, Poole, & Coverdale, 2003; Thomas, 2009). **Horizontal violence** involves interpersonal conflict, harassment, intimidation, harsh criticism, sabotage, and abuse among nurses, and may occur because nurses feel oppressed by other dominant groups, such as physicians or institutional administrators. Kelly (2000) reported that some nurses have characterized the violence perpetrated by nurses against other nurses who excel and succeed as the **tall poppy syndrome**. This perpetration creates an ostracizing nursing culture that discourages success.

Thomas and her research team (2009) studied the causes and consequences of nurses' stress and anger. In their interviews, nurses voiced horizontal and vertical violence as common sources of stress. Thomas (2009) stated, "One of the most disturbing aspects of our research data on nurses' anger is the vehemence of their anger at each other" (p. 98). Thomas (2009) identified common characteristics of horizontal violence as:

- Subtle nonverbal behaviors, such as rolling eyes, raising eyebrows, or giving a cold shoulder
- Sarcasm, snide remarks, rudeness
- Undermining or sabotaging
- Withholding needed information or assistance
- Passive-aggressive (behind the back) actions
- Spreading rumors and destructive gossip
- False accusations, scapegoating, blaming (p. 98)

Horizontal violence in nursing is counterproductive for the profession. Nurses can strengthen a sense of community among nurses by working to heal the disharmony. Nurses need to support other nurses' successes rather than treating colleagues as tall poppies that must be cut down.

There are occasions when unpleasant but nonmalicious action must be taken with regard to nursing colleagues. In addition to advocating for patients' unmet needs, nurses are advocates when they take appropriate action to protect patients from the unethical, illegal, incompetent, or impaired practice of other nurses (ANA, 2001). When nurses are aware of these situations, they need to obtain appropriate guidance from supervisory personnel and institutional policies; then, they need to confront the offending nurses in a constructive, compassionate way. Though action needs to be taken to safeguard patients' care, the manner in which a nurse handles situations involving unethical, incompetent, or impaired colleagues must not be a matter of gossip, condescension, or unproductive derogatory talk.

Thomas (2009) suggested that individual nurses need to self-reflect at the end of the workday by examining their actions and the dialogue they had with others. All nurses, those who follow through with daily self-reflection and those who do not, need to "make a commitment to supportive colleagueship" and "refuse to get caught up in workplace negativism" (p. 109).

Nurses on the 'Net

Many people who use the Internet have already experienced, to some degree, the consequences of unethical or illegal behavior, such as being the target of someone else's devious actions. There is no doubt that computers influence our personal and professional lives on an everyday basis, and so nurses and nursing students need to understand the potential for unethical and illegal behaviors.

Matters in Moral Spaces

The potential for professional boundary crossings exist as lines and moral spaces become blurred. **Moral space** is defined as "what we live in . . . any space formed from the relationships between natural and social objects, agents and events that protect or establish either the conditions for, or the realization of, some vision of the good life, or the good, in life" (Turnbull, 2003, p. 4). Respect for one another's moral spaces takes a serious commitment by those who use the Internet. Dozens of ethical codes of conduct exist for users of the Internet, but no matter how many codes exist or what population they serve, the codes are of no use if they are not practiced or if people are lacking in moral integrity. Nurses and nursing students must remain devoted to respecting human beings in all interactions and actions, even social networking. Some of the issues that can violate the principle of autonomy are matters of respect for human beings, self-determination, trustworthiness, confidentiality, and privacy.

Social Networking and Cellular Phones

Nurses are increasingly using social networks to befriend others who have common interests or to keep in touch with long-time friends. Facebook, Twitter, YouTube, and cellular phones have become highly important as communication methods for healthcare professionals, as they have for everyone. Two broad views exist on the degree of value and use of social networking, cell phones, and other media.

On the positive side, nurses and physicians have found value in sharing professional information and knowledge with patients or other nurses and physicians. Some nurses and physicians see social networking as unavoidable, but also as a means of providing minute-by-minute information and updates about healthcare trends and treatments. In 2011, the American Nurses Association published a booklet on the principles of social networking for nurses. The ANA highlighted how these social networking principles fit with the ANA's three foundational documents, one of which is the *Code of Ethics for Nurses with Interpretive Statements* (2001). The ANA (2011) stated that social networks "provide unparalled opportunities for rapid knowledge exchange and dissemination among many people" (p. 3).

Physicians also see value in the use of social networks to take care of routine work, such refilling prescriptions, answering questions, and sharing informational websites. In 2011, the American Medical Association (AMA) issued a policy statement on professionalism in the use of social media. The AMA stated that social media support "personal expression, enable individual physicians to have a professional presence online, foster collegiality and camaraderie within the profession, [and] provide opportunity to widely disseminate public health messages" (para. 1).

On the negative side, questions of confidentiality and privacy arise when nurses, physicians, and patients share information with each other on social networks or cellular phones. The public nature of any social communication poses ethical and legal problems, and solutions are usually labeled by employers and other leaders as unclear, gray, complicated, and uncertain.

The growing number of employee violations is driving employers to initiate disciplinary courses of action against personnel who engage in inappropriate behaviors on social network sites and cellular phones and to reenforce old policies or enforce new ones. If the codes of ethics and current hospital policies were followed, new policies on social networking and cellular phone use would not be required. Lee Thomas, Federal Secretary of the Australian Nursing Federation, acknowledged her concern by saying, "Social networking is instant and fun (so I'm told) but people are increasingly using these mediums to complain about employers, fellow staff members and among our colleagues [and] even patients" (2011, p. 23).

In two horror stories, nurses were suspected of patient exploitation and violations of confidentiality and privacy. One occurred in 2010 at Tri-City Medical Center in Oceanside, California. Five nurses were fired and a sixth nurse was disciplined for violating confidentiality. According to a spokesperson at the medical center, there was enough substantial information to warrant the firings of the five nurses, as the fired nurses discussed patient cases on Facebook ("Five nurses fired," 2010).

In an even more repulsive story in Louisiana, Lee Zurik, Investigator for Fox 8 Live WVUE-TV, stated that St. Tammany Parish Hospital emergency room (ER) nurses were reported by Reba Campbell, ER technician, for allegedly exploiting, making fun of, and taking cell phone pictures of unconscious patients on at least two different occasions. The most recent case involved an overweight man who overdosed on pain and anxiety medications. According to Zurik, Campbell stated:

> Clancy [one of the three reported nurses] and the other nurse walks in and puts these glasses on the patient and starts to make fun of him. That wasn't funny enough, so they took charcoal that we dumped down his throat and painted his face like a football player and said, "Welcome to St. Tammany Parish Hospital ER. This is your initiation for trying to kill yourself." (Zurik, 2011, para. 10)

Then two other nurses pulled out their phones. Campbell stated the nurses were "taking pictures with their two cell phones of this patient, unconscious, painted like a clown with charcoal and glasses on his face" (Zurik, 2011, para. 12). The nurses evidently had taken pictures of unconscious patients before, because the co-workers had been observed sitting at a desk and ranking the best pictures of different patients. One of the nurses even texted the photos on her cellular phone to a physician who named one patient picture as best in a text reply to the nurse. The attorney representing the unconscious charcoaled patient named the hospital and three nurses in the lawsuit. Of the three nurses and the physician, only one nurse has been fired.

Not related to and before those two incidents occurred, Thomas and her research team (2009) had interviewed nurses across the United States to find meaning in their layers of stress and anger over unethical, harmful, and dehumanizing treatment of patients as part of a larger study to uncover reasons for nurses' stress and anger. One of the themes that she discovered was "I feel morally sick." Nurses described situations they had observed as repugnant; they felt physically sick, disgusted, and nauseated, and believed they were powerless to do anything about those abhorrent situations. Thomas's interpretation of the narratives was that the nurses were experiencing moral distress as a result of their stress and anger. Moral distress is defined in a previous section of this chapter.

The nurses' narratives in Thomas's study were depictions of their terrible real-life experiences and feelings regarding stories not related necessarily to social networking. Unethical and illegal events have always been described and exposed by concerned healthcare personnel, but the digital age has brought many incidents to new levels of public exploitation. Sadly, social networking potentially could be a means for nurses to express frustrations in relation to their workplace, coworkers, and patients, but no matter what reasons exist for sharing and divulging information, nurses who do so violate their professional boundaries and most likely will have their license suspended or revoked. Information-sharing of any privileged information amounts to illegal, inappropriate, and unethical violations. Many nurses and physicians are seeing these concerns as a valid worry and accordingly are taking action collectively through professional organizations. The American Nurses Association (2011) published six principles of social networking for nurses. Where patients and nurses and all surrounding issues are concerned in health care, the commitments of privacy and confidentiality serve as the foundation for these six principles of social networking.

The Association of Pediatric Hematology/Oncology Nurses (APHON) recently issued a position statement on ethical guidelines for social networking ("Association of Pediatric Hematology/Oncology Nurses," 2011). In their social media policy, the AMA (2011) advised that physicians should weigh all of the issues of online presence, such as violations of patient confidentiality, privacy, and relationships. Other professional nursing organizations are already following suit as more issues of confidentiality, privacy, and exploitation have surfaced.

BOX 3.12 ETHICAL FORMATIONS: DOS AND DON'TS OF SOCIAL NETWORKING

Do

- Know your professional and legal responsibilities to maintain privacy and confidentiality.
- Know and follow your employer's policies on social networking.
- Educate yourself about privacy settings on the sites you use.
- Keep in mind that colleagues, as well as current and future employers, could access your posts, photos, and other activity.
- Remember, your employer has the right to access your online activity on work computers.

Don't

- Disclose any information about patients in your care.
- Upload photos or video of you, patients, or coworkers in a clinical setting.
- Make disparaging comments about patients, your employer, or coworkers.
- Discuss or post stories of clinical events, even if they are shocking or would be of interest to friends.

Source: Quoted from College and Association of Registered Nurses in Alberta. (2010). Dos and don'ts of social networking . . . avoid a social networking nightmare. *Alberta RN, 66*(6), 22–23.

Employers and professional organizations worldwide are taking measures to prevent ethical and legal violations in patient care. The College and Association of Registered Nurses of Alberta (CARNA, 2010) offered some "Dos and Don'ts" of social networking. These guidelines serve as an excellent reminder to nurses everywhere to observe their code of ethics. Refer to Box 3.12 for these guidelines.

Nurses and physicians serve as role models, whether or not they want this role. The newcomers to the healthcare professions emulate the conduct of the role modelers, both the positive and negative behaviors. It is imperative that existing nurses influence new nurses and other personnel in a positive manner. In most of the codes of ethics for nurses, including the ANA code, there is explicit discussion about nurses maintaining respect, confidentiality, and privacy; those same concepts are applicable to social networking and cellular phone use.

KEY POINTS

- Nursing ethics is defined as the examination of all kinds of ethical and bioethical issues from the perspectives of nursing theory and practice.
- To practice nursing ethically, nurses must be sensitive enough to recognize when they are facing seemingly obscure ethical issues in their everyday work.
- Within the 2001 ANA code are nine moral provisions that are nonnegotiable with regard to nurses' work. Detailed guidelines are found in the accompanying interpretive statements of each provision.

KEY POINTS (continued)

- A clear patient focus in the code obliges nurses to remain attentive and loyal to each patient in their care.
- A theme common to the ANA (2001) and ICN (2006) codes is a focus on the importance of compassionate patient care aimed at alleviating suffering.
- Boundaries facilitate a safe space in a relationship, because they give each person in the relationship a sense of legitimate control, whether the relationships are between the nurse and patient, the nurse and physician, the nurse and administrator, or nurse and nurse.
- Nurses with moral integrity act consistently with their personal and professional values.
- Nurses' moral distress occurs when institutional constraints prevent them from acting in a way consistent with their personal and professional values that make up their moral integrity.
- Nurses' work involves hard choices that sometimes result in avoidance of patients, emotional and physical suffering, painful ambiguity, contradiction, frustration, anger, and guilt.
- Research reveals a link between moral distress and the concepts of incompetent or poor care, unsafe or inadequate staffing, overwork, cost constraints, ineffective policy, futile care, unsuccessful advocacy, the current definition of brain death, objectification of patients, and unrealistic hope.
- Truthtelling means that nurses should not intentionally deceive or mislead patients.
- No matter how disappointing the news will be to patients and families, nurses must evaluate the situation carefully with wisdom and contemplation before making any decision on the degree of information disclosure.
- When nurses have the moral courage to do what they believe is the right thing in a particular situation, they make a personal sacrifice of possibly standing alone but will feel a sense of peace in their decision.
- Patient advocacy, an essential element of ethical nursing practice, requires that nurses embrace the ideals of the promotion of well-being and uphold the rights and interests of their patients.
- Nurses ingrained with the ideals of socialized power seek goals to benefit others with the intent to avoid harm or negative effects.
- Nurses' genuine attention to cultural diversity and the diversity within each culture promotes ethically competent care, which is essential in everyday nursing practice.
- For a successful nurse–physician relationship, three essential features need to be present: competence, respect, and trust.
- Nurses often treat other nurses in hurtful ways. Many refer to this treatment as horizontal violence.

KEY POINTS (continued)

- Social networking invokes questions of confidentiality and privacy when nurses, physicians, and patients share information with each other. The public nature of social communication poses ethical and legal problems, and solutions are usually unclear.
- The growing number of employee violations arising in social network sites worldwide is driving employers to initiate disciplinary courses of action against their personnel and to enforce new policies to prevent inappropriate behaviors.

CASE STUDY: JILL BECOMES DISHEARTENED

www

Jill is a 28-year-old, attractive, intelligent, and technically competent RN who has worked for 5 years in a medical–surgical unit of a small hospital. She has been well liked by her professional colleagues, and she habitually makes concerted attempts to deliver compassionate care to her patients. Recently, she left her job and began working in the busy surgical intensive care unit (ICU) at a local county hospital. Jill changed her job because she wanted to gain more-varied nursing experience. She was very excited and enthusiastic about her new job, but shortly after Jill began working in the ICU, she began to question her career decision. The more experienced nurses in the ICU are what Jill describes as "abrupt" and "exasperating" when she asks for help in learning ICU patient care and procedures. Jill states that the ICU nurses seem to be "testing my resolve to stick it out" and seem to want her to fail at learning how to work in the ICU. Many of the surgeons who regularly have patients in the ICU are described as being demanding and impatient with the ICU nursing staff. In addition to being intimidated by the ICU nursing staff, Jill says that she also is very intimidated by the physicians and was chastised by one of them for asking what he called "a stupid question." There is an "air of unhappiness" among all of the nurses throughout the hospital. Jill says working at this hospital is like no other situation that she has been involved with since becoming a nurse.

1. What do you believe are the underlying causes of the ICU nurses' treatment of Jill? Do you believe that it is likely that Jill's treatment has anything to do with her personal characteristics?
2. What could Jill do to try to improve her situation?
3. What are the possible implications in Jill's delivery of care that could arise because of the treatment that she is experiencing?
4. Do you believe that the "air of unhappiness" among all of the nursing staff at the hospital might be directly or indirectly affecting the treatment that Jill is receiving? Might it be affecting patient care hospital-wide? Give your rationale.
5. If Jill wants to make positive changes at the hospital, what can she do?
6. What qualities of an ethical nurse will Jill demonstrate when developing the strategies and proposing her plan to hospital administrators for making positive changes? Give your rationale.

References

American Association of Critical-Care Nurses. (2004). *The four A's to rise above moral distress: ask, affirm, assess, act.* Retrieved from http://www.aacn.org/WD/Practice/Docs/4As_to_Rise_Above_Moral_Distress.pdf

American Association of Critical-Care Nurses. (2008). *Position statement: Moral distress.* Retrieved from http://www.aacn.org/WD/Practice/Docs/Moral_Distress.pdf

American Medical Association. (2006). *Opinion 8.082: Withholding information from patients.* Retrieved at http://www.ama-assn.org/ama/pub/physician-resources/medical-ethics/code-medical-ethics/opinion8082.page

American Medical Association. (2011). *AMA policy: Professionalism in the use of social media.* Retrieved from http://www.ama-assn.org/ama/pub/meeting/professionalism-social-media.shtml

American Nurses Association. (2001). *Code of ethics for nurses with interpretive statements.* Silver Spring, MD: Author.

American Nurses Association. (2011). *ANA's principles for social networking and the nurse: Guidance for registered nurses.* Silver Spring, MD: Author.

Aristotle. (2002). *Nicomachean ethics* (C. Rowe, Trans.). New York: Oxford University Press.

Association of Pediatric Hematology/Oncology Nurses (APHON) releases position statement on use of social media by its members. (2011, June 7). *Newswise.* Retrieved from http://www.newswise.com/articles/association-of-pediatric-hematology-oncology-nurses-aphon-releases-position-paper-on-use-of-social-media-by-its-members

Beauchamp, T. L., & Childress, J. F. (2009). *Principles of biomedical ethics* (6th ed.). New York, NY: Oxford University Press.

Bennett, W. J. (Ed., with commentary). (1993). *Honesty.* In W. J. Bennett, (Ed.), *The book of virtues: A treasury of great moral stories* (pp. 597–662). New York, NY: Simon & Schuster.

Bu, X., & Jezewski, M. A. (2006). Developing a mid-range theory of patient advocacy through concept analysis. *Journal of Advanced Nursing, 57*(1), 101–110.

Butts, J. B. (2011). PRISMS—Acronym for key action verbs for strategies to promote patient advocacy. Personal Collection. Ellisville, MS.

Churchman, J. J., & Doherty, C. (2010). Nurses' views on challenging doctors' practice in an acute hospital. *Nursing Standard, 24*(40), 42–47.

College and Association of Registered Nurses of Alberta. (2010). The tech report: Dos and don'ts of social networking . . . avoid a social networking nightmare. *Alberta RN, 66*(6), 22–23.

Corley, M. C. (2002). Nurse moral distress: A proposed theory and research agenda. *Nursing Ethics, 9*(6), 636–650.

Corley, M. C., Minick, P., Elswick, R. K., & Jacobs, M. (2005). Nurse moral distress and ethical work environment. *Nursing Ethics, 12*(4), 381–390.

Davis, A. J., Fowler, M. D., & Aroskar, M. A. (2010). *Ethical dilemmas & nursing practice* (5th ed.). Boston, MA: Pearson.

Edson. M. (1999). *Wit.* New York, NY: Faber & Faber.

Ehrenreich, B., & English, D. (1973). *Witches, midwives, and nurses: A history of women healers.* New York, NY: The Feminist Press.

Erichsen, E., Danielsson, E. H., & Friedrichsen, M. (2010). A phenomenological study of nurses' understanding of honesty in palliative care. *Nursing Ethics, 17*(1), 39–50.

Esterhuizen, P. (2006). 30th anniversary issue: Is the professional code still the cornerstone of clinical nursing practice? *Journal of Advanced Nursing, 53*(1), 104–113. (Original work published 1996)

Five nurses fired for Facebook postings. (2010, June 7). *10News.com.* Retrieved from http://www.10news.com/news/23857090/detail.html

Fry, S., & Johnstone, M. J. (2002). *Ethics in nursing practice: A guide to ethical decision making* (2nd ed.). Oxford, UK: Blackwell Science.

Fry, S. T., Veatch, R. M., & Taylor, C. (2011). Introduction. In S. T. Fry, R. M. Veatch, & C. Taylor (Eds.), *Case studies in nursing ethics* (4th ed.) (pp. xv–xxix). Sudbury, MA: Jones and Bartlett.

Hakesley-Brown, R., & Malone, B. (2007). Patients and nurses: A powerful force. *The Online Journal of Issues in Nursing, 12*(1). Retrieved from http://www.nursingworld.org/MainMenuCategories/ANAMarketplace/ANAPeriodicals/OJIN/TableofContents/Volume122007/No1Jan07/tpc32_416093.aspx

Hamric, A. B. (2000). What is happening to advocacy? *Nursing Outlook, 48*(3), 103–104.

Hanks, R. G. (2007). Barriers to nursing advocacy: A concept analysis. *Nursing Forum, 42*(4), 171–177.

Holm, S. (2006). What should other healthcare professions learn from nursing ethics. *Nursing Philosophy, 7*, 165–174.

International Council of Nurses. (2006). *The ICN code of ethics for nurses*. Geneva, Switzerland: Author.

Jameton, A. (1984). *Nursing practice: The ethical issues*. Englewood Cliffs, NJ: Prentice-Hall.

Johnstone, M. J. (2008). *Bioethics: A nursing perspective* (5th ed.). Chatswood, AU: Saunders Elsevier.

Jones, J. M. (2011). Nurses top honesty and ethics list for 11th year. *Gallup 2010*. Retrieved from http://www.gallup.com/poll/145043/nurses-top-honesty-ethics-list-11-year.aspx

Katz, J. R. (2007). *A Career in nursing: Is it right for me?* St. Louis, MO: Mosby Elsevier.

Kelly, C. (2000). *Nurses' moral practice: Investing and discounting self*. Indianapolis, IN: Sigma Theta Tau International Center Nursing Press.

Kidder, R. M. (2005). *Chapter 1: Moral courage*. Retrieved from http://www.globalethics.org/resources/Chapter-1-Moral-Courage-by-Rushworth-M-Kidder/27/

Laabs, C. (2011). Perceptions of moral integrity: Contradictions in need of explanation. *Nursing Ethics, 18*(3), 431–440.

Lachman, V. D. (2007). Moral courage: A virtue in need of development? *MedSurg Nursing, 16*(2), 131–133.

Lipson, J. G., & Dibble, S. L. (2005). Introduction: Providing culturally appropriate health care. In J. G. Lipson & S. L. Dibble (Eds.), *Cultural and clinical care* (pp. xi–xviii). San Francisco, CA: University of California, San Francisco Nursing Press.

Loprinzi, C. L., Schapira, L., Moynihan, T., Kalemkerian, G. P., von Gunten, C., & Steensma, D. (2010). Compassionate honesty. *Journal of Palliative Medicine, 13*(10), 1187–1191.

Malloy, D. C., Hadjistavropoulos, T., McCarthy, E. F., Evans, R. J., Zakus, D. H., Park, I., . . . Williams, J. (2009). Culture and organizational climate: Nurses' insights into their relationship with physicians. *Nursing Ethics, 16*(6), 719–733.

McCue, C. (2011). Using the AACN framework to alleviate moral distress. *The Online Journal of Nursing Issues, 16*(1). Retrieved from http://www.nursingworld.org/MainMenuCategories/ANAMarketplace/ANAPeriodicals/OJIN/TableofContents/Vol-16-2011/No1-Jan-2011/Articles-Previous-Topics/AACN-Framework-and-Moral-Distress.aspx

McKenna, B. G., Smith, N. A., Poole, S. J., & Coverdale, J. H. (2003). Horizontal violence: Experiences of registered nurses in their first year of practice. *Journal of Advanced Nursing, 42*(1), 90–96.

Pendry, P. S. (2007). Moral distress: Recognizing it to retain nurses. *Nursing Economics, 25*(4), 217–221.

Plante, T. G. (2004). *Do the right thing: Living ethically in an unethical world*. Oakland, CA: New Harbinger.

Ponte, P. R., Glazer, G., Dann, E., McCollum, K., Gross, A., Tyrrell, R., . . . Washington, D. (2007). The power of professional nursing practice—An essential element of patient and family centered care. *The Online Journal of Issues in Nursing, 12*(1). Retrieved from http://www.nursingworld.org/MainMenuCategories/ANAMarketplace/ANAPeriodicals/OJIN/TableofContents/Volume122007/No1Jan07/tpc32_316092.aspx

Pullon, S. (2008). Competence, respect, and trust: Key features of successful interprofessional nurse-doctor relationships. *Journal of Interprofessional Care, 22*(2), 133–147.

Purnell, L. (2002). The Purnell model of cultural competence. *Journal of Transcultural Nursing, 13*(3), 193–196.

Purnell, L. (2011). Models and theories focused on culture. In J. B. Butts and K. L. Rich (Eds.), *Philosophies and theories for advanced nursing practice* (pp. 525–568). Sudbury, MA: Jones and Bartlett.

Redman, B. K., & Fry, S. T. (2000). Nurses' ethical conflicts: What is really known about them? *Nursing Ethics, 7*, 360–366.

Robb, I. H. (1916). *Nursing ethics: For hospital and private use.* Cleveland, OH: E. C. Koeckert. (Original work published 1900)

Schluter, J., Winch, S., Holzhauser, K., & Henderson, A. (2008). Nurses' moral sensitivity and hospital ethical climate: A literature review. *Nursing Ethics, 15*(3), 304–321.

Spector, R. E. (2004). *Cultural diversity in health and illness* (6th ed.). Upper Saddle River, NJ: Pearson-Prentice Hall.

Spence, D., & Smythe, L. (2007). Courage as integral to advancing nursing practice. *Nursing Praxis in New Zealand, 23*(2), 43–55.

Stein, L. I. (1967). The doctor-nurse game. *Archives of General Psychiatry, 16*(6), 699–703.

Stein, L. I., Watts, D. T., & Howell, T. (1990). The doctor-nurse game revisited. *Nursing Outlook, 38*(6), 264–268.

Thomas, L. (2011). Social networking opens a pandora's box. *Australian Journal of Nursing, 18*(9), 23.

Thomas, S. P. (2009). *Transforming nurses' stress and anger: Steps toward healing* (3rd ed.). New York, NY: Springer.

Tschudin, V. (2006). 30th anniversary commentary "Is the professional code still the cornerstone of clinical nursing practice?" *Journal of Advanced Nursing, 53*(1), 112–113.

Turnbull, D. (2003). Genetics and disability: Exploring moral space. *Journal of Future Studies, 7*(4), 3–14.

Vaartio, H., Leino-Kilpi, H. Salanterä, S., & Suominen, T. (2006). Nursing advocacy: How is it defined by patients and nurses, what does it involve and how is it experienced? *Scandinavian Journal of Caring Science, 20*, 282–292.

Volker, D. L. (2003). Is there a unique nursing ethic? *Nursing Science Quarterly, 16*(3), 207–211.

Wright, D., & Brajtman, S. (2011). Relational and embodied knowing: Nursing ethics within the interprofessional team. *Nursing Ethics, 18*(1), 20–30.

Zurik, L. (2011, May 27). Lee Zurik investigation: ER horror story. Retrieved from http://www.fox8live.com/news/local/story/Lee-Zurik-Investigation-ER-horror-story/NIh3JgoWZ0qd2RiliUFiag.cspx

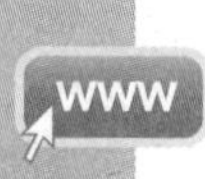

For a full suite of assignments and additional learning activities, use the access code located in the front of your book to visit this exclusive website: http://go.jblearning.com/butts. If you do not have an access code, you can obtain one at the site.

Part II

Nursing Ethics Across the Life Span

Reproductive Issues and Nursing Ethics

Janie B. Butts

You and I are persons. More specifically, we are human persons—persons who are members of the species Homo sapiens. *But what does it mean to say that someone is a person? And what is the significance of being human?*

—*David DeGrazia,* Human Identity and Bioethics, *2005*

OBJECTIVES

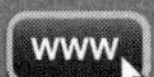

After reading this chapter, the reader should be able to:

1. Explore the maternal–fetal conflict as it relates to rights, autonomy, nursing, health care, and medical treatment.
2. Explain ways in which the Federal Abortion Ban could affect the maternal–fetal relationship.
3. Discuss the views for full moral status of an embryo or fetus.
4. Contrast the issues of abortion from both sides of the debate: pro-choice groups and pro-life groups.
5. Compare the ethical issues for each of the three major types of assisted reproductive technology.
6. Discuss the rationale for couples to make informed choices about pregnancy and the types of assisted reproductive technology in terms of genetic screening, testing, and counseling.
7. Discuss the ethical considerations for maternal substance abuse.
8. Integrate Bergum's relational ethics into the essential interpretational aspects of the American Nurses Association *Code of Ethics for Nurses with Interpretive Statements* (2001) for the care of childbearing women.

Maternal–Fetal Conflict

Tran (2004) defined **maternal–fetal conflict** as a conflict that occurs "when a pregnant woman's interests, as she defines them, conflict with the interests of her fetus, as defined by the woman's physician" (p. 76). A maternal–fetal conflict can occur when a pregnant woman's treatment is hazardous to the fetus or when a pregnant woman does not comply with a physician's recommendations that are traditionally believed to nurture the fetus's growth and development. This ethical issue is concerned with each person's right to life versus the possibility of bringing harm to one person when treating the other of the two biologically connected persons. In years past, when physicians and nurses cared for a pregnant woman, they considered the mother and fetus as one patient unit with intricate detail. Everything about the care and treatment of the whole patient was weighed according to the perceived benefits of the whole compared with perceived combined burdens. The dual care concept has become a prominent consideration that has progressed simultaneously with the development of fetal medicine and treatment (Iris, Amalia, Moshe, Arnon, & Eyal, 2009). Society, nurses, and physicians share the goal of optimal pregnancy outcomes; that is, physicians and nurses are supposed to consider the best care and medical treatment possible for each person separately and distinctly. With this dual care frame of mind, however, several ethical dilemmas surrounding a person's rights arise. Ludwig (2008) posed these questions:

- What accounts for the rising awareness of the maternal–fetal conflict?
- What happens when medical therapy is indicated for one patient, yet contraindicated for the other?
- When does the fetus or newborn become a person?
- People have rights. Does a fetus have rights?
- What if maternal decisions seem to be based on unusual beliefs?
- What about obtaining court orders to force pregnant women to comply?

Issues Related to the Maternal–Fetal Conflict

Federal Abortion Ban

The National Right to Life Committee (NRLC) and other pro-life groups (also known as anti-choice groups) have campaigned for years for equal rights and protection for the unborn fetus, based on the viewpoint that the fetus is a human life—one that, if not a person yet, has the potential to be a person. On November 5, 2003, President George W. Bush signed into law the Federal Abortion Ban Act of 2003.

According to the NRLC (2003), the Federal Abortion Ban, also initially known as the Partial Birth Abortion Ban Act of 2003, was placed into law to prohibit physicians from performing partial-birth abortions and thereby "killing fetuses." **Partial-birth abortion** is a nonmedical term that refers to late-term or third-trimester abortions by way of a procedure called intact dilation and extraction (abbreviated as intact D & E). In other words, a **late-term abortion** consists of physicians delivering a live fetus vaginally, yet only partially, for the sole purpose of terminating a pregnancy by way of an intact D & E. The term *partially* means that for head presentation, the entire head must be outside the mother's vagina before the fetus can be terminated, and for breech presentation, any part of the fetus's trunk past its navel must be outside the mother's vagina before the fetus can be terminated.

Several states have agreed with the American Civil Liberties Union (ACLU, 2006) by striking down the federal partial-birth abortion ban, ruling it unconstitutional, whereas other states are pushing for the abortion ban to apply as early as 12 to 13 weeks gestation, a push that is viewed by the ACLU as deceptive. The time line of 12 to 13 weeks bleeds into the first trimester of pregnancy, meaning that no longer could the term partial-birth abortion be used; rather, the term abortion must be applied.

The U.S. Supreme Court reviewed the Federal Abortion Ban because of the strikedowns by several states, even though some states are continuing to support the ban, which leaves unresolved issues, anger, and moral fanaticism on each side of the argument. The public anxiously awaited the final decision, and on April 18, 2007, under the direction of Chief Justice John Roberts, the U.S. Supreme Court announced a 5 to 4 decision to uphold the Federal Abortion Ban. According to the ACLU (2007), the U.S. Supreme Court's decision of upholding the ban undermines the core tenet of *Roe v. Wade*: that a woman's health must remain unrivaled. No health exception for women was written in the law. In a written dissent, Justice Ruth Bader Ginsburg made a strong criticism by warning the majority justices that they are placing women's health in danger and undermining women's battle for equality. Justice Ginsburg stated, "the Act, and the Court's defense of it, cannot be understood as anything other than an effort to chip away at a right declared again and again by the Court—and with increasing comprehension of its centrality to women's lives" (as cited in ACLU, 2007, para. 5). For a condensed timeline of the Federal Abortion Ban, please refer to the Planned Parenthood Action Center (2010); for an overview of state policies on abortion, see the Guttmacher Institute (2011).

Civil Liberties

Historical records have indicated that multiple and complex ethical, legal, and political issues have arisen, including criminalization of pregnant women. Courts have ordered physician-sanctioned cesarean deliveries for the sake of the fetus against the mother's wishes; pregnant women have been prosecuted for their abuse of alcohol and other drugs; and courts have ordered pregnant women to receive blood transfusions in life-threatening or other conditions even when the women were refusing blood transfusions for religious beliefs (ACLU, 1997; Chandis &

Williams, 2006). Issues of abortion and forced treatments tap into questions of whether the fetus is viewed as a person, has a right to life, or is viewed as having equal moral status to the mother versus a pregnant woman's right to bodily integrity and right to privacy, dignity, and choice.

It is important for the reader to know the ACLU's opinion of government officials tampering with women's rights during pregnancy. In a 1997 article titled "Coercive and Punitive Governmental Responses to Women's Conduct During Pregnancy," the ACLU created strong statements, as highlighted in the two quoted passages in Box 4.1.

Since the latter part of the 20th century, there have been astounding advances in reproductive technologies, so much so that the technologies have sparked public, ethical, and political scrutiny concerning a woman's private choice (autonomy) versus public regulation and law (Harris & Holm, 2000). Nurses sometimes feel as if they are caught in the middle and do not know how to manage the care related to the maternal–fetal conflict. In Provisions 1, 2, and 5 of the *Code of Ethics for*

BOX 4.1 ETHICAL FORMATIONS: AMERICAN CIVIL LIBERTIES UNION

Women's Reproductive Rights Violated

A decade ago [meaning the 1980s], we saw a rash of cases in which government officials zealously embraced a misguided mission to protect fetuses by attempting to control the conduct of pregnant women.... Inevitably, such actions backfire: women who fear the government's "pregnancy police" will avoid prenatal care altogether, and both they and their fetuses will suffer as a result.

The ACLU ... defended many of the women who were subject to coercive or punitive state actions. We won case after case, and attempts to bully and punish pregnant women eventually diminished.

Recently, however, we have seen this dangerous trend revive. (Introduction)

Coercive and punitive treatment of pregnant women violates the civil liberties of individual women and fosters distrust of health care providers. . . . An influential 1988 Illinois Supreme Court decision, *Stallman v. Youngquist,* warned courts not to make "mother and child . . . legal adversaries from the moment of conception until birth." Rejecting a child's claim of damages from its mother, the court wrote:

> Holding a mother liable for the unintentional infliction of prenatal injuries subjects to State scrutiny all the decisions a woman must make in attempting to carry a pregnancy to term, and infringes on her right to privacy and bodily autonomy.

Although we may not always approve of a woman's conduct during pregnancy, we must insist that women be offered educational, social, and medical services that can persuade them to make the wisest and healthiest choices. Coercion is both a counterproductive and an illegal alternative. (Section 4)

Source: Quoted from American Civil Liberties Union. (1997). Coercive and punitive governmental responses to women's conduct during pregnancy. Retrieved from http://www.aclu.org/reproductiverights/gen/16529res19970930.html

Nurses with Interpretive Statements, the American Nurses Association (ANA), (2001) has clarified nurses' roles in regard to appropriate ethical behavior and action toward patients. (See Appendix A for the ANA *Code of Ethics*, as well as Box 4.8 at the end of this chapter.) Included in these three provisions are concepts to which nurses are ethically bound, such as the respect for human dignity, the patient's right to self-determination, a commitment to the patient's interest, the respect of privacy and confidentiality, and the protection of the patient's rights. Individual nurses need to make certain that they follow these ethical guidelines in a nonjudgmental and caring way. Protecting the woman's rights and decisions and maintaining dialogue of the highest quality among the woman, her family, and other healthcare professionals are most critical because of the deeply sensitive issues that women face in reproduction, procreation, or abortion. The manner in which nurses interact and intervene with these patients often will affect their own health and emotional outcomes.

Reproductive Rights

Women's decisions to have a baby, not to have a baby, or to have an abortion are among the most critical decisions she will make in her life. Although a woman may involve significant others, this type of decision is intensely personal and is one that she will hope to make on her own without coercion or mandates from healthcare professionals or federal or state governments.

One of the ethical questions is, "Does a woman have a right to have a child?" Infertility, for instance, is not a life-threatening disorder, but it does cause undue suffering and shame to millions of women and couples. A legal question is, "If there is a right to reproduce, should it include the right to unlimited and scarce resources?" As technology advances, more questions begin to surface; for example, should fertility medicine be regulated? Healthcare professionals must attempt to resolve the question of how society should strike a balance among the various options of procreation, reproduction, testing, and maternal rights.

Many times, legal rights and moral rights overlap because of the policies that are legislated to laws enforcing certain rights. **Moral rights** include liberty rights and claim rights (Mahoney, 2007). **Liberty rights**, sometimes called negative rights, are those rights a person can impose on others without a fear of someone or some group preventing those rights from being exercised. Liberty rights include freedom of speech, autonomy, privacy, and others as stated in the first 10 amendments of the U.S. Constitution. Health care in the United States is a liberty right.

Claim rights, sometimes called positive or welfare rights, are those rights owed to people through active and positive steps taken by others or groups to ensure the claim is met. There are two population exceptions in the United States to healthcare liberty rights—poor people and elders—and they fall under claim rights. Social federal and state programs help to ensure that claim rights are fulfilled and preserved.

If there is a right to reproduction, is it a liberty right, a claim right, or both? In addition, does an unborn fetus or child have healthcare rights? Answers to these questions remain unclear, but most experts agree that all healthcare rights are of critical importance to everyone. Reproductive rights are about human rights, quality health care, choice, liberation from enforced sexual pleasures and abuse, and population growth and distribution.

Moral Standings of Humans

> *Whatever factor signals the end of full moral standing would seem to be relevant as a marker of when full moral standing begins. . . . The moral problems with manipulation of sperm and egg cells are often believed to be less troublesome than those arising from manipulating a late-term fetus or postnatal infant. It is important to know why this is so. It must be that, no matter how we attribute moral status to sperm and egg cells, we view them as having a moral standing that is different from the late-term fetus or postnatal infant. If we can identify what it is that is responsible for this perceived shift in moral status, perhaps we can understand better when full moral standing accrues.*
>
> —*Robert Veatch (2003, p. 40)*

When the phrase "moral standing of humans" is mentioned, what comes to mind? In Veatch's (2003) quotation, he has suggested that whatever it is that causes moral standing to end is what makes it begin. On this topic, he pondered a general question: Could any of the physiological or neurological criteria be the signals of the beginning and ending of moral standing in humans, such as the criteria used for higher brain death, whole-brain death, or the cardiac definition of death? There is no specific way for people to determine which, if any, one criterion determines when full moral standing begins and ends. The question of when full moral standing begins and ends requires complex considerations.

Full moral status has been recognized as persons with privileges and the capacity to reason, make autonomous decisions, and consider themselves as the unique subjects of their own interests and experiences. DeGrazia (2008) stated, "to have moral status is to bear direct or independent moral importance" (p. 183). There are numerous views on the point at which full moral status begins. These views include, but are not limited to:

- Full moral status begins at conception—a fundamentalist or strong right-to-life view of potentiality or Future-Like-Ours Argument (see definition of FLOA in the next paragraph).
- Full moral status begins when humans come into existence, or become sentient beings—a biological view.

- Full moral status is acquired when the being becomes a person, or when personhood can be established—a person essentialism view
- Full moral status is based on the amount of accrued possession of interests, which was detailed in 1974 by Feinberg as the interest principle, and what is now known as the time-relative interest account.

The Future-Like-Ours Argument to Determine Moral Status

In 2004, the President's Council on Bioethics (PCB) issued a report titled *Monitoring Stem Cell Research*. Based on the report, President Bush took a strong stance that is based on two underlying assumptions: each person originates as a single-cell zygote at the time of conception, and full moral status is acquired at origination. Based on this stance, many people believe that the single-cell zygote has full moral status because it has the "potential" to become a sentient being. A stronger argument that stems from potentiality is the Future-Like-Ours Argument (FLOA), which was presented in detail by Marquis (1989). The FLOA is used as a strong contention against abortion because pro-life groups argue that a fetus has the potential to become a person with a future like other living human beings experiencing life, as well as the possibility of its fullest actualization, lifespan, and the possibility of rational decision-making abilities. This argument includes the potential for a fetus, once born, in the future to experience having a spouse, children, other family members, friends, successful careers, and all that life has to offer.

The Biological Approach to Determining Moral Status

The biological stance is a reasonable, scientific-based approach for determination of moral status. Many philosophers and bioethicists (e.g., DeGrazia, 2006; Steinbock, 1992) have contended that the sentience of the fetus is integral to determination of moral status. To have sentience requires the fetus to have the capacity of feelings.

With the biological view, there is evidence that the single zygote cell is *derived* from the sperm and ovum, but the cell has not come into existence or being yet, meaning that beings originate as nonsentient entities. The single zygote cell does not come into being or existence until the cell has completed the division process, at which time the entity becomes a uniquely individuated human organism (DeGrazia, 2006). During the 2-week division process after the formation of the single-cell zygote, there is a potential through various biological processes for the embryo to develop into twins, either by fraternal or identical twinning (or multi-embryos), or through a unique occurrence called fusion when two embryos can actually fuse into one embryo. Based on this scientific information, the single-cell zygote cannot be uniquely individuated until the division process is completed, and "if not uniquely individuated, the zygote is not yet a unique member of our basic kind (according to the biological view): human organism" (DeGrazia, 2006, p. 51).

Interest Approach to Moral Status

The possession of interests is a requirement for moral status according to Feinberg (1974), who approached the interest argument from the function of rights, or having interests at stake. If the sentient being has interests at stake, those interests must be considered when there is moral deliberation about that being. If no interests have been incurred, interests cannot be considered in a moral deliberation. Without interests, rights cannot be assumed. Steinbock (2006) suggested that Feinberg was making a conceptual link between a being's interests and consciousness. In other words, only conscious beings can have a stake in something; nonconscious beings do not have any interests of their own. Steinbock stated:

> Embryos are not mere things. They are alive and have the potential to become beings with interests—indeed to become people, like you and me. But their potential to become persons does not give them the moral status or the rights of actual persons. Early embryos, indeed early-gestation fetuses, have no consciousness, no awareness, no experiences of any kind, even the most rudimentary. . . .Within even the precursor of a nervous system . . .or without consciousness, they cannot have desires; without desires, they cannot have interests. (p. 29)

However full moral standing is defined, these perplexing issues will not be resolved because of the profound level of disagreements to the following questions: When do we come into existence, or sentience? Does life begin at conception? Do sentience and full moral standing occur simultaneously? How does personhood fit with the full moral standing conception? Is there a supreme entity in charge of society?

Abortion

> *Science cannot resolve moral conflicts, but it can help to more accurately frame the debates about those conflicts.*
>
> —*Heinz R. Pagels,* The Dreams of Reason, *1988*

Because pro-choice and pro-life (also known as anti-choice) debaters justify their claims and arguments on each side, the dilemma is deadlocked with no hope in the future for resolution. These diametrically opposed sides have ethical, political, legal, and religious implications. Opposition even occurs regarding the use of labeling groups. The opposing groups have historically been labeled as pro-choice and pro-life, but as both sides tightened their reigns on their beliefs and values, the pro-choice groups began labeling pro-life groups as anti-choice. The rationale behind this decision was that pro-life groups were making claims that pro-choice groups did not value life. The pro-choice groups strongly believe that if the term *pro-life* could be replaced by the term *anti-choice*, the insinuations and accusations made by pro-life groups that pro-choice groups did not believe in the value of life itself would be diminished. The current status of this controversy is unchanged.

Pro-life groups refer to themselves as pro-life, and pro-choice groups refer to pro-life groups as anti-choice. The author of this chapter takes the stance that this argument of labels is largely irresolvable and therefore will use the terms pro-choice and pro-life because of the widespread use of these terms in the media.

Abortion, especially in the first trimester, is legal in many countries, including the United States, but intense moral and political scrutiny, even legal action, has continued to surface since the *Roe v. Wade* decision of January 22, 1973. In *Roe v. Wade*, the U.S. Supreme Court ruled that states could not make any laws that banned abortions in the first or second trimester, except for certain reasons—such as the woman's health must be at risk—in the second trimester. In the third trimester, states can make laws banning abortions; unless a third-trimester abortion is critical to a woman's survival, the woman is required to follow her state law.

In 1971, 2 years before the *Roe v. Wade* decision, Judith Jarvis Thomson (1971), a philosopher, wrote a classic and well-known article titled "A Defense of Abortion," which served as a foundation for the abortion debate. At the very beginning of her article, she agreed that every person has a right to life and that this right is extended to fetuses. Then, to make her argument, she stated that she was pretending that a fetus is a person because it in fact becomes a human person at some time before birth. However, her conclusive premise was that, even assuming that the fetus has a right to life, the fetus morally could not infringe on the mother's own right to control her own body or use her body to stay alive.

The definition of **abortion** includes two meanings: a woman giving premature birth before the fetus is capable of sustaining life, as in a miscarriage or spontaneous abortion, or a woman's intentional termination of a pregnancy. The latter definition is the core of the pro-choice and pro-life debate. The debaters argue with political fervor and bitterness, sometimes resulting in violence, about the legality, rightness, or wrongness of a woman's choosing to terminate her pregnancy, but in the pro-choice view, abortion is almost always permissible and can be justified.

From 1973 to December 2006, there were more than 50 million registered abortions in the United States (Guttmacher Institute, 2011). Documented reasons for abortions include: rape, incest, physical life of mother, physical health of mother, fetal health, mental health of mother, and personal choice; personal choices included too young, not ready for responsibility, too immature, economic, to avoid adjusting life, mother single or in poor relationship, and enough children already.

The Central Ethical Dilemma

The central ethical dilemma of the abortion debate is about rights: the right to life of the fetus or the woman's right to control her own body by choosing whether to carry a pregnancy to term, have a baby, and parent it. The fetus (or embryo) as person or nonperson and a fetus (or an embryo) with or without moral status remain at the center of most of the pro-choice and pro-life rights debates.

Pro-Choice View

With the pro-choice view, a common argument is that abortion is legally permissible, regardless of the morality involved. A woman has a basic right to make up her own mind about choices of pregnancy or abortion, and her right always prevails over any other right, including any fetal rights. At the core of the pro-choice stance is the right of privacy based on the U.S. Constitution, U.S. Declaration of Independence, and the worldwide Universal Declaration of Human Rights. Sentience, moral status, and personhood are among the various arguments used in the pro-choice view.

To the pro-choice group, abortion is morally as well as legally permissible. Many people contend that a fetus that cannot survive outside a woman's body is not considered viable; therefore, a fetus cannot override the woman's right to choose an abortion when the fetus is not viable outside the womb. With this pro-choice view, there are various opinions on the beginning of life. Two of those opinions are (1) the fetus does not have human life until the mother is in the 17th week of gestation, and (2) the fetus with sentience and moral status has human life at the 7th month of gestation, when its nervous system has fully developed.

There are two types of **emergency contraception** (EC). EC is defined as postcoital birth control measures that prevent pregnancy. One type is RU486, or mifepristone. This drug is available by prescription as an alternative to a surgical abortion procedure and can be administered up to 50 days from conception. After taking mifepristone, the fetus and other tissues are aborted.

The other EC is called the Plan B morning-after pill. In August 2006, the FDA approved the over-the-counter sale of Plan B for women ages 17 and over (Plan B must be prescribed by a primary care provider if the person is under age 17). Plan B has been a popular drug among adolescents because the drug can actually prevent implantation of a fertilized egg if taken within 72 hours of intercourse.

Pro-choice groups believe that if a woman and fetus are warranted as having equal moral standing, as believed by pro-life groups, a woman's rights are weakened, causing the woman and the fetus to be at odds with each other. Some pro-life groups argue that, in special circumstances, the woman may have an abortion, such as in cases of incest or rape or if the infant is severely deformed. These circumstances are often viewed as a double standard, meaning abortion is accepted when the procedure is subjectively needed. Even today, the argument continues as to when a fetus becomes a person—whether it is at conception, when the heartbeat develops, when the nervous system develops, when it is considered viable outside the womb, or when the baby begins the process of thinking. From the personhood perspective, people should have rational thinking and possess the highest possible moral importance.

Pro-Life View

On the side of the pro-life group, the personhood view stems from a fundamental understanding that the embryo or fetus is a person. Most pro-life groups argue that life and full moral status begin at conception and that abortion is immoral and murderous and should be illegal. According to this view, the embryo, from the time of conception and throughout the development of the fetus, has the same right to life that is due each person living outside of the womb. Historically, unless a mother's life was threatened, the embryo (or fetus) was protected because it is worthy of respect yet vulnerable to murder and harm. This protection begins at the time of conception, but especially applies in the second and third trimesters.

Most pro-life groups believe that life begins at conception as a single-cell zygote, and moral status is acquired at conception; the belief is taken based on faith values and cultural origins rather than scientific, biological evidence. Opinions vary among pro-life groups as to when personhood begins in lieu of conception. Among the times given are:

- After the ovum splits into two cells a few hours after conception
- 12 days after conception, when the fertilized ovum has attached itself to the uterine lining
- 2 weeks from conception, when the yellow streak develops, which is the neural tube that protects the backbone and prevents splitting into two embryos (before the yellow streak develops, the embryo may split into identical twins)
- 3 weeks from conception, as the fetus begins to develop body parts
- 4 weeks from conception, when the heartbeat begins (it should be noted that when 3D and 4D ultrasounds, the HDI 3000 and HDI 4000 systems, are performed in high-risk pregnancies, heartbeats are detected very early)
- 6 weeks from conception, as the first brain waves are sensed
- 2 months, and again at 3 months, from conception when the fetus begins to resemble a human being (again, the detailed 3D and 4D ultrasounds produce very clear pictures of fetal development, such as thumb-sucking and smiling)
- 4 months from conception, when the fetus has its own characteristics that could be differentiated from other fetuses
- 24 weeks from conception, when the fetus is said to become viable
- 26 weeks from conception, when the fetus's higher brain begins to function
- At birth, only after delivery and breathing is separate from the woman's body

Pro-life groups sometimes quote several passages from the Bible, but the Catholic Church's position about abortion is a little more complex (Harris & Holm, 2003). According to the Catholic Church, the whole issue regarding the morality of abortion stems from the greater question of when the fetus receives a soul. Because many interpretations of the Bible exist, the Catholic Church has taken a general stance on this moral issue, as Harris and Holm stated: "because killing is such a grave moral wrong, one should act cautiously and presume that there may be ensoulment from conception. . . . Abortion and the destruction of embryos should therefore be treated as the killing of an ensouled being" (p. 122). (See Box 4.2.)

Speaking Out

The legal and moral debates about abortion and women's reproductive rights continue. The National Abortion and Reproductive Rights Action League (NARAL) and the Pro-Choice America and the National Right to Life Committee (NRLC) each have representatives who speak out.

NARAL Pro-Choice America (2011) published, "In addition to President Obama, we worked with our allies in the 111th Congress to improve women's access to reproductive-health care. The U.S. House is now under anti-choice control. Pro-choice lawmakers are now more crucial than ever to stop an extreme anti-choice agenda."

Speaking on behalf of NRLC, Gans and Balch (n.d.) stated, "It is incumbent upon each of us in the pro-life movement to learn (and it most definitely can be learned) how to persuasively talk about life issues . . . and never, never miss the opportunity to speak on behalf of those who have no voice. It literally can be the difference between who will live and who will die."

BOX 4.2 ETHICAL FORMATIONS

- If almost all abortions during the first trimester are considered legally permissible, how should one view a woman's taking a prescribed dose of mifepristone (RU486) to abort a fetus? Would you view this drug as morally or legally permissible? Both? Neither? Explain your answer.
- After reading all the arguments on rights and human life in this section, what do you believe about abortion? Address your views to the following points and use an ethical framework (theory, approach, or principle) to justify your answers:
    - □ Your moral and legal views on abortion
    - □ When you think a human life begins
    - □ When you think a human life becomes a person

Please describe these points clearly so that you will clarify your own beliefs and values regarding these issues. Remember that there is not one right answer. These views are your opinions based on your values, an ethical theory, and the readings in this book and other sources.

- If you are giving nursing care to a woman who just received a partial-birth abortion by way of an intact D & E, first describe your own beliefs concerning partial-birth abortion, and then identify nursing strategies that you would use in caring for this patient.

Many times, women who are pro-choice and believe in women's reproductive rights receive abortions but do not necessarily want the procedure. They may find themselves in situations of unintended pregnancy where they must have an abortion for reasons already described in this section. Just because a woman believes in her right to choose does not mean that her intentional decision to have an abortion and lose her fetus will not be emotionally traumatizing to her (Burke, 2002). Sometimes women feel restricted from expressing their grief because they fear that no one wants to hear about it. They may believe that they cannot discuss the abortion or loss of their fetus with anyone because it needs to be kept a deep, dark secret. Some women may believe that they do not have permission to grieve for the loss of their fetus, and therefore they experience extreme sorrow, which is a type of grief called **disenfranchised grief**. When one is not allowed to grieve or must hide it, the grief process is prolonged and far worse. "Such 'impacted' [disenfranchised] grief can even become integrated into one's personality and touch every aspect of one's life" (Burke, 2002, p. 51). (See Box 4.3.)

Reproductive Technology

> *On July 25, 1978, Louise Joy Brown, the world's first successful "test-tube" baby, was born in Great Britain. Though the technology that made her conception possible was heralded as a triumph in medicine and science, it also caused many to consider the possibilities of future ill-use. . . . The most important question was whether this baby was going to be healthy. Had being outside the womb, even for just a couple of days, harmed the egg? . . . Today [26 years later], the process of "in vitro" fertilization is considered commonplace and utilized by infertile couples around the world.*
>
> —*Jennifer Rosenberg, 2007*

The Browns tried to conceive for 9 years before they tried in vitro fertilization. Lesley Brown's fallopian tubes were blocked. Reproductive failure can be emotionally and financially devastating to couples. Because of infertility, 1% of all infants born in the United States are conceived with assisted reproductive technology (ART) (Centers for Disease Control and Prevention [CDC], 2011). In many Western countries ART accounts for 1% to 3% of annual births.

Infertility is generally defined as a woman's not being able to become pregnant after the couple has tried for 1 year. The term **assisted reproductive technology** (ART) refers to the handling and management of sperm and eggs and every kind of fertility treatment or drug used for the purpose of retrieving eggs to be used in the treatment. Treatments not included under the ART umbrella include those in which only sperm are managed, such as artificial insemination; surgical procedures

BOX 4.3 ETHICAL FORMATIONS: DISENFRANCHISED GRIEF—FORBIDDING THE GRIEF OF ABORTION

From the words of Tina . . .
If you regret an abortion, nobody wants to hear about it. After all, there's nothing anyone can do to fix the problem. So you have to tell yourself what happened was good—and everyone around you tells you the same thing. After that, I knew I would never bring up the subject again. (p. 55)

From the words of Kathy . . .
Dear Mom, I'm sorry I never told you the truth about my abortion for so long. I told you I was having minor surgery—female problems. Remember? . . . And what really kills me the most is that you and Daddy came to see me that night in the hospital. . . . I was so scared—scared you'd find out what really happened that day. Man, I was hurting inside. And there you two were standing at the foot of my bed extending your love and concern. Mom, didn't you notice I couldn't even look you in the eyes? And over the years the times I turned from you whenever the abortion issue was raised? I can still see your face the moment I finally told you. Eight years later . . . you never looked up at me . . . [and] you sat quietly and gently spoke to me. Just as long as I kept my shameful secret, you were willing to keep it too. . . . Oh how I wish you had been able to talk about it . . . to cry with me, to help me get through that horrible time. You knew it all . . . but we never talked. I was so desperately alone. (pp. 55–56)

Source: Quoted from Burke, T. (with Reardon, D.). (2002). *Forbidden grief: The unspoken pain of abortion.* Springfield, IL: Acorn.

on women or men; or drugs that involve infertility when eggs are not going to be retrieved.

The three types of ART are:

1. In vitro fertilization (IVF): Extracting the woman's eggs, fertilizing them with sperm, and then transferring the embryo through the cervix into the uterus
2. Gamete intrafallopian transfer (GIFT): Transferring unfertilized eggs and sperm into the woman's fallopian tubes via a very small abdominal incision
3. Zygote intrafallopian transfer (ZIFT): Fertilizing eggs in the laboratory with sperm, and then transferring the zygote into the fallopian tubes

Embryos resulting from IVF can be frozen until the time comes that one or more of them are needed. The embryo is then unfrozen and implanted without significant risks to the fetus.

The concerns over the future of human life and family structure, human cloning, the low success rate of ART, and the cost of reproductive technology give society enough reason to ask a most basic ethical question: Should reproductive technology be used at all (Munson, 2004)? The cost of reproductive technology is one that is a global concern because of scarce medical and healthcare resources. In the Center for American Progress report on future choices of ART, Arons (2007) stated

> Americans of all viewpoints will be challenged by the questions raised by assisted reproductive technologies. . . . Assisted reproductive technologies bring to the fore important questions about who we are as individuals and families and whom society deems entitled to reproduce and parent. And these questions are not going to go away. While some might like to stop the clock so they can hash out the ground rules, others keep right on playing. (Para. 12, 6)

As stated previously in the section on reproductive rights, reproductive health in the United States is currently a liberty right, one that a couple may pursue without interference from any governmental agency, provided there are no laws against what is being pursued. How should private insurance companies and other reimbursement agencies weigh the priorities of healthcare resource allocation and distribution for those who are dying and critically ill against those who believe they have an autonomous right to a child? Most reimbursement agencies do not pay for many of these expensive reproductive medical procedures. But what does the future hold for autonomy and rights to reproductive services? How will distributive justice be managed?

In addition, there are specific ethical issues about reproductive technologies other than the broad ones already mentioned. These issues are divided into five groups: (1) the risks resulting from technology; (2) surrogacy (for donor eggs, embryo donation, or carrying fetuses); (3) the handling of surplus reproductive products, such as eggs or embryos that will not be used; (4) the implications of sperm sorting or gender selection; and (5) genetic modification and enhancement (Frankel, 2003; Wachbroit & Wasserman, 2003).

The first group of ethical issues involves risks created as a result of technology. Examples include ART and freezing embryos. One risk is multiple-infant live births. Of almost 39,000 births achieved using ART, 33% were considered multiple-infant live births (CDC, 2011). The ethical principles include beneficence, nonmaleficence, and justice—promoting human good for the woman or the couple who strongly desires a baby, doing no harm to the fetuses, and distribution and allocation of resources during the process and after the births.

The second group of ethical issues involves third-party involvement through donor eggs and embryos and carrying fetuses through surrogacy. **Surrogacy** is a particularly good example, such as when a man can fertilize the woman's egg but the woman cannot carry the fetus to term for some reason. In this case, the couple may ask a surrogate woman to carry the fetus to term, a process called **gestational surrogacy**. Other types of surrogacy include **traditional surrogacy**, in which the surrogate uses her own eggs and is artificially inseminated with semen from the prospective father and carries the fetus to birth; **egg donation**, in which a woman donates her eggs for in vitro fertilization with specific semen; and **embryo donation**, when a couple with a history of past successful pregnancy and delivery donates embryos to prospective couples seeking parenthood by way of in vitro fertilization and implantation.

The ethical issues regarding surrogacy are many. Who "owns" the infant once it is delivered by the surrogate? Who is the mother—the woman who produced the egg or the one who carried the fetus to term and delivered it? Is the meaning of family integrity or biological relationships at stake, or does it matter? Other concerns are legal issues: finding a legal way to pay the surrogate woman for her time and effort because the selling of children usually is illegal, avoiding treating babies as commodities, and avoiding exploitation of financially needy women (Munson, 2004; Wachbroit & Wasserman, 2003). As the population increases, so will surrogacy. The principles involved are autonomy and nonmaleficence. These principles involve the issues of a couple's feelings about the right to choose; the surrogate's right to choose to be a surrogate; and doing no harm to the outcome of the child, the family biological structure, and individual freedoms.

The third group of ethical issues consists of **surplus reproductive products** resulting from technology. For example, because the success rate is low for in vitro fertilization, a woman may have stored many frozen eggs in an attempt for a successful pregnancy. Once the woman is pregnant, what happens to the remaining eggs? Many of the eggs are fertilized, but only a very few are implanted. What happens to these embryos? For people who believe that life begins at conception, is destroying the remainder of the fertilized eggs (embryos) considered murder? Beliefs about the right to life, the point at which life and full moral standing begin, and the question of whether destroying embryos is murder are at the center of this debate, as well as the principles of autonomy and nonmaleficence.

The fourth group of ethical issues is called **sperm sorting** or **gender selection**, which is advanced technology enabling persons to create the kind of child they want to have, to balance the family, or to prevent X-chromosome-linked or other genetic diseases (Harris & Holm, 2003). The medical procedure through which sperm sorting is accomplished is called **preimplantation genetic diagnosis** (PGD). Family balancing, or evening out gender representation in children, is a concept used to help justify and promote the use of gender selection prior to implantation. The principles to be considered in sperm sorting, family balancing, and gender selection include autonomy, beneficence, nonmaleficence, and justice.

Occurring in 1 of every 1,000 live births overall, more than 500 X-linked chromosome diseases have now been identified, including hemophilia, Duchenne muscular dystrophy, and X-linked mental retardation. Other genetic diseases that can be identified through PGD include Fanconi's anemia, thalassemia, sickle-cell disease, neurofibromatosis, and many others (University of Minnesota Cancer Center, 2010). Sperm sorting highly increases a couple's chance of having an unaffected child. In Box 4.4, Adam and Molly Nash and their parents' decision to use PGD are highlighted.

The last ethical issue, the fifth group, is **inheritable genetic modification** (IGM), which is a procedure used to modify genes along the germ lines that are transmitted to offspring (Frankel, 2003). Stem-cell research could help prevent

BOX 4.4 ETHICAL FORMATIONS: A REFLECTION ON MOLLY AND ADAM NASH

Adam Nash was born in Colorado on August 29, 2000. He had been an embryo that was sorted, screened, and selected from at least 12 embryos from the Nash couple, Lisa and Jack, for the purpose of tissue matching for the critically ill daughter, Molly.

Molly Nash was born to the Nash parents on July 4, 1994, with Fanconi's anemia, a fatal autosomal recessive bone marrow failure (aplastic anemia), which is only treatable with a bone marrow transplant from a sibling's umbilical cord blood. At that time, the success rate of a bone marrow transplant from an unrelated donor was only 42%, but from a sibling, the success rate increased to 85%.

The Nash parents, with support of physicians, made the decision to have preimplantation genetic testing on their embryos in the hopes of saving their only child. In the process, 12 of Lisa's eggs were fertilized by Jack's sperm via in vitro fertilization; 2 of the embryos had Fanconi's anemia and were discarded. Of the remaining 10 embryos, only one matched Molly's tissue. This one became Adam Nash.

Source: Grady, D. (2000, October 4). Baby conceived to provide cell transplant for his dying sister. *New York Times*, p. 24.

genetic diseases from ever occurring in families through the generations by modifying the germ lines of the embryos. Genetic traits in the embryo can be enhanced with IGM. What if researchers could help a couple create the perfect baby? In 1932, Aldous Huxley suggested in his book *Brave New World* that genetics and reproductive technology would be society's worst nightmare because of the government's involvement in these activities (as cited in Frankel, 2003).

Consider the following ethical questions regarding the Nash case:

- Were the Nashes justified in creating Adam for the purpose of helping Molly get well? In other words, should humans be used as a means to an end? Explore the connection of Kant's deontology theory and the Nashes' situation.
- What could have potentially happened to the nine remaining embryos?
- How was it justified to discard the two embryos that had Fanconi's anemia and keep the one that became Adam? Consider your beliefs regarding when life begins and the moral equality of each life.

What is the future of genetic modification? No one knows exactly, but Huxley's 1932 prediction for the future of genetic technology is strikingly different from Frankel's forecast. Frankel (2003) stated:

> But as we begin the twenty-first century, the greater danger, I believe, is a highly individualized marketplace fueled by an entrepreneurial spirit and the free choice of large numbers of parents that could lead us down a path, albeit incrementally, toward a society that abandons the lottery of evolution in favor of intentional genetic modification. The discoveries of genetics will not be imposed on us. Rather, they will be sold to us by the market as something we cannot live without. (p. 32)

BOX 4.5 ETHICAL FORMATIONS

- Do you believe that destroying a fetus or embryo is murder? Explain your thoughts.
- Ben and Lynn want to select the gender of their next baby. They currently have a girl, and this time they want a boy to balance the family. Do you think the destruction of their remaining embryos would be for an inconsequential reason—family balancing? Explain your thoughts based on an ethical framework—theory, approach, or principle.
- Do you think that family balancing and the prevention of genetic diseases are reasons that should be considered equal in moral weight in a sperm sorting procedure with resultant destruction of extra embryos? Explain your thoughts.
- Explore your own feelings regarding sperm sorting that involves PGD and genetic modification that involves IGM. Write down your feelings about these two procedures.
- What are ethical strategies that you as a nurse might use if you were caring for two couples using gender selection (sperm sorting), one seeking family balancing and one preventing X-linked mental retardation? Be specific when listing these strategies.

When these genetic issues are mentioned, emotions flare between people divided in their opinions. One side's view is of how great society's future will be with the new developments. The other side's view is that science should not be interfering with nature or God's work. Not only do these genetic issues spark extreme emotions, they also are the most complex of all the ethical issues that people in society face today. The prospect of designing, altering, enhancing, or ending the life of fetuses or embryos is challenging.

The standard principles of autonomy, beneficence, nonmaleficence, and justice should be addressed in the ethics involved with all PGD and other genetic manipulations such as IGM. However, the issues seem much more complex than just principle-driven or even theory-driven justifications. Genetic manipulation is essentially an unexplored territory that leaves nurses and other healthcare professionals in moral distress. Frankel's (2003) statement with regard to IGM, which could be applied to all genetic manipulation, is the question of "whether we will shape it or be shaped by it" (p. 36). (See Box 4.5.)

Issues of Other Reproductive Services

Prenatal care is critical to the future health of the child. There are numerous prenatal health issues, but only the critical ethical issues of genetic counseling and testing and maternal substance abuse are included in this section.

Genetic Screening and Testing

Thousands of genetic diseases have been discovered, and that number increases every day (Munson, 2004). Genes that are causally linked to biochemical, cellular, and physiological defects are responsible for these genetic diseases. DNA testing can identify some of these diseases in the fetus, and many new technologies are available. For example, today, Down syndrome can be detected at 10 to 14 weeks of gestation by performing a chorionic villus sampling of the products of conception, or by an older method of amniocentesis, which cannot be performed until 16 to 18 weeks of gestation. Diseases such as sickle cell, phenylketonuria (PKU), and Tay-Sachs can be screened with high accuracy. As an example, let us look at sickle-cell disease, an autosomal recessive disease. If one parent has the disease and the other is not affected, all four children will be carriers. However, if both parents are carriers, there is a chance that one in four children will have the disease, which makes for a 25% chance overall.

Genetic screening involves professionals counseling individuals or couples about their risk for genetically linked diseases (Munson, 2004). Genetic screening can be useful for couples with a background of genetic disease, such as sickle-cell anemia, because of its inheritance pattern. As Munson pointed out, however, once couples have this information, they often have no idea what to do with it. Should couples decide not to have children at all based on this 25% chance? Should couples take their chances and get pregnant anyway with the 25% risk and, if so, should the woman be allowed to have a prenatal genetic test with only a 25% risk involved? If she found out that her fetus had a recessive disease, would she need to consider an abortion? If she would not consider having an abortion, what would be her next step? Last, should there perhaps have been no reason for the prenatal genetic test in the first place?

Couples need to consider these questions before wandering down the path of expensive prenatal testing. There is the possibility that a woman can have embryo selection, sometimes called sperm sorting, via in vitro fertilization before implantation of the embryo. As previously discussed, however, embryo selection means that the remaining embryos will be discarded, diseased or not, unless the couple donates them to other couples or for research purposes. Even when used for research, the embryos are destroyed after they are used.

There are a variety of prenatal tests that allow for a close inspection of tissue and bone, including ultrasound, radiography, and fiber optics. **Prenatal genetic diagnosis** is accomplished through an examination of the fetal DNA. Prenatal genetic diagnosis is commonly performed through amniocentesis at 15 weeks of pregnancy or later or by chorionic villus sampling (CVS), which is performed between 10 and 12 weeks of pregnancy (American Academy of Family Physicians, 2010). The CVS test carries a risk for fetal foot or toe deformities; with amniocentesis, a risk of miscarriage exists. The most common test used for prenatal genetic diagnosis is a blood test for alpha fetoprotein. It is performed several weeks after conception and predicts such disorders as spina bifida or anencephaly with high accuracy.

Knowing when to test and when not to test could pose an ethical conflict for healthcare professionals. Many women want to know prior to delivery that everything is all right, and often they believe that genetic testing will provide a certain degree of personal control and comfort. Should women have prenatal tests performed for what would seem like trivial reasons to other people? Will the woman's insurance company pay for these tests? What if she has no insurance but still wants these? Does she have an autonomous right to testing just because the technology is available?

Many experts hold two basic views: (1) that prenatal testing should be done if the woman strongly believes in her right to have the procedure and wants it performed, and (2) that the costs of the prenatal testing are very small compared to the costs of raising a child with a genetic disease or debilitating disorder (Munson, 2004). These decisions reach to the very core of family values and biological structure.

Stem-cell research offers considerable hope for correction of genetic diseases, but until the time comes for its full use, couples must make their decisions based on the technology available to them. Testing is appropriate when a couple can depend on accurate information, make an informed choice and decision, and live with the outcome once the decision about prenatal testing is made (see Box 4.6).

Maternal Substance Abuse

Maternal substance abuse is detrimental to a fetus or newborn. However, according to research, some pregnant women who abuse drugs do not seem to understand the potential harm that they are inflicting on their unborn children (Perry, Jones, Tuten, & Svikas, 2003). As one would expect, the women who are unaware of the danger that they are posing to their unborn children are those women who are abusing drugs but who do not seek help. This same group of women also was found to be more likely to believe that having a small baby is a

BOX 4.6 ETHICAL FORMATIONS

- Do you think that a couple has a right to have a child with a prenatally diagnosed disabling genetic disease? Explain your thoughts.
- Do you think that physicians and nurses should inform couples that are thinking about having a baby about all the genetic tests that are available to them? Why or why not? Explain your thoughts.
- Do you think a mother has a right to know the results of her prenatal genetic tests, whether positive or negative? Explore both sides based on the literature and then justify your answer based on an ethical framework—theory, approach, or principle.
- What approaches would you take as a nurse caring for a pregnant mother carrying a fetus with Down syndrome? Consider all the options.

positive occurrence. The results of this research underscore the need for wide-scale community education programs about maternal drug abuse. Nurses can be a valuable resource in this effort.

Maternal drug screening is not performed routinely, and testing a woman or an infant without informed consent is considered to be a violation of a patient's right to privacy (Keenan, 2006). If healthcare providers perform maternal or newborn testing without the mother's consent and the test results are positive, any decision to restrict or remove parental rights would be based on illegally obtained evidence.

The handling and treatment of maternal drug abuse varies from state to state, but it is important to remember the violations of women's rights (liberty rights) that have occurred in some states. Possible violations may include:

- Prosecution of a pregnant woman who abuses drugs
- Charging a pregnant woman with drug possession if she is arrested for drug abuse prior to fetal viability
- Charging a pregnant woman with distribution of drugs to a minor if she is arrested for drug abuse after the fetus is considered viable
- Reduction of parental rights

Nurses have an ethical responsibility to recognize maternal substance abuse. Although nurses might personally find a pregnant woman's substance abuse morally objectionable, compassion is warranted. A family, rather than an individual person, is wounded by the woman's abusive behavior. Action is sometimes taken based on state laws to protect a fetus or child who is at risk from maternal substance abuse, but nurses must consider that a woman's decision or desire to seek treatment might result in a violation of the woman's rights. A woman's decision to obtain help often involves limited trust toward healthcare providers (see Box 4.7).

Nursing Care of Childbearing Women

Ethical and legal issues in reproductive health are incredibly complex and challenging, but at the same time they encourage us with the promise of correcting genetic diseases. Sometimes the possibilities inherent in new genetic technologies,

BOX 4.7 ETHICAL FORMATIONS

- If you were a maternal-child nurse, after considering the ACLU's statement regarding women's rights, what action would you take if you suspected that a pregnant patient at the clinic where you work was abusing drugs? What information would you need to guide your actions?
- What would you do if you suspected that the woman will avoid the clinic in the future if you address the abuse issue?

including human cloning, cause people to become apprehensive or fearful. First, nurses caring for childbearing women must be educated and remain current with reproductive ethics. Nurses need to understand and respect the beliefs and practices about pregnancy and childbearing of various cultures.

Nursing management for childbearing women is focused on the ethical relationship between the nurse and the woman. Refer to Box 4.8 regarding the essential aspects of the 2001 ANA *Code of Ethics for Nurses with Interpretative Statements*. Related to the *Code of Ethics for Nurses* is the relational care that is explained by Bergum (2004), who emphasized that the nurse should always ask, "What is the 'right thing to do' for oneself and others" (p. 485). The nurse–patient relationship, as Bergum has experienced it, is a moral entity. Relational ethics is an action ethic that is created within the moral space of a relationship (Jopling, 2000; Bergum, 2004). A moral space is where the relationship is created, where nurses display responsibility, and where they respond to others. Nurses must be morally responsible to the childbearing women for whom they care, whether they are caring for them clinically, educating them, or overseeing their care. In so doing, nurses need to remember the dual care framework for pregnant women: woman and fetus.

Bergum (2004) identified four themes to define relational ethics: environment, embodiment, mutual respect, and engagement. No matter what ethical issue is of concern, nurses need to focus on the quality of the moral relationship between the nurse and patient. In relational ethics, the first theme, environment, is a living system. It is important to understand how the whole environment is affected by actions that each person takes. The living environment is in every nurse, and every action that is taken by nurses affects the outcome of the healthcare system as a whole. For example, the goal of a healthcare agency for a woman who had a partial-birth abortion could be to discharge her after 1 day. The patient and agency depend on the responsible and competent actions of nurses and others to meet the goal of a 1-day discharge.

Embodiment is the second theme, and is defined as having a scientific knowledge, a compassion for human life, and experiencing feeling and emotion for another person. For example, if after a prenatal genetic test a 16-week-pregnant woman has just been told that her fetus has Down syndrome, the nurse would understand the science behind the test and know the aftercare procedure. The nurse would have a mindful reality of the woman's pain and suffering and therefore have compassion for her.

Mutual respect is the third theme in relational ethics. Mutual respect is a way for people to exist together and have equal worth and dignity; it often is difficult to attain, but it is the central theme of relational ethics. In the example of the woman and her fetus with Down syndrome, mutual respect could be initiated by the nurse's regard for the woman's feelings, values, beliefs, and attitudes. The word

BOX 4.8 ETHICAL FORMATIONS

Essential aspects from the *Code of Ethics for Nurses with Interpretive Statements* on the care of childbearing women:

- The need for health care is universal, transcending all individual differences (1.1, p. 7).
- Respect for human dignity requires the recognition of specific patient rights, particularly the right of self-determination (1.4, p. 8).
- Each nurse has an obligation to be knowledgeable about the moral and legal rights of all patients to self-determination. The nurse preserves, protects, and supports those interests by assessing the patient's comprehension of both the information presented and the implications of decisions (1.4, p. 8).
- Nurses must examine the conflicts arising between their own personal and professional values, the values and interests of others who are also responsible for patient care and healthcare decisions, as well as those of patients (2.2, p. 10).
- In situations where the patient requires a personal opinion from the nurse, the nurse is generally free to express an informed personal opinion as long as this preserves the voluntariness of the patient and maintains appropriate professional and moral boundaries (5.3, p. 19).
- It is essential to be aware of the potential for undue influence attached to the nurse's professional role (5.3, p. 19).

mutual means to have a reciprocal and interactive focus. Based on this concept, the woman would need to reciprocate that respect toward the nurse.

The fourth theme, relational engagement, is when the nurse and patient can find a few minutes to interact about something that is important to them. The nurse needs to understand the patient's circumstances and vulnerability. An example of engagement for the woman and her fetus with Down syndrome can be accomplished by the nurse's engaging in a conversation with the woman about her feelings concerning the diagnosis and options for her and her fetus.

Dialogue is in the center of the moral space, at the focus of relational ethics, and is the venue for the four themes to emerge. Depersonalization and coldness often surround the healthcare systems that women use. Nurses must give personalization to childbearing women by practicing relational ethics. On relational ethics and the moral life, Bergum (2004) stated:

> With relational space as the location of enacting morality, we need to consider ethics in every situation, every encounter, and with every patient. If all relationships are the focus of understanding and examining moral life, then it is important to attend to the quality of relationships in all nursing practices, whether with patients and their families, with other nurses, with other health care professionals, or with administrators and politicians. (p. 485)

KEY POINTS

- There are different variations of how organizations and people view the moral standing of the fetus. Generally, the degree to which moral standing is placed on the fetus influences maternal rights—the greater the degree of moral standing of the fetus, the more restraint of maternal rights. The central ethical dilemma regarding abortion is about rights—the right to life of the fetus or the woman's right to control her own body. The U.S. Supreme Court justices upheld the Federal Abortion Ban on April 18, 2007 (ACLU, 2007). This ban initially was known as the Partial-Birth Abortion Ban of 2003.
- Most women who have abortions agree that they could not have a baby, carry a fetus, or raise a family for personal or health reasons. Some women, though they may strongly believe in maternal rights, experience disenfranchised grief because they believe that they do not have permission to grieve the loss of their fetus, thus they experience extreme sorrow.
- Assisted reproductive technology (ART) has been a miracle and a relief for women or couples who experience infertility. There are three types of ART: in vitro fertilization (IVF), gamete intrafallopian transfer (GIFT), and zygote intrafallopian transfer (ZIFT). Ethical issues regarding ART include the risks resulting from technology; surrogacy (donor eggs, embryo donation, or carrying fetuses); the handling of surplus embryos and fetuses; implications of sperm sorting, gender selection, and family balancing; and genetic modification and enhancement—the dream of creating a perfect child.
- Preimplantation genetic diagnosis (PGD) is a procedure that allows implantation of a selected gender or a perfect or near perfect embryo. Many genetic diseases can be detected through gene technology, screening, and genetic diagnosis. Knowing when to test and when not to test could be an ethical difficulty for all people concerned with the issue. Maternal rights should be respected, but weighing maternal rights against burdens of costs may be a hard choice for couples and providers of care.
- Maternal substance abuse, including alcohol and other drugs, can be detrimental to the fetus or newborn infant. There tends to be lack of education from providers of care or a deficit of pregnant women in comprehending the adverse effects of substance abuse. Maternal and infant drug screening is not performed on a routine basis and may not be done without express informed consent. Nurses have a moral responsibility to educate their patients and recognize maternal substance abuse. However, a woman's decision to obtain help is her decision, and that decision is dependent upon the degree of trust that she has developed with her providers of care.
- Nurses should incorporate and apply essential concepts from the ANA *Code of Ethics for Nurses with Interpretive Statements* (2001) and Bergum's (2004) relational ethics. Bergum's themes of relational ethics are environment, embodiment, mutual respect, and engagement. Dialogue is in the center of the moral space, and serves as the venue in which Bergum's four themes can emerge.

CASE STUDY: PARTIAL-BIRTH ABORTION (INTACT D & E)

www

Ms. Mason, age 34 and 19 weeks into her pregnancy, received a prenatal genetic diagnosis of Huntington's disease for her fetus via amniocentesis. The day after the diagnosis, the physician explained two options to Ms. Mason: carrying the fetus to term or having a late-term abortion to terminate the pregnancy. The physician explained how the procedure would be performed. Mr. and Ms. Mason were devastated and needed a few days to process the information. When they returned to the clinic, the Masons informed the physician and nurse that they had decided to have the partial-birth abortion. They made a decision not to have any more children, even after the physician had explained the possibility of embryo selection (sperm sorting) for future children.

1. The day that the physician explains the options to Ms. Mason, you try to establish a genuine ethical relationship with her so that the two of you can have a deeper understanding of the situation. As a nurse, what specific approaches will you use for this relationship?
2. Based on the reading, what ethical issues are at stake? Explain.
3. You are in the room with the physician on the day that the Masons return with their decision to have the abortion. As a nurse, what approaches will you take with the Masons on this day? Consider your own values and beliefs about abortion, especially partial-birth abortion, in light of the fetus having Huntington's disease.
4. If they had chosen to have this baby, the Masons would need to think about who would care for their impaired child in the case of their deaths. A person with Huntington's disease is not usually afflicted with symptoms until his or her mid-30s. Financial demands would also be a problem. Explore the ramifications of a decision to keep the fetus and raise the child, especially with the Masons knowing that the outcome would be severe impairment in the child's middle 30s.
5. How can the Masons justify having an abortion when Huntington's disease does not usually affect a person until the middle 30s, well after the child has reached maturity?
6. Explain how each principle—autonomy, beneficence, nonmaleficence, and justice—can guide or be applied in this case. How can you justify each principle?

References

American Academy of Family Physicians. (2010). Prenatal diagnosis: Amniocentesis and CVS. Retrieved from http://familydoctor.org/online/famdocen/home/women/pregnancy/fetal/144.html

American Civil Liberties Union. (1997). Coercive and punitive governmental responses to women's conduct during pregnancy. Retrieved from http://www.aclu.org/reproductiverights/gen/16529res19970930.html

American Civil Liberties Union. (2006). U.S. Supreme Court to hear argument in federal abortion ban challenges. Retrieved from http://www.aclu.org/reproductiverights/abortionbans/27305prs20061108.html

American Civil Liberties Union. (2007). Case summaries: U.S. Supreme Court upholds Federal Ban on Abortion methods: Ruling undermines women's health and equality. Retrieved from http://www.aclu.org/reproductiverights/abortionbans/29778res20070518.html

American Nurses Association. (2001). *Code of ethics for nurses with interpretive statements.* Washington, DC: Author.

Arons, J. (2007). Future choices: Assisted reproductive technologies and the law. Retrieved from http://www.americanprogress.org/issues/2007/12/future_choices.html

Bergum, V. (2004). Relational ethics in nursing. In J. L. Storch, P. Rodney, & R. Starzomski (Eds.), *Toward a moral horizon: Nursing ethics for leadership and practice* (pp. 485–502). Toronto, Canada: Pearson-Prentice Hall.

Burke, T. (with Reardon, D. C.). (2002). *Forbidden grief: The unspoken pain of abortion.* Springfield, IL: Acorn.

Centers for Disease Control and Prevention. (2011). Assisted reproductive technology. Retrieved from http://www.cdc.gov/art/

Chandis, V., & Williams, T. (2006). The patient, the doctor, the fetus, and the court-compelled cesarean: Why courts should address the question through a bioethical lens. *Medicine and Law, 25*, 729–746.

Degrazia, D. (2005). *Human identity and bioethics.* New York, NY: Cambridge University Press.

DeGrazia, D. (2006). Moral status, human identity, and early embryos: A critique of the president's approach. *Journal of Law, Medicine, & Ethics, 34*(1), 49–57.

DeGrazia, D. (2008). Moral status as a matter of degree? *The Southern Journal of Philosophy, 46*, 181–198.

Feinberg, J. (1974). The rights of animals and unborn generations. In W. T. Blackstone (Ed.), *Philosophy & environmental crisis* (pp. 43–68). Athens: University of Georgia Press.

Frankel, M. S. (2003). Inheritable genetic modification and *A Brave New World*: Did Huxley have it wrong? *Hastings Center Report, 33*(2), 31–36.

Gans, O., & Balch, M. S. (n.d.). Defending the pro-life position, and framing the issue by the language we use. Retrieved from http://www.nrlc.org/abortion/facts/abortionresponses.html

Guttmacher Institute. (2011). Facts on inducted abortions in the United States. Retrieved from http://www.guttmacher.org/pubs/fb_induced_abortion.html

Guttmacher Institute. (2011). State policies in brief: Abortion. Retrieved from http://www.guttmacher.org/statecenter/spibs/index.html

Grady, D. (2000, Oct. 4). Baby conceived to provide cell transplant for his dying sister. *New York Times*, p. 24.

Harris, J., & Holm, S. (2000). Introduction. In J. Harris & S. Holm (Eds.), *The future of human reproduction: Ethics, choice, & regulation* (pp. 1–37). Oxford, UK: Clarendon.

Harris, J., & Holm, S. (2003). Abortion. In H. LaFollette (Ed.), *The Oxford handbook of practical ethics* (pp. 112–135). Oxford, UK: Oxford University.

Iris, O., Amalia, L., Moshe, M., Arnon, W., & Eyal, S. (2009). Refusal of treatment in obstetrics—A maternal-fetal conflict. *Journal of Maternal-Fetal and Neonatal Medicine, 2*(7), 612–615.

Jopling, D. A. (2000). *Self-knowledge and the self.* New York, NY: Routledge.

Keenan, C. (2006). Maternal versus fetal rights: Part 1. In S. W. Killion & K. Dempski (Eds.), *Quick look nursing: Legal and ethical issues* (pp. 144–145). Sudbury, MA: Jones and Bartlett.

Ludwig, M. J. (2008). Ethics in medicine: Maternal-fetal conflict. Retrieved from http://depts.washington.edu/bioethx/topics/matern.html

Mahoney, J. (2007). *The challenge of human rights: Origin, development, and significance.* Oxford, UK: Blackwell.

Marquis, D. (1989). Why abortion is immoral. *Journal of Philosophy, 86*, 183–202.
Munson, R. (2004). *Intervention and reflection: Basic issues in medical ethics* (7th ed.). Belmont, CA: Wadsworth-Thomson Learning.
National Abortion and Reproductive Rights Action League Pro Choice America. (2011). The difference pro-choice leaders make. Retrieved from http://www.prochoiceamerica.org/about-us/successes/pro-choice-leaders.html
National Right to Life Committee. (2003). Final language Partial-Birth Abortion Act as approved by both houses of Congress. Retrieved from http://www.nrlc.org/abortion/pba/partial_birth_abortion_Ban_act_final_language.htm
Perry, B. L., Jones, H., Tuten, M., & Svikas, D. S. (2003). Assessing maternal perceptions of harmful effects of drug use during pregnancy. *Journal of Addictive Diseases, 22*, 1–9.
Planned Parenthood Action Center. (2010). History of the federal abortion ban. Retrieved from http://www.plannedparenthoodaction.org/positions/history-federal-abortion-ban-637.htm
President's Council on Bioethics. (2004). Monitoring stem cell research: A report of the President's Council on Bioethics. Washington, DC: Author. Retrieved from http://www.bioethics.gov/reports/stemcell/index.html
Roe v. Wade: The 1973 Supreme Court decision on state abortion laws. (2001). In R. M. Baird & S. E. Rosenberg, J. (2007). *First test-tube baby—Louise Brown. Your Guide to 20th Century History*. Retrieved from http://history1900s.about.com/od/medicaladvancesissues/a/testtubebaby.htm
Steinbock, B. (1992). *Life before birth: The moral and legal status of embryos and fetuses*. New York, NY: Oxford University Press.
Steinbock, B. (2006). The morality of killing human embryos. *Journal of Law, Medicine, & Ethics, 34*(1), 26–34.
Thomson, J. J. (1971). A defense of abortion. *Philosophy and Public Affairs, 1*(1), 47–66.
Tran, L. (2004). Legal rights and the maternal-fetal conflict. *BioTeach Journal, 2*, 76–80.
University of Minnesota Cancer Center. (2010). Umbilical cord blood transplantation program. Retrieved from http://www.cancer.umn.edu/research/programs/transbioucb.html
Veatch, R. (2003). *The basics of bioethics* (2nd ed.). Upper Saddle River, NJ: Prentice Hall.
Wachbroit, R., & Wasserman, D. (2003). Reproductive technology. In H. LaFollette (Ed.), *The Oxford handbook of practical ethics* (pp. 136–160). Oxford, UK: Oxford University.

For a full suite of assignments and additional learning activities, use the access code located in the front of your book to visit this exclusive website: http://go.jblearning.com/butts. If you do not have an access code, you can obtain one at the site.

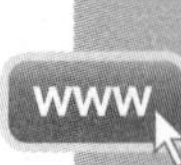

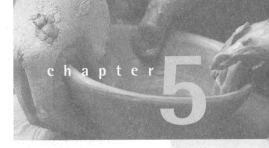

chapter 5

Infant and Child Nursing Ethics

Karen L. Rich

Heaven lies about us in our infancy.
—*William Wordsworth, "Intimations of Immortality," 1807*

OBJECTIVES

After reading this chapter, the reader should be able to:

1. Discuss issues of vulnerability as they relate to the care of infants and children.
2. Understand ethical issues regarding the universal vaccination of children and the nurse's role.
3. Identify issues of social justice as they apply to infants and children.
4. Evaluate ethical factors regarding refusing treatment for infants and children.
5. Discuss landmark cases in the ethical and legal care of infants and children.
6. Understand the nurse's role as an advocate in the care of infants and children.

Mothering

In the book *Ethics for the New Millennium*, the Dalai Lama (1999) emphasized the importance of the ethic of compassion. Empathy, which is one's "ability to enter into and, to some extent, share others' suffering" (p. 123), represents compassion (*nying je*) at a basic level. The Dalai Lama stated that compassion can be developed, going beyond empathy to the extent that it arises without effort and "is unconditional, undifferentiated, and universal in scope" (p. 123). Compassion is a desire to separate another being from suffering. Compassion also is a sense of intimacy toward all feeling and perceiving beings (Dalai Lama, 1999). Persons with this well-developed level of compassion include in the scope of their compassion even those beings that may harm them. According to the Dalai Lama, this profound form of intimacy and compassion can be likened "to the love a mother has for her only child" (p. 123).

All animals are born into an initial condition of vulnerability and dependence. Human infants and children "arrive in the world in a condition of needy helplessness more or less unparalleled in any other animal species" (Nussbaum, 2001, p. 181). Historically, Western ethics generally has ignored human vulnerability and its resultant consequence of creating a need for humans to depend on one another (MacIntyre, 1999). However, some feminist philosophers, such as Virginia Held (1993) and Sara Ruddick (1995), have used the underlying premise of human dependence as the foundation for their views of ethics. In fact, feminist philosophers have proposed that the caring that occurs between a mother and her vulnerable and dependent child can be used as a model for all moral relationships. This model is similar to the model of compassion discussed by the Dalai Lama.

In considering how a feminist approach to ethics is relevant to the care of infants and children, nurses can think in terms of what Tong (1997) called a care-focused feminist ethics approach; this type of approach to ethics supports feminine values, such as "compassion, empathy, sympathy, nurturance, and kindness" (p. 38), that often have been marginalized in male-dominated societies. These values and virtues also are ones that are traditionally associated with good mothering.

There have been heated debates about the differences between the types of moral reasoning engaged in by males and females (see *Care-Based Versus Justice-Based Reasoning* in Chapter 1). However, Stimpson (1993) noted that "crucially, both women and men can be feminists" (p. viii). In accepting and using the feminine model of social relationships that exist between mothers and children, Stimpson stated "a moral agent, female or male, will be [what Held (1993) called] a 'mothering person'" (p. viii).

Held (1993) proposed the concept of "mothering person" as a gender-neutral term used to describe the type of mothering that would occur in a society without male domination. Held stated that there are good reasons to believe that mothering should be a practice performed by both women and men. Ruddick (1995) defined a mother as one who is capable of doing maternal work and

> a person who takes on responsibility for children's lives and for whom providing child care is a significant part of her or his working life. [She continued] I am suggesting that, whatever difference might exist between female and male mothers, there is no

> reason to believe that one sex rather than the other is more capable of doing maternal work. (pp. 40–41)

When providing ethical care to infants and children, nurses support mothers and mothering persons, both females and males, who share in the unconditional compassion toward their children as described by the Dalai Lama.

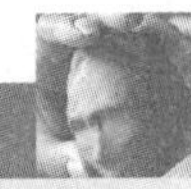

www Ethical Reflections

- Engage in a debate with your colleagues using the following positions: (1) mothering is an inherently female trait, and (2) mothering is not an inherently female trait.
- What can nurses do to include fathers in the "mothering" of children?
- Discuss the Dalai Lama's statement about compassion being similar "to the love a mother has for her only child." Why do you agree or disagree with this statement?

Foundations of Trust

> *A boy bathing in a river was in danger of being drowned. He called out to a passing traveler for help, but instead of holding out a helping hand, the man stood by unconcernedly and scolded the boy for his imprudence. "Oh sir!" cried the youth, "pray help me now and scold me afterwards."*
>
> —AESOP, *AESOP'S FABLE*

"Children are vulnerable, often frightened small people" (Ruddick, 1995, p. 119). An infant's development of basic trust versus basic mistrust is the first of Erik Erikson's (1950/1985) eight stages of psychosocial development. According to Ruddick, it is the responsibility of mothers to establish the feeling of trust between themselves and their children, because children's trust ideally is founded on the nurturance and protectiveness of their mothers. Unless there are unusual circumstances, parents are entrusted with the autonomy to make decisions for their minor children. This autonomy is an endorsement of the trust that societies place in parents' ability and desire to provide care that is consistent with the best interests of their children. Although parents generally have autonomy privileges in decision making for their children, children have their own basic dignity as human beings. Kahlil Gibran (1923/2000) described an interesting perspective on the soul, or spirit, of children and parental rights (see Box 5.1).

Because most children depend on their mothering persons to be trustworthy, mothering persons often are wary when they are judging healthcare policies and choosing the people they entrust to meet their children's healthcare needs. Trust becomes an even greater issue when mothering people are not able to choose their children's healthcare providers, as is usually the case with nurses. Justified maternal wariness includes a cautious trust of nurses and other healthcare professionals who interact with and treat one's children. However, it is natural, and often a source of comfort, for parents to believe that healthcare professionals have a more complete grasp of the medical facts and probabilities related to their child's health care than they themselves have in many instances. Consequently, parents depend on and

BOX 5.1 ETHICAL FORMATIONS: GIBRAN, "ON CHILDREN"

Your children are not your children. They are the sons and daughters of Life's longing for itself. They come through you but not from you, and though they are with you yet they belong not to you. You may give them your love but not your thoughts, for they have their own thoughts. You may house their bodies but not their souls, for their souls dwell in the house of tomorrow, which you cannot visit, not even in your dreams. You may strive to be like them, but seek not to make them like you. For life goes not backward nor tarries with yesterday. You are the bows from which your children as living arrows are sent forth. The archer sees the mark upon the path of the infinite, and He bends you with His might that His arrows may go swift and far. Let your bending in the archer's hand be for gladness; for even as He loves the arrow that flies so He loves also the bow that is stable. (pp. 17–18)

Source: Gibran, K. (2000). *The prophet.* New York, NY: Alfred A. Knopf. (Original work published 1923)

trust healthcare professionals to support or guide them in making difficult healthcare decisions for their children. Sometimes this trust is similar to the unavoidable trust that was discussed in Chapter 2.

Universal Vaccination

Because of the grave threat of nonpreventable infectious diseases, people living before and during the early 1900s would have been delighted to have a wide array of available vaccines. However, due to successful public health advances in the 20th and 21st centuries, many people in the United States have not personally encountered some of the diseases that are now vaccine-preventable. Therefore, some people take for granted the benefits of available vaccines. According to the National Network for Immunization Information,

> most parents today have not seen a child paralyzed by polio, or choking to death from diphtheria, or brain damaged by measles. Fear of vaccine-preventable diseases has diminished while concerns about vaccine safety have increased—even though a number of the vaccines are even safer than decades ago as a result of medical research. (NNii, 2009, para. 3)

States vary in regard to mandatory childhood vaccination laws, sometimes called "school laws" (Centers for Disease Control [CDC], 2007). Every state allows vaccination exemptions for medical reasons, which are are based on documented medical information received from physicians, usually related to a child's allergy to vaccine components or an immune deficiency. If parents have sincere religious beliefs that are contrary to the acceptance of immunizations for their children, religious exemptions are allowed by all states except Mississippi and West Virginia (Institute for Vaccine Safety Johns Hopkins

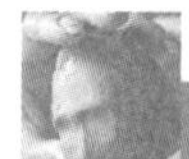

Ethical Reflections

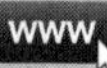

- With your colleagues, use the Socratic method discussed in Chapter 1 to analyze the concept of nurse–family trust.
- What factors and behaviors might influence mothering persons' trust of the nurses who care for their children?
- What factors and behaviors might influence nurses' trust of mothering persons?
- Discuss the different forms of paternalism (see Chapters 2 and 8) as they relate to the ethical care of children.

Bloomberg School of Public Health, 2011). Twenty states allow personal belief exemptions for parents' religious, philosophical, and other nonmedical objections to vaccines.

When exemptions are obtained, children can attend school without immunizations in most states, although parents or guardians may be judged liable in a civil case if, because of their child's lack of immunization, a vaccine-preventable communicable disease is transmitted to another person. Also, if parents follow the CDC's (2007) recommended guidelines to protect unvaccinated children, these unprotected children may miss months of school, as the CDC recommends that unvaccinated children remain at home during vaccine-preventable disease outbreaks, which may occur in waves spanning a number of weeks.

Some parents who are opposed to a program of universal vaccination seek ways to achieve natural immunity for their children. A popular method that is sometimes used to try to achieve natural immunity for children is having children attend "exposure parties." Groups of well and previously uninfected children are brought together with a child or children who are currently believed to be infectious with a specific vaccine-preventable disease, such as chicken pox, rubella, or measles (NNii, 2004a, 2004b, 2007). These parties are not without risks to children, including the most obvious result of having one's child endure sometimes dangerous and unnecessary illnesses (see Box 5.2).

The American Nurses Association (ANA)'s (2011) 1997 position statement about childhood immunization is still current:

> The ANA recognizes the importance of immunizations to the health of individual children and the community as a whole, and of the pivotal roel [sic] nursing plays in assuring immunizations. The fulfillment of the immunization goal is a major undertaking that cannot be realized without the full endorsement of all professional nurses. For that reason, ANA will strive to attain the highest rate of immunization coverage in order to insure maximum protection overall for the general population. (ANA, 2011, para. 2)

In 2011, the ANA released a public service announcement (PSA) about nurses' roles in promoting immunizations. The theme for the campaign was nurses' power to protect people and to bring immunity to every community, which is a theme that is consistent with the role of nurses as trusted patient advocates. Box 5.3 contains nonconfrontational suggestions for healthcare professionals to use if parents resist immunizations for their children.

Children Underserved by Healthcare Systems

Children are particularly vulnerable people because they must depend on others for their life-sustaining needs, including their health and well-being. Childhood vulnerability is heightened for some children because of conditions such as poverty and unfavorable social or family situations. Evidence suggests that healthcare professionals often do not adequately meet the nonmedical needs of vulnerable children

BOX 5.2 ETHICAL FORMATIONS: RISKS OF MEASLES VERSUS RISKS OF THE MEASLES VACCINE

Risks of Measles

- Measles is a serious disease caused by a highly contagious virus that spreads when people touch or breathe in infectious droplets passed by coughing and sneezing.
- Measles begins with fever, followed by cough, runny nose, and conjunctivitis ("pink eye").
- Infection of the middle ear, pneumonia, croup, and diarrhea are common complications.
- Measles encephalitis (an infection of the brain) occurs in 1 per 1,000 cases of natural measles, frequently resulting in permanent brain damage in survivors.
- Approximately 5% of children (5 out of 100) with measles will develop pneumonia.
- Of every 1,000 children who get measles in the United States, 1 to 2 die from the disease.
- Death is more common in infants, in malnourished children, and among immunocompromised persons, including those with leukemia and HIV infection.

Risks of the Vaccine

- MMR is an attenuated (weakened) live virus vaccine. It prevents measles, mumps, and rubella.
- Nearly all (over 80%) children who get the MMR vaccine will have no side effects.
- Most children who have a side effect will have only a mild reaction, such as soreness, redness, or swelling where the shot was given; mild rash; mild to moderate fever; swelling of the lymph glands; and temporary pain, stiffness, or swelling in the joints.
- In about 5 to 15% of children given MMR, a fever in excess of 103°F may occur—usually beginning about 7 to 12 days after they receive the vaccine.
- About 15% of women who receive MMR will develop acute arthritis or swelling of the joints. This condition is usually very short lived.
- In rare cases (about 3 children out of 10,000 given MMR, or 0.03% of recipients), a moderate reaction such as seizure related to high fever may occur.
- In rare cases (about 1 child out of 30,000 given MMR), a child may develop temporary low platelet count, which can cause bleeding.
- In extremely rare cases (less than 1 child out of 1,000,000 given MMR), children have a serious reaction, such as lowered consciousness, coma, or hypersensitivity (anaphylaxis)—swelling inside the mouth, difficulty breathing, low blood pressure, and rarely, shock.

Source: National Network for Immunization Information. (2004a). Measles parties. Retrieved from http://www.immunizationinfo.org/issues/exposure-parties/measles-parties

(Barreto, Perez, & Halfon, 2007). Providers fail to inquire about family conditions such as homelessness, social problems, substance abuse, and poverty because they are unsure about resources that are available or believe that they have no way to help families solve these problematic issues. By failing to provide interventions to improve serious nonmedical problems during childhood, healthcare providers unintentionally may compound these problems, such as contributing to an increased risk of developmental delays, substance and physical abuse, and emotional disorders among children and their families.

BOX 5.3 ETHICAL FORMATIONS: OVERCOMING VACCINATION RESISTANCE

- Ascertain exactly what is bothering the parent about vaccinations.
- Clearly state your recommendation and rationale.
- Voice your respect for the parent's views.
- Develop a mutually acceptable plan.
- If possible, administer vaccines that protect against the diseases for which the child is most at risk, based on the child's age and immunization history, and the prevalence of the disease in your community.
- Be sure to repeat your recommendations when you subsequently see the child and parent; parents may reconsider their decisions.

Source: Adapted from Dias, M., & Marcuse, E. K. (2000, July). When parents resist immunization. *Contemporary Pediatrics.* Retrieved from http://www.dshs.state.tx.us/immunize/forms/resist.pdf

More than 8 million children in the United States are uninsured (childrensdefense.org, 2011; State Health Access Data Assistance Center [SHADAC] & Urban Institute, 2005), though most of these children are eligible for Medicaid or State Children's Health Insurance Program (SCHIP) services (SHADAC & Urban Center, 2005). Healthcare providers need to screen underserved children who are particularly vulnerable to "the 'double jeopardy' of childhood poverty" (Barreto et al., 2007, p. 174). A two-pronged assessment should be conducted that focuses on "the types and impacts of higher levels of exposure to risk factors as well as assessing available levels of resources and health services (protective and health-promoting factors)" (p. 174) for children affected by poverty. Ethical practice in the nursing care of children includes nurses' willingness to address social problems that often are very difficult to solve, such as immigration, homelessness, and poverty, that continue to have a major impact on the health of children in the United States.

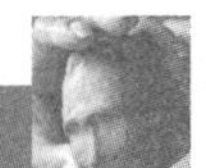

www Ethical Reflections

- Do you believe that exposure parties are unethical? Defend your answer.
- Review the ethical theories and approaches in Chapters 1 and 2. Which theories and approaches are particularly relevant to ethics and immunization issues and laws?
- Research some of the reasons that parents refuse immunizations for their children and gather specific information about exposure parties. Imagine that you are a public health nurse working at a county health department. A mother brings her newborn in for a well-baby checkup. The baby's mother tells you that she has heard that exposure parties are a good way to immunize children. How would you respond to the mother's comment?

Children of Immigrant Families

The 2010 census revealed that children of immigrants represent one in four people under the age of 18, and that these children "are now the fastest-growing segment of the nation's youth, an indication that both legal and illegal immigrants as well as minority births are lifting the nation's population" (Yen, 2011, para. 3). According to the Center for Health and Health Care in Schools (2005), "the poverty rate of children in immigrant families is 21%" (para. 2). Because of welfare law changes in 1996, during their first 5 years in the United States, immigrants are not eligible to receive assistance from the Temporary Assistance to Needy Families (TANF) and Medicaid programs that serve the poor (Borjas, 2011; Center for Health and Health Care in Schools, 2005); however, eligibility for these programs has been opened in some states through state-funded programs. Food stamp access is also restricted among immigrant families.

Children born in the United States to non-U.S. citizen immigrant mothers automatically are granted U.S. citizenship at birth; however, some governmental officials are critics of readily providing healthcare benefits to these so-called anchor babies (babies that provide a reason for noncitizen parents to remain in the United States) (Globe Editorial, 2006). These critics have created federal policies that involve lengthy bureaucratic red tape that often prevents these infants from rapidly receiving Medicaid coverage for health care. Although these children are "known to" the Medicaid program because the program pays the hospital bills generated from their births, the government requires additional paperwork for continued Medicaid coverage. This additional paperwork often frightens parents who fear deportation.

Consequently, many of these so-called anchor babies, who are U.S. citizens and thus eligible for healthcare programs, do not receive immunizations and other primary and secondary preventive services. Ironically, creating barriers to early health care for these children often causes more taxpayer expense because money subsequently must be spent to treat preventable diseases. The American Academy of Pediatrics (1997) proposed 10 recommendations for pediatricians to help children of immigrant families. These recommendations, which also are useful for nurses, are shown in Box 5.4.

Global Problems of Poverty and Infectious Diseases

Statistical data regarding the unmet needs of infants, children, and adolescents worldwide should concern all compassionate people, but especially nurses. Of special significance is the fact that about two-thirds of the deaths accounted for in these statistics are the result of conditions for which there are low-cost prevention measures or treatment. Data taken directly from the World Health Organization (WHO, 2008) website include the following:

- Nearly 10 million children under the age of 5 die each year—more than 1,000 every hour—but most could survive threats and thrive with access to simple, affordable interventions.
- The risk of death is highest in the first month of life. Preterm birth, birth asphyxia, and infections cause most newborn deaths.

BOX 5.4 ETHICAL FORMATIONS: RECOMMENDATIONS FOR CHILDREN OF IMMIGRANT FAMILIES

1. Oppose denying needed services to any child residing within the borders of the United States.
2. Take advantage of educational opportunities and resources to achieve a better understanding of immigrant cultures and the healthcare needs of immigrant children and families.
3. Tolerate and respect cultural differences in attitudes and approaches to child-rearing.
4. Be aware of the special health problems for which immigrant children are at risk, such as vaccine-preventable diseases, tuberculosis, syphilis, and parasitic diseases; poor nutritional status; delayed growth and development; poor dental health; poor mental health; and school problems.
5. Be educated about the unique stresses that immigration may place on children and families and about resources that provide services in the family's language.
6. With the approval of the child's parent or legal guardian, recognize and support the extended family in healthcare activities.
7. Follow up with continuing health supervision, mental health, and social services for any screening received by immigrants and refugees before they entered the United States.
8. Develop linguistically and culturally appropriate services in concert with public health, social services, and school systems in local communities.
9. Define the healthcare needs of immigrant children.
10. Support and participate in locally developed, community-based activities that increase access to health care for immigrant children (pp. 155–156).

Source: Adapted from American Academy of Pediatrics Committee on Community Health Services. (1997). Health care for children of immigrant families. *Pediatrics, 100,* 153–156.

- Pneumonia is the prime cause of death in children under 5 years of age. Nearly three-quarters of all cases occur in just 15 countries. Addressing the major risk factors—including malnutrition and indoor air pollution—is essential to preventing pneumonia, as are vaccination and breastfeeding. Antibiotics and oxygen are vital tools for effectively managing the illness.
- Diarrheal diseases are a leading cause of sickness and death among children in developing countries. Breastfeeding helps prevent diarrhea among young children.
- Treatment for sick children with Oral Rehydration Salts (ORS), combined with zinc supplements, is safe, cost-effective, and saves lives.
- One African child dies every 30 seconds from malaria. Insecticide-treated nets prevent transmission and increase child survival.
- Over 90% of children with HIV are infected through mother-to-child transmission, which can be prevented with antiretrovirals, as well as safer delivery and feeding practices.
- About 20 million children under 5 worldwide are severely malnourished, which leaves them more vulnerable to illness and early death.

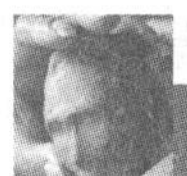

Ethical Reflections www

- What is social justice? (see Chapters 1 and 11)
- Consider the problems of global poverty and infectious diseases as they affect children and relate them to social justice. What can nurses do to improve social justice for the world's population of children?
- Do you believe that many members of the world population avert their eyes from the healthcare plight of innocent children? Support your answer.
- Review critical theory in Chapter 1. Read additional literature, as needed. How can critical theory be applied to the worldwide healthcare disparities involving children?
- What other ethical theories and approaches discussed in Chapters 1 and 2 apply to the worldwide disparities in health care for children? Explain.

Abused Children

Child abuse, which includes physical, sexual, and emotional abuse, as well as neglect, is a form of family violence (Ramsey, 2006). Family violence is an "action by a family member with the intent to cause harm to or control another family member" (Allender & Spradley, 2005, p. 908). The most common form of child abuse falls under the category of neglect (Ramsey, 2006). Although all states have mandatory child abuse reporting laws, it is believed that abuse is significantly underreported.

The ethical responsibility of nurses in the care of children includes the responsibility to be alert to the signs of abuse and to report abuse appropriately. Nurses, along with all other healthcare professionals, are considered mandatory reporters of possible abuse (Ramsey, 2006). Situations that signal possible abuse include:

- Conflict between the explanation of how an incident occurred and the physical findings, such as poorly explained bruises or fractures
- Age-inappropriate behaviors or behaviors that signify poor social adjustment, such as "aggressive behavior, social withdrawal, depression, lying, stealing, thumb sucking" (Ramsey, 2006, p. 59), and risk-taking (sexual promiscuity, reckless driving, etc.)
- Alcohol and other drug abuse
- Problems in school
- Suicidal ideation

The usual responsibility of handling a patient's treatment confidentially is waived in the instance of suspected child abuse, even when the person reporting the abuse is the patient (Ramsey, 2006). Abuse does not need to be confirmed as factual in order to be reportable. The identification of suspected abuse should be promptly reported to the agency designated by each state. There is legal protection in most states for professionals, including nurses, who are reporting suspected abuse in good faith, though healthcare professionals may be exposed to legal sanctions if they fail to report suspected abuse to the appropriate agencies.

Surrogate Decision Making

Children are legally incompetent individuals who, in most cases, must have surrogate decision makers for important life decisions, including healthcare decisions. Ethicists have established standards that are accepted as being ethically appropriate for guiding healthcare decisions made on behalf of infants and children. The most commonly accepted ethical standard that underlies surrogate decision making for children is based on a standard of best interest. When using the **best interest standard**, surrogate decision makers base their decisions on what they believe will provide the most benefits and the least burdens for the child. The best interest standard is a quality-of-life assessment, and when using it a surrogate decision maker must determine the highest net benefit among the available options, assigning different weights to interest the patient has in each option and discounting or subtracting inherent risks or costs. The best interest standard protects another's well-being by requiring surrogates to assess the risks and benefits of various treatments and alternatives to treatment, making it inescapably a quality-of-life criterion (Beauchamp & Childress, 2009, p. 138).

The standard of best interest is similar to the standard of substituted judgment, but the two standards are distinctly different. The aim of the **standard of substituted judgment** is for a surrogate to make decisions that abide by the previously known (either verbalized or inferred) treatment preferences that persons had when they were able to express those preferences (i.e., when they were competent) at a time when persons are no longer able to express treatment preferences (i.e., when they are no longer competent). Thus, some ethicists argue that only a standard of best interest is appropriate when decisions are made for children because decisions are being made for persons who have never been legally competent; consequently, there is no history of known preferences from children based on their competent thinking.

In using the best interest standard, parents must sacrifice their personal goals for their child in favor of the child's needs and interests. Parents are put in a difficult situation when they must be uncompromising in trying to attend to one child's best interest when it may conflict with the best interest of another child or children within the same family (Ross, 1998).

Refusal of Treatment

Parents sometimes refuse treatment for their children, and children themselves may, in some cases, be deemed to have decisional capacity to refuse treatment based on religious beliefs or other reasons. In general, religious and cultural beliefs are given respect in healthcare matters and are protected through liberties granted by the U.S. Constitution (Jonsen, Siegler, & Winslade, 2006, 2010). Serious consideration must be given to the wishes of maturing children who are judged to have good insight about the benefits and burdens of their healthcare treatment. The following factors should be taken into consideration and carefully weighed when evaluating the extent of autonomy to be granted to minor children in refusing health care, keeping in mind, however, that efforts need to be made not to undermine the relationship between children and their mothering person(s) (Jonsen et al., 2006):

- The support for the child's request by the child's mothering person(s)

- The severity of the child's condition, such as a child with a terminal and irreversible condition who refuses additional painful treatment versus a situation, such as meningitis, in which the child's condition is acute and reversible
- The consequence of direct harm to the child that potentially could result from the child's decision and the child's realistic understanding of the possible consequences
- Fear, distress, or parental pressure as a motivation for the child's decision

Parental autonomy with regard to a child's healthcare treatment is usually given wide latitude (Jonsen et al., 2006, 2010; Ross, 1998); however, some parental refusals are considered to be abusive or neglectful. State laws protect children from parental healthcare decisions based on religious or other beliefs that can result in serious risk or harm to the child (Jonsen et al., 2006). Nevertheless, many states do not prosecute parents for abuse or neglect if they try to refuse treatment based on religious beliefs. In general, the following principles are followed in overriding parental autonomy in the treatment of children:

- The parent or parents are not given the right of parental autonomy if they are deemed to be incapacitated or incompetent because of factors such as substance abuse, certain psychiatric disorders, minimal ability to comprehend the best interest of the child, or habitual physical abuse.
- As is done when considering respect for the autonomy of a child, the severity of the child's condition and the direct harm to the child that could result from nontreatment should be evaluated. The child should be treated even against the wishes of the parents to prevent or cure serious disease or disability.
- Blood transfusions should be given to a child of a Jehovah's Witness when transfusions are needed to protect the child from the serious complications of disease or injury. Court authority need not be sought in an emergency situation, as legal precedent protects the safety of the child (see Box 5.5).

When analyzing the ethical path to take in regard to refusals of treatment for children, consultation may need to be sought from mental health practitioners or an ethics committee.

Impaired and Critically Ill Children

When neonatal intensive care units (NICUs) were developed in the 1960s, the goal was to increase the likelihood that premature babies would survive. Many medical and technological advances followed, and researchers are still making strides in neonatology today. NICUs are often complicated and scary places for parents who are grappling with the trauma of having a severely impaired or terminally ill neonate. Parents frequently must make life-and-death decisions about their infants

BOX 5.5 ETHICAL FORMATIONS: PROTECTION OF VULNERABLE CHILDREN

In the words of a Supreme Court decision about the authority of a Jehovah's Witness parent, "Parents may be free to become martyrs themselves, but it does not follow that they are free ... to make martyrs of their children" (*Prince v. Massachusetts*, 1944).

Source: Jonsen, A. R., Siegler, M., & Winslade, W. J. (2006). *Clinical ethics: A practical approach to ethical decisions in clinical medicine* (6th ed.). New York, NY: McGraw-Hill, p. 98.

within a context that would be highly stressful even in the best of circumstances. NICUs are often emotionally charged places for nurses, too, as they watch the miracles of life play out before them while they also share in the experience of a family's deepest suffering.

Quality of Life

In considering quality-of-life determinations for newborns and children, it is important to refer back to the ethical foundation involved with surrogate decision making for children—that is, the standard of best interest. There are at least two differences between how quality-of-life decisions are judged for infants and children as opposed to how they are judged for adults (Jonsen et al., 2010). Adults are either able to verbalize preferences that reflect their personal evaluations about the quality of their lives or other people have a general idea of those preferences when an adult becomes incapacitated. In contrast, "[i]n pediatrics, the life whose quality is being assessed is almost entirely in the future, and no expression of preferences is available" (Jonsen et al., p. 158).

Healthcare professionals must be aware of any tendencies they may have to judge the quality of life of pediatric patients as lower than the children, to the best of their ability, or their mothering person(s) would judge it. Nurses are not in a position to make major, ethics-laden treatment decisions in the care of infants and children; even advanced-practice nurses, such as nurse practitioners who work in NICUs, work in collaboration with other healthcare professionals. However, all nurses who work with children are potentially very influential in the healthcare decisions made by parents and other healthcare providers. Practical wisdom, in the tradition of Socrates, Plato, and Aristotle, and the good character of nurses are essential elements in the compassionate care of children.

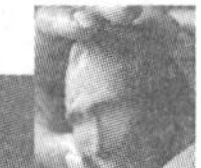

www Ethical Reflections

- Identify specific issues of social justice related to the high-technology health care provided to premature infants. For example, should healthcare professionals consider "How small is too small?" when planning and providing care for a fetus or neonate?
- What information and approaches can be used to analyze the ethics of decision making about age-based distribution of healthcare resources?
- How should scarce healthcare resources be used? For technologically advanced intensive care services for the very young? For technologically advanced intensive care services for the very old? For prevention and health promotion? Support your position(s).
- Who should decide about how scarce healthcare resources should be distributed? Why?

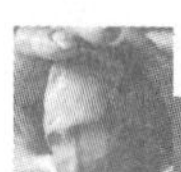

Ethical Reflections

- Discuss criteria and methods that healthcare providers can use to evaluate the motives, requests, and behaviors of mothering persons in regard to making quality-of-life decisions for their seriously impaired children. Use the story of Ashley in Box 5.6 as a case study. Ashley's parents asked physicians to stunt her growth so that her small size would make it easier for them to physically care for her.
- Apply ethical theories, approaches, and decision-making models in analyzing this case.
- Do you agree or disagree with the child receiving hormones to stop her growth? Support your answer.
- Another parent–child ethics case that has been widely debated in the media is the case of Terri Schiavo. Research the specific events of this case.
- Because Terri was an adult rather than a legally incompetent child, compare and contrast relevant quality-of-life determinations.
- Evaluate the ethics-related parent–child issues involved with this case. What type of decision-making standard were Terri's parents using?
- What is the standard that is most accepted by ethicists in a case like Terri's? Why?

Withholding and Withdrawing Treatment

A comprehensive discussion of end-of-life issues is provided in Chapter 9. This discussion generally can be used as a basis for considering decisions about withholding and withdrawing treatment for children; infants, however, fall into a special class of persons in regard to withholding and withdrawing treatment.

Anyone seriously interested in the study of nursing and healthcare ethics realizes that it is difficult to separate ethics from related laws, governmental regulations, and public policies. In evaluating the ethical care of infants in terms of withholding and withdrawing treatment, it is helpful to understand the history and circumstances involved with several landmark cases. Some of these cases help to summarize and clarify the usual actions that are expected to be taken with regard to the treatment of infants, although conclusions about the ethical directions provided by these cases are by no means without dispute. The following discussion is based on public information about these cases and a history provided by Pence (2004).

1971: Johns Hopkins Cases

In the 1970s, two infants with Down syndrome were "allowed to die" at Johns Hopkins Hospital, based on what some people believe were the selfish motives of the parents (Pence, 2004). A third infant with Down syndrome was referred to Johns Hopkins shortly thereafter because of the hospital's reputation for allowing the other two infants to die. However, at this point the hospital staff presented a more balanced view of the infant's prognosis that resulted in a different outcome: the third baby was treated and lived.

1984: Child Abuse Prevention and Treatment Act Amendments (Baby Doe Rules)

The 1984 Child Abuse Prevention and Treatment Act Amendments, also referred to as the Baby Doe rules, are based on the case of Infant Doe, who was born in Indiana in 1982. "'Baby Doe' cases arise when parents of impaired neonates or physicians charged with the care of these neonates question whether continued treatment is worthwhile and consider forgoing treatment in order to hasten death" (Pence, 2004, p. 216).

Many of the events in the short life of Infant Doe greatly influenced the precedent that has set the direction for the treatment of impaired newborns. Infant Doe was born on April 9, 1982, and died 6 days

BOX 5.6 ETHICAL FORMATIONS: "PILLOW ANGEL"

The father's plea was heartfelt and most unusual. Stop the physical growth of my developmentally disabled little girl [with static encephalopathy], he asked a panel of doctors, so that we may be better able to care for her as years go by.

Strapped in a wheelchair, the daughter, a charming dark-haired 6-year-old named Ashley . . . "There's no question this little girl's world is her family," says a doctor who attended that session. "Any concerns were put to rest by watching [the parents and the child]." Which is one reason the medical staff at Seattle's Children's Hospital agreed to the father's 2004 request, deciding that it was ethical to remove Ashley's uterus and breast buds and begin hormone treatments to stop her growth.

Today Ashley is a 9-year-old girl with the mind of a baby, who will never grow into a fully developed woman. Her family . . . initially kept their decision private. But an article published in a medical journal [in October 2006] brought an outcry of public criticism about their choice. . . . For doctors, stopping Ashley's growth presented two issues: Would the novel treatment improve her life? And would it cause harm?

[As cited by Morehouse, Ashley's parents shared the following statements on their website:]

We call [Ashley] our Pillow Angel since she is so sweet and stays right where we place her—usually on a pillow . . .

Source: Morehouse, M. (2007, January). Girl, interrupted. *People*, 69–70.

later (Pence, 2004). The controversy surrounding the care of Infant Doe was based on disagreements about whether treatment should be withheld because the infant had Down syndrome and a tracheo-esophageal fistula. The obstetrician who delivered Infant Doe discouraged the parents from seeking surgical correction of the fistula and indicated that the baby might become a "mere blob." Based on the obstetrician's recommendations and their own beliefs, the parents refused care for their infant. Hospital staff and administrators disagreed with this decision and appealed the decision to a county judge. No guardian ad litem was appointed for the baby, and an unrecorded, middle-of-the-night hearing was conducted by the judge at the hospital. The meeting resulted in the judge's support of the parents' decision. The hospital staff appealed the decision unsuccessfully all the way to the Indiana Supreme Court. They were in the process of taking the case to the U.S. Supreme Court when Infant Doe died.

The specific details of what followed these events are interesting but are beyond the scope of this chapter. However, the ultimate outcome was that the media attention given to the Infant Doe case precipitated action by the Reagan administration, specifically the U.S. Justice Department and the U.S. Department of Health and Human Services (DHHS) (Pence, 2004). **Baby Doe rules** were published by the federal government and became effective on February 12, 1984. The rules were based on Section 504 of the Rehabilitation Act of 1973, which forbids discrimination based entirely on a person's handicaps. The Baby Doe rules provide for a curtailment of federal funds to institutions that violate the regulations.

BOX 5.7 ETHICAL FORMATIONS: THE CASE OF INFANT DOE

The U.S. Civil Rights Commission reviewed the Infant Doe case in 1989, along with other Baby Doe cases, and "the commission concluded that [the obstetrician's] evaluation was 'strikingly out of touch with the contemporary evidence on the capabilities of people with Down syndrome.'"

Source: U.S. Commission on Civil Rights, as cited by Pence, G. (2004). *Classic cases in medical ethics.* Boston, MA: McGraw-Hill, p. 220.

According to Pence (2004), "this interpretation by the Justice Department created a new conceptual synthesis: imperiled newborns were said to be handicapped citizens who could suffer discrimination against their civil rights" (p. 221; see Box 5.7) It is noteworthy that the federal Second Circuit Court of Appeals issued a ruling within 10 days of the Baby Doe rules that made the new rules essentially unenforceable. This ruling was based on the case of Baby Jane Doe.

Baby Jane Doe: Kerri-Lynn

Baby Jane Doe, Kerri-Lynn A., was born in 1983 at St. Charles Hospital in Long Island, New York. She was transferred to the NICU at the University Hospital of the State University of New York (SUNY) at Stony Brook because of her complicated condition at birth. Kerri-Lynn was born with spina bifida, hydrocephalus, an impaired kidney, and microcephaly (Pence, 2004). Her parents were lower middle-class people who had been married for only 4 months when Kerri-Lynn was conceived. After Kerri-Lynn was born, there was disagreement among the medical staff and other people about whether she should be treated or provided with comfort measures (food, hydration, and antibiotics) and allowed to die. The parents decided in favor of withholding aggressive treatment.

The controversy resulted in legal proceedings that eventually included the involvement of the Justice Department and the DHHS. Leaders within these agencies wanted to send representatives to review Kerri-Lynn's medical records to ascertain whether the Baby Doe rules were being violated. However, the parents and the hospital objected to allowing the government representatives to review the records. Ultimately, a federal appeals court, and then the U.S. Supreme Court, ruled in favor of the parents and the hospital in the case of *Bowen v. American Hospital Association et al.* in 1986 (Pence, 2004).

This ruling essentially removed the enforcement potential from the Baby Doe rules. The rules cannot be enforced if the government has no authority to review the individual medical records of infants to determine if the rules are being violated. The Supreme Court explained that because the parents do not receive federal funds for the provision of medical care, their decisions are not bound by Section 504 of the Rehabilitation Act (Pence, 2004). Baby Jane Doe's parents later allowed the recommended surgery to be performed (see Box 5.8). The attorney who represented her parents reported in 1998 that Kerri-Lynn was 15 years old and living with her parents.

BOX 5.8 ETHICAL FORMATIONS: THE CASE OF KERRI-LYNN

In 1994, B. D. Colen was a lecturer in social medicine at Harvard University. He provided an update on Kerri-Lynn:

> Now a 10-year-old . . . Baby Jane Doe is not only a self-aware little girl, who experiences and returns the love of her parents; she also attends a school for developmentally disabled children—once again proving that medicine is an art, not a science, and clinical decision making is best left in the clinic, to those who will have to live with the decision being made.

Source: Pence, G. (2004). *Classic cases in medical* ethics. Boston, MA: McGraw-Hill, p. 226.

Although "in reality [the Baby Doe regulation] does not apply directly to physicians, nurses, or parents, it does get the attention of many" (Carter & Leuthner, 2003, p. 484). The 1984 Child Abuse Prevention and Treatment Act (Baby Doe rules) generally provides three reasons to withhold treatment from newborns; confusion remains, however, about whether the rules are an attempt to mandate nutrition, hydration, and medications for all neonates. This confusion, in addition to the compassion that most people feel toward a dying or severely impaired child, is one reason that healthcare professionals experience moral uncertainty in relation to decisions about withholding and withdrawing treatment from neonates. The 1984 act states:

> The term "withholding of medically indicated treatment" does not include the failure to provide treatment (other than appropriate nutrition, hydration, or medication) to an infant when, in the treating physician's . . . reasonable medical judgment:
>
> 1. the infant is chronically and irreversibly comatose,
> 2. the provision of such treatment would
>   a. merely prolong dying,
>   b. not be effective in ameliorating or correcting all of the infant's life-threatening conditions, or
>   c. otherwise be futile in terms of the survival of the infant, or
> 3. the provision of such treatment would be virtually futile in terms of the survival of the infant and the treatment itself under such circumstances would be inhumane. (U.S. Child Protection and Treatment Act of 1984 as cited by Carter & Leuthner, 2003, p. 484)

According to Carter and Leuthner (2003), the language in these rules that addresses situations in which aggressive treatment of infants is not required can be interpreted to mean two different things with regard to nutrition: "(1) every infant should always be provided with medical means of nutrition [or] (2) every infant should receive nutrition appropriate for his/her medical situation" (p. 484).

Carter and Leuthner proposed that the Baby Doe rules should not be interpreted to restrict or prevent the withdrawal of nutrition. However, interpretations of the rules with regard to withholding and withdrawing nutrition, hydration, and medications vary among healthcare providers and institutions, and, as mentioned previously, healthcare providers experience moral uncertainty regarding these rules. When situations arise that precipitate discussions about withholding and withdrawing nutrition and hydration from newborns, the involvement of an ethics committee is recommended. It also may be helpful for healthcare professionals serving on an ethics committee to obtain consultation from ethicists who specialize in pediatric care.

1993: In the Matter of Baby K.

Although the Baby Doe rules provided a basis for the right of parents to refuse treatment for their severely disabled newborns, the ruling left the unanswered question of whether parents also have the right to insist on treatment for their newborns when medical staff believe the treatment would be futile or useless. The landmark case that provided a precedent for this type of situation involved Baby K., born with anencephaly in 1992. Baby K.'s mother insisted that a hospital provide maximum treatment for her child, including ventilator support. Hospital physicians disagreed with the mother's wishes and proposed that warmth, nutrition, and hydration were all that should be required in Baby K.'s care. The case was taken to the legal system for resolution. In reviewing this case, judges noted that medical assessments indicated that Baby K. was not being subjected to care requested by her mother that would cause the baby pain or suffering. Judges serving on the U.S. Court of Appeals for the Fourth Circuit ruled in favor of the mother and ordered the hospital to provide the level of care that Baby K.'s mother requested (In the Matter of Baby K, 1993).

The Influence of Nurses: Character

Those who stand for nothing, fall for anything.

—*Alexander Hamilton*

The good character or virtuous behavior of nurses, other healthcare professionals, and parents is not the only character that is relevant to the well-being of children. A child's own character development is important, too. School nurses are in a special position to help with this, and any nurse who works with children would do well to keep in mind the importance of influencing the development of a child's good character and educating others about this development. Ryan and Bohlin (1999) suggested that children need to be engaged in "heart, mind, and head" to know "who [they] are" and "what [they] stand for" (pp. xvi–xvii).

The search for the meaning of life overshadows almost all human endeavors in people young and old. In the fast-paced world of the 21st century, parents are busy trying to provide their families with necessities and physical comforts, and children are often busy playing video games and watching television—there is scarcely time to ponder the greater mysteries of life. Ryan and Bohlin (1999) proposed that "detached from a conception of the purpose of life, virtues become merely nice ideals, empty of meaning" (p. 39). They suggested that adults should not fear stimulating children to ponder the age-old question about why they were born. Many children, but particularly children who are ill, think about the meaning of life even when they do not know how to articulate their feelings. Nurses can provide these children with a kind hand and a warm heart during frightening times.

Almost any time is a good time to take the opportunity to educate children in the development of moral and intellectual virtues; as the old saying goes, "It is never too early." Stenson (1999) proposed that there are three ways to help children internalize virtuous habits and strengths of character when they are on their journey from infancy to adulthood. Those three means of internalization, and the order in which they occur, are:

> 1. By example: Children learn from what they witness in the lives of parents and other adults they respect (and thus unconsciously imitate).
> 2. Through directed practice: Children learn from what they are repeatedly led to do or are made to do by parents and other respected adults.
> 3. From words: Children learn from what they hear from parents and other respected adults as explanations for what they witness and are led to do. (Stenson, 1999, p. 207)

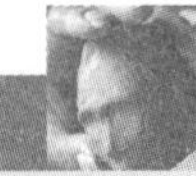

www Ethical Reflections

- Box 5.9 contains examples from the ANA's (2001) *Code of Ethics for Nurses with Interpretive Statements.* How are these examples relevant to nursing ethics in the care of infants and children?
- What other provisions and statements in the ANA's *Code of Ethics for Nurses* are particularly pertinent to the nursing care of infants and children? (See Appendix A) Discuss these provisions and provide examples of how they apply to nursing practice.

BOX 5.9 ETHICAL FORMATIONS: *CODE OF ETHICS FOR NURSES*

- Nursing care is directed toward meeting the comprehensive needs of patients and their families across the continuum of care (1.3, p. 7).
- Prior to implementation, all research should be approved by a qualified review board to ensure patient protection and the ethical integrity of the research (3.3, p. 13).
- Nurses have the duty to question and, if necessary, to report and to refuse to participate in research they deem morally objectionable (3.3, p. 13).
- Nurses are faced with decisions in the context of the increased complexity and changing patterns in the delivery of health care (4.1, p. 16).
- The nurse has responsibility to be aware not only of specific health needs of individual patients but also of broader health concerns such as world hunger, environmental pollution, lack of access to health care, violation of human rights, and inequitable distribution of nursing and healthcare resources (8.1, p. 23).

Nurses are patient advocates, but they also are role models. Nurses may never know when the example that they show to children and their mothering person(s) may influence the future of a child or may influence the future of nursing.

CASE STUDY: TO FEED OR NOT TO FEED?

www

Baby S. is a neonate admitted to the NICU at the county hospital where you work as the nurse manager. Mrs. S. had an amniotic fluid embolus during her delivery, and Baby S. experienced anoxia. Consequently, Baby S. had an Apgar score of 0 at birth. The baby was "successfully" resuscitated but remains unconscious. All of the baby's organs experienced hypoxic insult. Baby S. was placed on a ventilator and parenteral nutrition was later initiated. Mrs. S. is physically very weak and experiencing grief, along with her husband, over the condition of their infant. They have two other young children, ages 2 and 5 years old. Baby S. has been weaned from the ventilator but has remained unresponsive. Mr. and Mrs. S. have requested that the hospital staff discontinue their infant's nutrition and hydration. The NICU medical, nursing, and social work staff have not previously experienced a situation quite like the one that is occurring with the S. family.

Case Study Questions

1. You are meeting with the neonatologists, the NICU charge nurse, the infant's primary nurse, the hospital chaplain, and the social worker in the NICU. What do you contribute to the group's discussion with regard to how you believe the staff should proceed in providing the best care for Baby S. and her family?
2. How do the Baby Doe rules affect this case?
3. One of the staff RNs comments, "I think the mother and father are being selfish about their request to withdraw nutrition from Baby S. I think it is because they don't want to be bothered with taking care of her at home." How do you address these comments?
4. What surrogate decision-making standard should be used in this case? What influence should the interests of Baby S.'s siblings have in decision making in this case?
5. Caring for Baby S. and interacting with her family has caused a great deal of emotional and moral suffering for the NICU nursing staff (see *Moral Suffering* in Chapter 2). What behaviors might you expect to observe among the nursing staff? What do you do as the nurse manager to address this situation?
6. As would be expected, Mr. and Mrs. S. also are experiencing a great deal of moral suffering and grief. How would you handle your personal interactions with Mr. and Mrs. S., and what would you do to help educate your staff in working with families in a situation such as this one? What do you know or what information can you locate about the grief that parents experience when their infant is extremely impaired or dies? How would you try to help Mr. and Mrs. S.?

KEY POINTS

- The words *mother* and *mothering person* can be gender neutral.
- The best-interest standard is generally the ethical approach used in making difficult decisions about the healthcare treatment of children.
- Children and other people may be harmed when children are not immunized. Nurses must understand the best ways to interact with parents who refuse to have their children immunized.
- Ethical practice in the nursing care of children needs to include nurses' willingness to address social problems, such as those resulting from immigration, homelessness, and poverty, that often are very difficult to solve.
- Globally, many children become sick annually and die from preventable diseases and conditions.
- Nurses are "mandatory reporters" of child abuse. There is legal protection in most states for nurses who are reporting suspected child abuse in good faith.
- The ethics of allowing children themselves or their parents to refuse healthcare treatments is based on a number of factors. These factors include the severity of the potential harm to the child that may result from the refusal.
- The Child Abuse Amendments of 1984 are frequently referred to as the Baby Doe rules. Although these rules lack power in actual enforcement, they are influential in decisions regarding the withholding and withdrawing of supportive care involving infants.

References

Allender, J. A., & Spradley, B. W. (2005). *Community health nursing: Promoting and protecting the public's health* (6th ed.). Philadelphia, PA: Lippincott Williams & Wilkins.

American Academy of Pediatrics Committee on Community Health Services. (1997). Health care for children of immigrant families. *Pediatrics, 100*, 153–156. Retrieved from http://pediatrics.aappublications.org/cgi/content/full/100/1/153

American Nurses Association. (2011). *1997 Position statement: Childhood immunizations.* Retrieved from http://nursingworld.org/readroom/position/social/scimmu.htm

American Nurses Association. (2001). *Code of ethics for nurses with interpretive statements.* Silver Spring, MD: Author.

Barreto, P., Perez, V. H., & Halfon, N. (2007). Underserved children: Preventing chronic illness and promoting health. In T. E. King & M. B. Wheeler (Eds.), *Medical management of vulnerable and underserved patients: Principles, practice, and populations* (pp. 169–178). New York, NY: McGraw-Hill.

Beauchamp, T. L., & Childress, J. F. (2009). *Principles of biomedical ethics* (6th ed.). New York, NY: Oxford.

Borjas, G. (2011). Poverty and program participation among immigrant children. *The Future of Children, 21* (1), 247–266. Retrieved from http://futureofchildren.org/futureofchildren/publications/docs/21_01_11.pdf

Carter, B. S., & Leuthner, S. R. (2003). The ethics of withholding/withdrawing nutrition in the newborn. *Seminars in Perinatology, 27*(6), 480–487.

Center for Health and Health Care in Schools. (2005, February 25). *InFocus: An in-depth analysis of emerging issues in health in schools.* Retrieved from http://www.healthinschools.org/focus/2005/no1.htm

Centers for Disease Control and Prevention. (2007). *National Vaccine Program Office: Immunization laws.* Retrieved from http://www.hhs.gov/nvpo/law.htm

Childrensdefense.org. (2011). *Who are the uninsured children, 2010: Profile of America's uninsured children.* Retrieved from http://www.childrensdefense.org/child-research-data-publications/data/data-unisured-children-by-state-2010.pdf

Dalai Lama. (1999). *Ethics for the new millennium.* New York, NY: Riverhead Books.

Dias, M., & Marcuse, E. K. (2000, July). When parents resist immunization. *Contemporary Pediatrics*, 1–4. Retrieved from www.dshs.state.tx.us/immunize/forms/resist.pdf

Erikson, E. H. (1985). *Childhood and society* (35th ed.). New York, NY: W. W. Norton. (Original work published 1950)

Gibran, K. (2000). *The prophet.* New York, NY: Alfred A. Knopf. (Original work published 1923)

Globe editorial: Blaming the babies. (2006, November 11). *The Boston Globe.* Retrieved from http://www.boston.com/news/globe/editorial_opinion/editorials/articles/2006/11/11/blaming_the_babies

Held, V. (1993). *Feminist morality: Transforming culture, society, and politics.* Chicago, IL: University of Chicago.

In the matter of Baby K. 832 F. Supp. 1022 (E.D. Va. 1993).

Institute for Vaccine Safety, Johns Hopkins Bloomberg School of Public Health. (2011). *Vaccine exemptions.* Retrieved from http://www.vaccinesafety.edu/cc-exem.htm

Jonsen, A. R., Siegler, M., & Winslade, W. J. (2006). *Clinical ethics: A practical approach to ethical decisions in clinical medicine* (6th ed.). New York, NY: McGraw-Hill.

Jonsen, A. R., Siegler, M., & Winslade, W. J. (2010). *Clinical ethics: A practical approach to ethical decisions in clinical medicine* (7th ed.). New York, NY: McGraw-Hill.

MacIntyre, A. (1999). *Dependent rational animals: Why human beings need the virtues.* Chicago, IL: Open Court.

Morehouse, M. (2007, January). Girl, interrupted. *People*, 69–70.

National Network for Immunization Information. (2004a). *Measles parties.* Retrieved from http://www.immunizationinfo.org/issues/exposure-parties/measles-parties

National Network for Immunization Information. (2004b). *Rubella parties.* Retrieved from http://www.immunizationinfo.org/issues/exposure-parties/rubella-parties

National Network for Immunization Information. (2007). *Chickenpox parties.* Retrieved from http://www.immunizationinfo.org/issues/exposure-parties/chickenpox-parties

National Network for Immunization Information. (2009). *Immunization issues: Vaccine misinformation.* Retrieved from http://www.immunizationinfo.org/issues/general/vaccine-misinformation

Nussbaum, M. C. (2001). *Upheavals of thought: The intelligence of emotions.* New York, NY: Cambridge University.

Pence, G. E. (2004). *Classic cases in medical ethics: Accounts of cases that have shaped medical ethics, with philosophical, legal, and historical backgrounds* (4th ed.). Boston, MA: McGraw-Hill.

Ramsey, S. B. (2006). Abusive situations. In S. W. Killion & K. Dempski (Eds.), *Quick look nursing: Legal and ethical issues* (pp. 58–59). Sudbury, MA: Jones and Bartlett.

Ross, L. F. (1998). *Children, families, and health care decision-making*. Oxford, UK: Oxford University.

Ruddick, S. (1995). *Toward a politics of peace*. Boston, MA: Beacon Press.

Ryan, K., & Bohlin, K. E. (1999). *Building character in schools: Practical ways to bring moral instruction to life*. San Francisco, CA: Jossey-Bass.

State Health Access Data Assistance Center & Urban Institute (2005, August). *Going without: America's uninsured children*. Retrieved from http://www.rwjf.org/files/newsroom/ckfresearchreportfinal.pdf

Stenson, J. B. (1999). Appendix C: An overview of the virtues. In K. Ryan & K. E. Bohlin (Eds.), *Building character in schools: Practical ways to bring moral instruction to life* (pp. 207–211). San Francisco, CA: Jossey-Bass.

Stimpson, C. R. (1993). Series editor's foreword. In V. Held (Ed.), *Feminist morality: Transforming culture, society, and politics* (pp. vii–ix). Chicago, IL: University of Chicago.

Tong, R. (1997). *Feminist approaches to bioethics: Theoretical reflections and practical applications*. Boulder, CO: Westview.

World Health Organization. (2008). What are the key health dangers for children? Retrieved from http://www.who.int/features/qa/13/en/index.html

Yen, H. (2011, July 12). Census: Share of children in US hits record low. Retrieved from http://www.huffingtonpost.com/2011/07/12/census-share-of-children-_n_896396.html

For a full suite of assignments and additional learning activities, use the access code located in the front of your book to visit this exclusive website: http://go.jblearning.com/butts. If you do not have an access code, you can obtain one at the site.

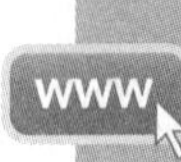

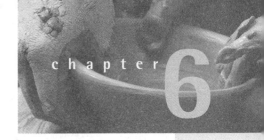

chapter 6

Adolescent Nursing Ethics

Janie B. Butts

In adolescence we are in many ways like empty but organic receptacles, fully formed though still growing waiting to be filled. And like receptacles we are capable at that stage of life of receiving with all our being, becoming one with what is within us.

—COLIN M. TURNBULL, THE HUMAN CYCLE

OBJECTIVES

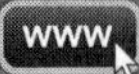

After reading this chapter, the reader should be able to:

1. Explore the phases of development of adolescence as they relate to unhealthy and risky behaviors.
2. Delineate the major risky behaviors in which adolescents engage, and include the major causes of death of adolescents as specified by the Centers for Disease Control and Prevention.
3. Discuss the rationale for the central ethical issues of adolescents in terms of family, peers, teachers, and healthcare professionals, including nurses.
4. Examine the significance of appropriate and inappropriate communication by health educators teaching adolescents a prevention program with health risk messages.
5. Discuss the benefits of health educators and nurses using theory-based health risk messages with a fear appeal to deliver education programs appropriately.
6. Describe the state of the research regarding the effectiveness of abstinence-only programs versus comprehensive sexual education programs, and include the three major ethical concerns when choosing a program among the abstinence-only or comprehensive sexual education programs.

7. Compare trust, privacy, and confidentiality and their significance regarding healthcare information, nursing care of adolescents, and adolescent decision-making capacity.
8. Discuss the other critical health issues that trigger ethical concerns, such as depression and suicidal ideation, alcohol and other drug use, sexual abuse, and eating disorders.
9. Explore the 10 stages of grief when adolescents learn of the sudden death of a peer or family member.
10. Delineate the 5 stages of grief that adolescents and others experience with their own dying process.
11. Discuss the moral framework of virtues that nurses need to incorporate in the care of adolescents, and include the major concepts from the ANA *Code of Ethics for Nurses with Interpretive Statements* (2001).

The Age of Adolescence

It is through good and bad experiences that adolescents learn to make life decisions and move toward independence. Through these interesting times, adolescents somehow develop their identity and their sense of sexuality. Many experts have defined adolescence as an age that occurs during the second decade of life and a period of transition that differs in length for each person (DiClemente, Hansen, & Ponton, 1996; Leffert & Petersen, 1999). Adolescence is a remarkable succession of physical, cognitive, emotional, moral, and psychosocial developmental changes.

Three separate phases, spanning 11 years, have been identified in the **adolescent developmental process** (Gullotta, Adams, & Markstrom, 2000; Leffert & Petersen, 1999). **Early adolescence** (ages 10–14) is a transitional period from childhood to middle adolescence and is usually marked by the onset of puberty. Adolescents begin puberty with experimentation and discovery. **Middle adolescence** (ages 15–17) is dominated by peer pressure, peer orientation, and stereotypical behaviors, such as following clothing trends and listening to music that is considered acceptable by peers. **Late adolescence** (ages 18–20) usually marks the transition from adolescence to adulthood. Adolescents generally begin to place more importance on their future and their life plans as they move into late adolescence.

Adolescents have a need to find out who they are and have a desire to push limits and test unknown waters. Many of the decisions that adolescents make are based on the values that they have adapted from the pressure of peer approval and the exposure to the quickly changing world around them. Mistakes and failures, but also successes, will occur along the way. Adolescents need to be encouraged to make autonomous decisions and express their values and preferences on a continuous basis so that they will evolve to maturity with a defined sense of self.

Risk-Taking Behaviors

There are more than 1.8 billion young people living in the world, the largest number of adolescents in history (United Nations Population Fund [UNFPA], 2011). Almost 65 million young people between the ages 10 and 24 live in the United States (Population Reference Bureau, 2011). Risk taking and the feeling of "it's not going to happen to me," or a feeling of invincibility, are the hallmarks of adolescence despite the new risks and newly discovered demands that have existed at no other time in history. The realities of massive social, economic, political, and cultural changes worldwide affect adolescents' development process.

Health risk behaviors include those behaviors that, according to Lindberg, Boggess, and Williams, "may threaten the well-being of teens and may prevent them from becoming fully functioning members of society" (2000, pp. 1–2). Adolescents who engage in one risky behavior have a tendency to engage in at least one or more other risky behaviors, especially paired behaviors such as smoking cigarettes and drinking alcohol or smoking marijuana and engaging in risky sexual activities.

In a literature review on adolescents and risk-taking behaviors, McKay (2003) and Cook, Dickens, and Fathalla (2003) found that the origin of most risk-taking behaviors is social and that these behaviors can result in injury from accidents, violence, and sexual abuse. The Centers for Disease Control and Prevention (CDC) has conducted the Youth Risk Behavior Surveillance System (YRBSS) numerous times in the past. In the 2009 YRBSS, the CDC (2010) reemphasized that risk-taking behaviors can often lead to death in adolescents. Three critical health behaviors have been identified and connected to the leading causes of death and disability among adolescents in the United States: injury due to violence (including suicide), use of alcohol and other drugs, and risky sexual activity (Centers for Disease Control [CDC], 2010). Refer to Box 6.1 for three different accounts of adolescent statistics from the YRBSS in 2009: (1) general statistics on adolescent health risks, (2) the risky behaviors that contributed to the leading causes of death for ages 10 to 24, and (3) the leading causes of death for ages 10 to 24. The reader should note that data from the 2009 YRBSS were taken only from U.S. high school students, grades 9 to 12, who were enrolled in and attending a high school.

Central Ethical Issues at a Glance

The age of adolescence brings with it overpowering family decision-making issues and health concerns, and as a result, complex healthcare ethical issues arise. Perplexing questions appear when people in society observe relationships between adults (or parents) and adolescents and begin to see that those relationships are disintegrating swiftly into disharmony. The ethical healthcare issues of adolescents are focused on rights—the rights that all people expect, especially people in the

BOX 6.1 ETHICAL FORMATIONS: HEALTH RISKS FACED BY ADOLESCENTS IN 2009

General Statistics on Adolescent Health Risks

- Almost 73% of high school students in the United States have consumed at least 1 alcoholic drink on at least 1 occasion.
- Almost 25% have engaged in binge drinking (5 or more drinks) on at least 1 occasion in the last 30 days.
- More than 1 in 5 high school students in the United States are current smokers.
- Almost 50% of high school students in the United States have tried smoking cigarettes.
- Nationwide, 46% of all students have engaged in sexual intercourse at least once and 34% currently are sexually active.
- Only 1 in 3 high school students participate in daily physical education classes.
- More than 1 in 3 children and adolescents are overweight or at risk of becoming overweight.
- More than 9 million cases of sexually transmitted diseases occur among young people ages 15–24 years.
- Nearly 5,000 cases of HIV/AIDS are reported each year among young people ages 15–24 years in areas with confidential reporting.
- Approximately 757,000 high school females reported having been pregnant in 2009.

Risky Behaviors That Lead to Major Causes of Death in Persons Aged 10 to 24 Years

- Unintentional injury and violence
- Tobacco use
- Alcohol and other drug use
- Sexual behaviors that contribute to unintended pregnancy or sexually transmitted infections (STIs), including HIV
- Unhealthy dietary behaviors
- Physical inactivity

Leading Causes of Death for Persons Aged 10 to 24 Years

- 30%: Motor vehicle crash
- 29%: Other causes, such as cancer and cardiovascular disease
- 15%: Homicide
- 14%: Other types of injury
- 11%: Suicide
- 1%: HIV infection

Source: Centers for Disease Control and Prevention. (2010). Youth risk behavior surveillance—United States, 2009. *Morbidity and Mortality Weekly Report, 59*(SS-5), 1–148. Retrieved from http://www.cdc.gov/mmwr/pdf/ss/ss5905.pdf

Western world. Some of those rights include the right of freedom to consent to or refuse treatment, the right to confidentiality and privacy of one's medical record, and the right not to be violated or taken advantage of because of membership in a vulnerable age group. Conducting research with adolescents is a concern because of that vulnerability, though research issues are not discussed in this chapter as nursing research books include information on the special concerns of vulnerable research subjects.

Certain central ethical themes regarding adolescents have become apparent:

- **Prevention education**: How, where, and to what extent adolescents receive information and education about prevention
  - Beneficence
  - Nonmaleficence
- **Trust, privacy, and confidentiality**: Limits of confidentiality; handling life-threatening illnesses and disorders
  - Respect for autonomy
  - Beneficence
  - Nonmaleficence
- **Consent**: Consenting to treatments without parental or guardian consent; refusal of treatment without parental or guardian consent
  - Respect for autonomy
  - Beneficence
  - Nonmaleficence
- **Research with adolescents**: A vulnerable population
  - Respect for autonomy
  - Beneficence
  - Nonmaleficence
  - Justice

Adolescent Relationships and Ethical Issues

Relationships are at the core of an adolescent's life. Because of the value that adolescents place on relationships, nurses need to remember that positive and negative relationship skills learned within a family continue with children into the adolescent stage. It is because of relationships that adolescents experience a complex set of patterns and feelings such as happiness, sadness, excitement, anger, fear, frustration, stress, and even loneliness (Urban Programs Resource Network, 2011).

Adolescents want and need to be heard and understood; parents want to give their opinions and be heard. Adolescents want relationships of their own with each other without interference from authority figures. On the other hand, healthcare and other professionals want to teach adolescents to prevent harm or illness or to manage disease, and media personnel want to grab adolescents' attention by whatever means necessary. Communication is the key issue in adolescent relationships. For instance, Box 6.2 contains two quotations from the United States: one from Dryfoos and Barkin (2006) on mentoring children and teens and one from a mother about her views on the role of communication.

One of the most common "lines" that nurses hear from adolescents is, "My parents don't listen to me!" Ironically, parents often say, "My kid won't listen to me!"

BOX 6.2 ETHICAL FORMATIONS: IMPORTANT MESSAGES FOR ADOLESCENTS

On Mentoring Children and Adolescents

One of my mantras is "every child must be attached to a responsible adult–if not a parent, then someone else." The need for close and consistent mentoring can change over time, but particularly in the early teen years, when communication with parents may be difficult, that someone else can play a significant role. Such a someone else can be a teacher, relative, friend, friend's parent, volunteer mentor, or youth worker [or nurse], preferably with some knowledge of youth development.

Source: Dryfoos, J. G., & Barkin, C. (2006). *Adolescence: Growing up in America today.* New York, NY: Oxford University Press.

From an Older Parent

My daughter used to be so wonderful. Now I can barely stand her and she won't tell me anything. I feel totally shut out. How can I find out what's going on?

Source: Wiseman, R. (2001). *Queenbees and wannabees: Helping your daughter survive cliques, gossip, boyfriends, and other realities of adolescence.* New York, NY: Three Rivers.

When it comes to other relationships involving adolescents, similar statements are sometimes made: "My school teacher doesn't listen to my complaints," "That nurse didn't understand my problem," and so on.

Attentive listening, meaning that the nurse is paying attention to what is being said and then giving a signal to the speaker that listening is occurring, is an effective technique for nurses when working with adolescents. Attentive listening helps nurses earn the respect of young people, which is a critical factor in nurse–adolescent relationships. Ways that nurses practice attentive listening include:

- **Focusing**: Making eye contact and not allowing the eyes to wander
- **Not interrupting**: Hearing the speaker in full before commenting and acknowledging the speaker by nods, smiles, or other expressions
- **Reflecting**: Summarizing the speaker's thoughts to clarify the meaning

Ethical Dilemmas Involving Prevention Education

Listening is important, but being the **giver of communication**—how, where, and to what extent—is a critical ethical concern for adolescent relationships of all kinds, especially in professional nurse–adolescent relationships. Beneficence and nonmaleficence are the principles that underlie the ethical management of prevention and health risk message programs involving this age group. Health risk messages are commonly defined as **fear appeals**, which are persuasive messages that arouse by fear by, "outlining the negative consequences that occur if a certain action is not taken" (Witte, Meyer, & Martell, 2001, p. 2). Sensationalists, political campaign personnel, religious leaders and preachers, and many other groups tend to use fear appeals. Health educators, nurses, physicians, and other related disciplines also commonly use fear appeals when there are health risks associated with a behavior.

If fear appeals are effective, the target population will be more likely to make healthy choices and practice safe behaviors.

Fear appeals also can be used incorrectly and can actually do more harm than good. Giving health risk messages without the integration of a theory can be time consuming and fragmented. A **theory** provides "an explanation of how two or more variables work together to produce a certain outcome(s)" (Witte et al., 2001, p. 3). A theoretical framework guides the development of a health risk message, which eliminates the guesswork and shortens the duration of the developmental phase. The goal of nurses for theory-based education programs or health risk messages is to teach young people the skills they need to make healthy choices and practice healthy behaviors. This aim is consistent with a beneficent approach because nurses promote human good through education. Most education programs for adolescents are theory-based, prevention-focused programs promoting health risk messages. Prevention education programs need to be focused not only on doing "good," but also on doing no harm—a nonmaleficence approach.

A theory-based, harm reduction program with health risk messages is an example of an approach that integrates beneficence and nonmaleficence. In using a harm reduction program, nurses teach adolescents to live safely with certain high-risk behaviors, such as by advocating participation in a needle exchange program for those addicted to intravenous or other needle-requiring drugs.

Another example is a prevention–intervention behavioral program providing theory-based health risk messages, one that Butts and Hartman (2002) has used in research: Becoming a Responsible Teen (BART), which was originally developed from research by St. Lawrence et al. (1995). St. Lawrence (1994) actually developed the BART training manual, an eight-session curriculum based on two theoretical frameworks: (1) Bandura's (1977) social learning and self-efficacy theory, and (2) Fisher and Fisher's (1992) information–motivation–behavioral skills model (IMB model). Today the **BART behavioral intervention program** remains a popular evidence-based program among health educators.

Nurses who are involved in prevention education need to use a theory-based curriculum and evaluate the program early in the planning phase. Questions to consider are:

- How much information is too much information?
- When and at what age will the information be presented?
- What types of information are appropriate?
- Where and how should the information be presented to be effective?

Nurses who give information to adolescents may potentially harm them if they choose a wrong or inappropriate prevention education program. This situation poses a critical ethical dilemma for nurses when they must choose among the many standardized and accepted programs that are available for adolescents. For example, nurses sometimes will need to choose between teaching sexual abstinence and teaching the use of safe sexual practices, or they could be asked to focus a program on religious beliefs. Choosing an age- or content-inappropriate program for a particular group or choosing information that could easily be misinterpreted could result in adolescents being misled, or an adolescent may perceive the health risk messages differently from the way the educator intended. Blunders could be critical to how adolescents will react to the information.

Even though alcohol and other drugs are harmful when abused or misused, a small glass of red wine is reported to actually protect the heart against disease (Gullotta et al., 2000). Messages such as this one can be quite confusing to adolescents. Another message that could be misleading is that in the United States, marijuana is an illegal drug for most people, but for others marijuana is legally used for medicinal purposes. As of 2011, 16 states and the District of Columbia have legalized the medicinal use of marijuana, and 5 states have pending legislation (ProCon.org, 2011). Additionally, adolescents sometimes receive conflicting and incorrect information because of others seeking political or monetary gain. For example, advertisers often show groups of attractive young people socializing and drinking beer; some companies intend to convey a subtle message that drinking beer makes one more attractive and popular. Another critical message that has caused considerable child and adolescent psychological problems such as anorexia nervosa or bulimia is the fashion industry's blatant promotion of super-thin models, conveying a message that one must be thin to be beautiful.

Previously, there were hundreds of adolescent prevention programs being used in the United States, but currently there are huge gaps in prevention education programs. The gaps could be symptoms of problems with prevention programs that consist of controversial or inadequate content, complacency in creating/instituting programs, and decreasing numbers of programs overall. For example, lack of teacher training, not enough material resources, inconsistent use of lesson plans, and failure to match lesson plans with the appropriate age are factors that have had large, negative ramifications for adolescent drug prevention programs across the country.

Prevention education programs are rapidly disappearing as drug use among adolescents increases, especially marijuana, Ecstasy, and LSD. In 2011, Feliz reported the University of Michigan's Monitoring the Future (MTF) findings from a large study of 46,000 teens from grades 8, 10, and 12. These adolescents reported a drastic decrease in exposure to drug prevention messages over the past 7 years, even though teens reported as a whole that drug prevention messages could be effective. The researchers of the MTF study have attributed lack of funding as one of several reasons for the disappearance of prevention programs. At the peak of the prevention education programs in the 1990s and early 2000s, drug use and other risky behaviors began a slight decline. The correlation between the slight decrease in drug use and the increase in the number of prevention education programs reveals the significance and positive influence that these programs have had on adolescents.

The CDC (2011) reported last year that high school students continue to engage in too many risky behaviors that lead to STIs, HIV, injury, addiction, depression, chronic disease, and suicide. Alcohol and other drug use among teens continues to be a life-threatening problem. Preteen drug use also remains a critical problem. Preteens abuse inhalants (inhaling, sniffing, huffing, or bagging substances) to get high at higher rates than do teens (McGuinness, 2006). For example, the use of inhalant substances increased in eighth graders from 22% to 26% and in sixth graders from 18% to 26% over 2 years. McGuinness reported that use of inhalant chemicals is a more common practice than marijuana use among adolescents ages 12 to 13 years. Furthermore, there are correlations between inhalant use, conduct disorder, depression, and suicidal behavior.

School nurses are often the ones who plan and implement programs, so they need to know the objectives and content and anticipate the message that will be heard by adolescents who participate in the program. Adolescents will usually assume that the message they hear is correct when school nurses conduct the prevention education program. If adolescents incorporate misinterpreted information into their viewpoints and behaviors, they could be at a higher risk of contracting STIs or HIV, developing a drug habit, sustaining alcohol- or other drug-related injuries, or developing suicidal ideation.

Abstinence-Only or Comprehensive Sex Education Programs

In the last two decades, examining how abstinence-only programs measure up to comprehensive sexual education programs has been a popular issue. In the 1990s and early 2000s, there was a much stronger religious and political focus on and plenty of funding for the teaching of sexual abstinence in schools, homes, and churches than in previous years, especially since the sexual revolution movement of the 1960s. Other than through fundamental religious teachings, sexual education was seldom taught in the United States before the HIV and AIDS epidemic began in the 1980s. Sexual abstinence–only programs are on the decline as funding is removed for these programs. Instead, funding is focused on comprehensive sexual education programs because research evidence supports their effectiveness.

The overall ethical concern about sexual education is complex, but generally nurses must evaluate at what point along the sexual abstinence–comprehensive sex education continuum the information conveyed becomes unethical, nonbeneficial, or even harmful. Adolescents need sexual education more than ever today. According to The Joint United Nations Programme on HIV/AIDS (UNAIDS, 2010), in many countries the HIV statistics are stabilizing and or showing a slight decline because HIV prevention programs are working. However, young people acquiring HIV remains a top concern in all countries. Most other STIs occur in young people as well.

Abortion rates among adolescents steadily declined in the 1990s, but the Guttmacher Institute (2011a) reported an increase in teen abortions; of the 757,000 teen pregnancies in the United States in 2010, 82% were unintended and more than 25% ended in abortion. The CDC (2010) reported in the 2009 YRBSS that a slight decline in pregnancy rates in adolescents occurred; reasons for this decrease include: pursuing and achieving higher levels of education and past comprehensive sexual education programs in schools, indicating that adolescents are slowly learning negotiation skills and effective contraceptive practices.

Three Major Ethical Concerns along the Continuum

Worldwide, adolescents continue to have unprotected sex. There are three major ethical concerns about the sexual abstinence–safe sex education continuum and adolescents. The first issue is that there is no clear definition of sexual abstinence today. Traditionally, adolescents have equated "having sex" with intercourse alone. Young people have sought more creative ways, other than coital sex, to express sexual intimacy, such as mutual masturbation, and oral and anal sex, because these types of sex have not been viewed as "traditional sex" (Remez, 2000). The term **sexual abstinence** in recent years has led to dissimilar and ambiguous opinions. A clear definition needs to be developed for, and then be communicated to, today's adolescents. Meanwhile, parents, educators, and others who teach sexual abstinence continue to say "just say no to sex," "don't have sex before marriage," or "delay the onset of sex." What do these statements mean exactly? Does abstinence mean not having vaginal penetration? Is oral or anal sex all right just as long as one does not participate in penis–vagina intercourse? Is abstinence referring only to a male and female relationship? What about same-sex relationships? How does abstinence apply in those situations?

The 1988 CDC recommendations for lowering the risk of contracting HIV and STIs remain current—not exchanging any bodily fluids, including saliva in exchanges such as French kissing, and using latex protection where indicated. Adolescents are at risk when they have unprotected sexual relations with body fluid exposures. Could abstinence be defined today as a person's being able to engage in any type of sexual activity just as long as the couple or group is protected with latex and does not exchange bodily fluids?

Without a clear definition, educators, parents, and other adults have only vague communication between themselves and adolescents about the meaning of sexual abstinence. What adolescents perceive as the definition of sexual abstinence and what adults are trying to teach as sexual abstinence most likely include a variety of different opinions. Ethically, this vagueness itself can be harmful, not beneficial, because the information may be misperceived. As a result, adolescents are left to their own interpretations. Misinterpreted information may lead to unprotected sex, which, in turn, may lead to an unwanted pregnancy, an STI, or infection with HIV.

A second issue is adolescent sexual intimacy, a reality that cannot be denied. In an in-depth study of intimacy and sexual abstinence, Hartwig (2000) contended that long-term abstinence damages individuals' development of their "capacity to love with greater depth and integrity" (p. 3). Although this depth of intimacy can be built upon by other means, Hartwig stated that intimate relationships through sex help people to move past fears and perplexities that sometimes cannot otherwise be overcome.

Early-stage adolescents, ages 13 to 15, may not be capable of managing the strong physical and emotional feelings that go with sexual relationships. Intimate relationships could be injurious to adolescents' emotional development in the short term, as well as having long-term effects. This issue is a challenge to educators and parents. Hartwig (2000) posed this question to adults: "How does one discourage premature sexual intimacy among those who intensely desire physical sexual intimacy and who often assume they are emotionally mature enough to form intimate relationships without shaming or vilifying sexual intimacy?" (p. 36).

According to Hartwig (2000), sometimes adolescents are restricted from learning to eliminate risks when they are exposed solely to abstinence-only programs. Adolescents need what Hartwig called a poetic approach to sexual education and sexual virtue, which complements and balances a moral approach. **Poetic intimacy** teachings must begin with young children. For adolescents, a process such as this one includes integrating the poetics of sexuality; examples include exposing adolescents to narratives that highlight tenderness and sensuality and teaching them to practice the use of graceful sexual language, not inappropriate and dirty language. If adolescents are not taught to manage sexual intimacy in a beneficial way, the ethical implication is that their developmental and emotional processes may be harmed. Developing this type of intimacy helps them come to terms with their sexual changes and feelings. Adolescents who learn graceful poetic intimacy develop ways to deepen their desire for intimacy without necessarily having sexual relationships, or they learn to make healthier choices when they decide to have sex.

A third issue is that there is controversy about whether abstinence-only programs have worked. The Guttmacher Institute (2011a) reported that abstinence-only programs may actually deter contraceptive use, which has the potential for increased unintended pregnancies. Even though leaders of schools and churches continue their efforts to teach abstinence-only programs, many adolescents are breaking the no-sex pledges that they make.

The Guttmacher Institute indicated a strong link between comprehensive sexual education programs and healthier sexual choices. By the late teen years, 7 of 10 adolescents have had sexual intercourse. Adults in the United States would like to see a comprehensive sexual education program implemented with curricula on healthy choices, abstinence, and strategies to be safe. Currently, 20 states and the District of Columbia mandate sex and HIV prevention education and another 12 states mandate only HIV prevention education. As pregnancy rates have slowly declined over the last decade for adolescents, STIs have remained alarmingly high and of deep concern to public health officials. In a January 2004 poll of 1,759 people in the United States, only 15% of adults thought that school officials should teach abstinence only and not provide information about contraception (Princeton Survey Research Associates, as cited in Bowman, 2004). Prevention is critical, but prevention must go beyond education. Adolescents need to be able to access healthcare services that provide them with family planning and STI treatment on a regular basis because many STIs are treatable and curable. Cervical cancer may follow if adolescents are not treated properly for STIs.

This third issue is one of great concern for nurses who work with adolescents. Inconsistency exists across programs. Ethically, nurses need to think about the possible harm that could be done as a result of the type of sexual education program they choose. Nurses need to evaluate the program early in the planning process by using the guidelines already mentioned in this chapter. It is important for nurses to think about the ways in which adolescents may perceive, interpret, or put into practice the content that is being presented to them. Once nurses can effectively focus on the adolescents who are receiving the message, they need to clarify the message, try to focus on what they are really saying to adolescents, and, most of all, attempt to clarify and anticipate as much as possible the message that adolescents are actually hearing. If a nurse takes time to focus on the audience and the content of the message, adolescents will realize that the nurse cares for them and is respecting them for their values and beliefs. As the nurse provides well-defined content and becomes an attentive listener, a reciprocal trusting and respectful relationship is more likely to develop. Some questions that school nurses should answer include:

- If a school nurse is planning a prevention education program for rural or urban middle school students on the issues of alcohol, other drugs, and sex, what are some considerations before or during the planning phase of the program?
- What is the most effective prevention program that can be used?
- What ethical considerations would be incorporated into program planning?
- What message do adolescents need to hear?
- What type of relationship should be established with the students?

Confidentiality, Privacy, and Trust

Confidentiality, privacy, and trust cannot be viewed as separate entities in a nurse–adolescent relationship. **Confidentiality** is linked with privacy and trust, and usually means that information given to someone is to be kept secret (Blustein & Moreno, 1999). **Privacy** used in this way means for someone to keep information secluded or secret from others. **Trust** means that adolescents sometimes explore their vulnerabilities with healthcare providers but, at the same time, believe that these providers will not take advantage of them. In other words, adolescents believe that the providers are reliable and dependable in managing their health and vulnerabilities. From an ethical standpoint, confidentiality, privacy, and trust are tightly woven with respect for autonomy, the adolescent's right to privacy, and the rights of service. Any breach of confidentiality, privacy, or trust is viewed as a violation of autonomy.

Trust is important to a healthy and respectful relationship. Once trust is broken and mistrust develops, it is very difficult for the informer (nurse) to regain trust. Adolescents will probably refuse to listen to anything that the nurse tries to convey. Trust is a basic need that must be developed in the first stage of life, according to Erik Erikson (1963). If trust is broken early in an individual's life, mistrust carries over to all of the person's relationships.

If adolescents do not trust the nurse, for example, they may not believe the nurse with regard to an informed consent (Blustein & Moreno, 1999). Adolescents may not listen to explanations. The most important way for nurses to gain the trust of adolescents is by relentlessly proving themselves: being consistent, giving correct information, keeping commitments, and showing concern and caring. These activities, combined, help indicate that nurses are trustworthy, meaning that nurses are dependable and authentic because they take responsibility for their own behavior and commit to their obligations (Gullotta et al., 2000).

Trust-Privacy-Confidentiality Dilemma

A legal, ethical, political, and practice issue surfaces when a trusting relationship may exist and the nurse is entrusted with an adolescent's confidential information. Sometimes the sensitive issue and the nature of the information is potentially harmful to the adolescent if it is not reported to proper authorities or others (University of Chicago, 2005). Adolescents are concerned about their privacy and what others think of them, especially their parents and peers. Nurses need to ensure that adolescents are examined privately and away from their parents and peers. Many times the physical and emotional health outcomes of risky behaviors force adolescents to seek medical treatment. Because of the sensitive issues involved and a potential for these issues to cause embarrassment, adolescents want to keep the information secret, especially from their parents.

Well-established research findings in the United States reveal that the likelihood of adolescents seeking health services for sensitive issues depends on how well their sensitive issues will remain confidential. Adolescents can seek family planning services at the state level, such as counseling and contraception through the Planned Parenthood Federation of America, which is a program that is federally funded by Title X of the Public Health Service Act, and be guaranteed confidentiality (Planned Parenthood Action Fund, 2010). Each state has a broad range of laws that stem from the federal laws concerning confidentiality and consent of adolescents. However, Title X will not provide funds for abortion for adolescents.

In the United States, the exception to adolescent autonomy over medical records involves the issue of abortion. Seventeen states require no parental involvement in an adolescent's decision to have an abortion. As of 2011, 36 states require some parental involvement in an adolescent's choice to have an abortion, with 21 states requiring parental consent, 11 states requiring only parental notification, and 4 states requiring parental consent and notification (Guttmacher Institute, 2011b). Even with required parental consent, the 36 states with this requirement have sought ways to work around complete parental involvement by having a judicial bypass, meaning that adolescents may obtain approval from a court to bypass parental involvement. Six of these states also permit family members other than parents, such as an aunt or a grandparent, to be involved in the abortion decision so that adolescents can avoid informing their parents. Most states allow for exceptions to the parental involvement law when abortions become a medical emergency or when an extraordinary situation exists, such as when the pregnancy was the result of sexual assault or incest.

Limits of Confidentiality

Nurses need to assure adolescents from the beginning of the interaction that confidentiality is an important component of the nurse–patient relationship. However, confidentiality must never be guaranteed; confidentiality can be breached in instances that place the adolescent or others at harm or danger—an exception called **limits of confidentiality** (University of Chicago, 2005). The nurse should assure the adolescent that confidentiality will not be breached *unless* harm or a potential threat to the patient or to known others is involved. In cases of potential harm, an adolescent must always be given a chance to disclose sensitive or controversial information to parents, guardians, or others involved, as appropriate. If the adolescent refuses to do so, nurses and other healthcare professionals are obligated to report the following information to state officials according to state laws:

- Suicidal ideation
- Homicidal ideation
- Physical abuse
- Sexual abuse
- Behaviors that put one at risk of physical harm (University of Chicago, 2005, para. 2)

Nurses must hold to these standards. Even if the situation is not considered a limit of confidentiality, the nurse should make every effort to involve the parents or guardians if the adolescent is younger than age 14, as the lines of confidentiality and consent are even more vague and unclear before the age of 14.

Consent Dilemma

Adolescents under the age of 18 can give consent for their own care in a broad range of circumstances and services. The minors who can consent are those who are over a certain age, mature, legally emancipated, married, in the armed forces, living apart from their parents, high school graduates, pregnant, or already parents (University of Chicago, 2005). They may also refuse treatment. An adolescent's right to consent to treatment or to refuse treatment is more frequently honored with certain types of services. These services include:

- Emergency care
- Family planning services, such as pregnancy care and contraceptive services
- Diagnosis and treatment of STIs or any other reportable infection or communicable disease
- HIV or AIDS testing and treatment
- Treatment and counseling for alcohol and other drugs
- Treatment for sexual assault and collection of the medical evidence for sexual assault
- Inpatient mental health services
- Outpatient mental health services

Deciding whether adolescents really have autonomous decision-making capacity is a consideration tightly linked to their personal self-directedness and characteristics, what Blustein and Moreno (1999) called **moral self-government**. The goal during adolescence is development of the moral self, as most adolescents' moral self is not yet fully formed. Blustein and Moreno stated that adolescents have an emerging capacity, which means that the moral self is evolving but it is not doing so evenly or consistently. Age and the stage of cognitive, emotional, and social development are factors that influence a person's ability to make mature decisions. An adolescent's capacity for decision making does not occur before the age of 15, and some experts have said that adolescents should not take part in significant autonomous decision making before age 14 (University of Chicago, 2005).

For many years, adults in the United States have valued the right to control their medical decisions. Adolescents are no different. In most states, these decisions are left up to healthcare professionals. If a valid consent between a nurse and an adolescent takes place, the initial phase should be more of a dialogue and educational exchange. During the consent process, the nurse's responsibility is to evaluate the adolescent's capacity for understanding and appreciating the process, especially with anticipated treatments or interventions. Consider the following scenario: Kelly, age 16, has come to a clinic where you work as a nurse. She has stated that she is at least 12 weeks pregnant but has not told anyone, not even her parents or boyfriend. She is fearful of losing her boyfriend if she tells him. She wants an abortion, has cash money, and does not want anyone to know about the pregnancy or the abortion. Explore the ethical issues surrounding this situation. Consider the trust-confidentiality-privacy dilemma and the consent dilemma. Identify specific nursing strategies that you must consider using with Kelly. The clinic is in a state that does not require direct parental involvement but does require consent by someone of legal age.

The consent process may be more than a single event in time, such as in cancer treatments. It could be that one or both parents were highly involved with the adolescent's initial treatment and consent, but later in the process, adolescents may develop considerable maturity and then have the capacity to consent or not consent to subsequent treatments. The adolescent's level of understanding and appreciation of the content of the consent may have progressively increased. Over time, the adolescent can take on more, if not all, of the responsibility in the decision-making process, and dialogue and education continue throughout the treatment. During the treatment and consent phases, documentation of the adolescent's progress in development of the moral self is essential.

Health Issues That Trigger Ethical Concerns

Many adolescent health issues cause nurses to have genuine ethical concerns. Some topics have already been discussed in this chapter, but there are others that are just as critical to adolescents' health and survival, such as depression and suicidal ideation, substance use and abuse, sexual abuse, and eating disorders. There are many other common, and equally critical, adolescent issues apart from the list covered in this chapter.

The same guidelines for privacy, confidentiality, and consent that were discussed in the last section apply to these critical health issues. The ethical principles involved with these issues are beneficence (doing good, such as with prevention education) and nonmaleficence (protecting adolescents from harm). The common ethical concern for nurses managing these four health problems is that they are all potentially harmful and may even lead to death if left undetected. In the majority of situations, these problems need reporting to the proper authorities or other people within the healthcare or school system, such as school officials, mental health counselors, or physicians. Because these conditions are harmful and fall into the category of limits of confidentiality, nurses should never promise privacy and confidentiality to adolescents when nurses have received such information. Nurses may not promise the adolescent that they will keep critical health information a secret or confidential, once disclosed by the adolescent. When the nurse first detects a health problem, protection and safety must come first.

Depression and Suicidal Ideation

Depression and **suicide** are closely linked. Because the age of adolescence is a time of great emotions and drama, depressive behavior may be hidden in daily displays of extremes. There are risk factors for adolescent suicidal ideation and attempts, many of which include family disturbances, familial tendency, sexual orientation conflicts, and socioenvironmental problems.

According to the American Association of Suicidology (2010), every year more than 34,000 Americans commit suicide, but more than 300,000 Americans are treated or hospitalized because of suicide attempts (McIntosh, 2010). Overall, the suicide rate has declined over the years, but it is important to note that for adolescents, ages 10 to 14 years, suicide rates have increased, with the 2007 final data highlighting 4,140 in the United States, which translates to 11.3 youth suicide deaths every day. Suicide remains the third leading cause of death in the United States for persons ages 15 to 24. Of the adolescent suicides, a high percentage of them had a psychiatric diagnosis.

Obtaining treatment for depression is essential for the prevention of suicide. Nurses may be fearful of making a mistake or missing signs of changes in adolescents. If a nurse finds an adolescent who is exhibiting behaviors that look suspiciously like signs of depression or **suicidal tendency**, the nurse must quickly identify the problem, ascertain the intention of the adolescent, and clearly explain the process of notification while offering hope and the prospect of a treatment plan. In 80% of youth suicides, adolescents had told someone about their suicidal ideation prior to the act.

Many state educational systems have initiated a program called **Gatekeepers** to spot suicidal youth. In Virginia, for instance, the trainers of the Gatekeepers first educated school nurse coordinators to be trainers, who provide training to other school nurses. Gatekeepers learn to recognize risky behaviors that may indicate suicidal ideation. Refer to Box 6.3 for warning signs of adolescent suicide. Consider the following scenario: A school nurse notices that a teacher in one class has a 15-year-old boy named Eric who keeps to himself and never talks to anyone. Lately, his behavior has become extreme: not eating in the cafeteria, keeping his head down at all times, and never making eye contact with anyone. He has completely withdrawn from any social interaction at school. The other teens are making fun of him and his behavior and say that he is acting strange. These actions against him just seem to make him go deeper into withdrawal. Based on the signs and symptoms, the school nurses believes him to be very depressed, and from the current literature, the school nurse gathers findings that he may be at risk for committing suicide. The school nurse then examines her moral obligations and the specific actions that should be taken in this situation. What are some strategies that the nurse should use in a plan to help Eric?

Alcohol and Other Drugs

Adolescents with a family history of substance or physical abuse are at high risk for developing substance abuse problems, along with those who are depressed, have low self-esteem, and feel like outcasts or that they do not fit in with their peers. An

BOX 6.3 ETHICAL FORMATIONS: ADOLESCENT SUICIDE—OBSERVABLE SIGNS AND SUBJECTIVE COMMENTS

Observable Signs

Change in eating and sleeping habits
Withdrawal from friends, family, and regular activities
Violent actions, rebellious behavior, or running away
Drug and alcohol use
Unusual neglect of personal appearance
Marked personality change
Persistent boredom, difficulty concentrating, or a decline in the quality of schoolwork
Frequent complaints about physical symptoms, often related to emotions, such as stomachaches, headaches, fatigue, and others
Loss of interest in pleasurable activities
Not tolerating praise or rewards
Giving away favorite possessions or throwing away valuable belongings
Becoming suddenly cheerful after a period of depression
Showing signs of psychosis

Subjective Comments

Complaints of being a bad person or feeling rotten inside
Verbal hints with comments such as "I won't be a problem for you much longer"
Comments such as "I want to kill myself" or "I'm going to commit suicide"

Source: American Academy of Child & Adolescent Psychiatry. (2008). *Facts for families, No. 10*: Teen suicide. Retrieved from http://www.aacap.org/cs/root/facts_for_families/teen_suicide

ethical issue raised with the use and abuse of alcohol and other drugs is the dilemma of balancing adolescents' **rights to autonomy**, **privacy**, and **freedom** to determine their own actions against the harmful effects of irresponsible use of alcohol and other drugs. When drug prevention programs were widespread in the past couple of decades, adolescents began talking more than ever about substance use and abuse (Banks, 1999). Dryfoos and Barkin (2006) delineated some early predictors of alcohol and drug abuse and protectors (see Box 6.4).

There is a federal government prevention campaign, called the Initiative on Underage Drinking, spearheaded by the National Institute on Alcohol Abuse and Alcoholism (NIAAA, 2010). Disturbingly, 5,000 adolescents under the age of 21 die each year from underage drinking. Statistics include 1,900 deaths from motor vehicle accidents, 1,600 from homicides, 300 from suicide, and the remaining numbers from injuries such as falls, burns, and drowning. Drinking continues to be a broad and widespread problem among adolescents. The Surgeon General is hoping that this program will help to reduce the amount of alcohol consumption by underage persons.

BOX 6.4 ETHICAL FORMATIONS: PREDICTORS AND PROTECTORS

Predictors of Drug Abuse

- Aggressiveness in early childhood
- Rebelliousness
- Unconventionality
- High-risk friends
- Parents who have problems or use drugs

Predictors of Alcohol Abuse

- Alcoholic parent(s)
- Restless, impulsive, aggressive behavior in early childhood
- Conduct disorder
- Depression
- Peers who drink
- Lack of parental monitoring, support, and supervision

Protectors

- Parents who talk to their teens, set expectations, and enforce consequences
- Close family ties
- Adult role models
- Participation in religious and other activities
- Positive attitudes toward school
- School achievement

Source: Jessor, R., Van Den Bos, J., Vanderryn, J., Costa, F., & Turbin, M. (1995). Protective factors in adolescent problem behavior: Moderator effects and developmental change. *Developmental Psychology, 31,* 923–933.

There is concern by many people that the campaign could backfire and cause teens to hide and drink, or go underground to drink, especially if parents are asked not to allow their underage children to drink (Underage Drinking Debate, 2006). Underground or **secret drinking** can lead to major unintended consequences. Another concern raised is the overmoralizing of the issue. Many professionals believe that moralizing should not be part of the message. **Underage drinking** is an illegal, but not necessarily immoral, act. The other issue is parenting—knowing what to teach and what not to teach. The consensus by most professionals is that parents should teach their children how to act responsibly and teach what is legal and illegal. There is a double standard; in other words, parents worry about their teens drinking alcohol but, at the same time, adults continue to be the largest consumers of alcohol (Dryfoos & Barkin, 2006).

School nurses need to take part in educating teens and parents on underage drinking. Striking a balance between a nurse's confidentiality regarding information learned and protecting the adolescent is a complex and difficult situation. The trust between the nurse and adolescent should not be broken unless there is evidence of impending physical harm, which is a limit of confidentiality.

Sexual Abuse

According to Banks (1999), **sexual abuse** is "an issue which is surrounded by apprehension and fear" (p. 157). Hundreds of thousands of minors are physically or sexually abused each year, most of the time within the family. Sexual abuse, however, may occur outside the home as well. All states have clear laws, policies, and guidelines for child protection from abuse.

Dating violence, though it always has been a problem, has come to the forefront in the last few years. Just as adults have and must solve romantic conflicts, so do adolescents. Middle to late adolescents are more apt than younger adolescents to be in a relationship involving violence that is usually related to anger, jealousy, emotional hurting, one partner's behavior, and one person trying to gain control over the other one (Wolfe, Jaffe, & Crooks, 2006). Males and females have communicated that jealousy is the main reason for aggression in a dating relationship. Other types of violence and abuse are evident within the adolescent population, such as gang violence, gay baiting and homophobic violence, bullying, harassment, and rape.

Nurses are responsible for critical event changes that are encountered during actual discussions with adolescents. Sexual abuse or other abuses are considered to fall under the limits of confidentiality. Nurses who work with adolescents must report any cases that they encounter to proper officials or health professionals. For example, a school nurse would report the abuse or violence to the principal, or a nurse in an emergency department would report sexual abuse to a physician, mental health worker, or social worker. Before explaining the severity of the situation to the adolescent, nurses should make every effort to help adolescents express their own feelings and reactions about their situation. The most effective prevention programs for risky behaviors, including violence, are those in which the content is focused on the risk factors associated with the problem area. Prevention programs must be multifaceted to be successful (Wolfe, Jaffe, & Crooks, 2006). Once the risk factors are addressed, the focus shifts to protective factors that provide adolescents with interpersonal relationship, conflict resolution, and decision-making skills. Interpersonal relationship skills are the focus of violence prevention programs.

Eating Disorders

Physical appearance is one of the most important aspects of self-image for all adolescents, but this is especially true for girls. Whitlock, Williams, Gold, Smith, and Shipman (2005) reported that as many as 50 to 75% of adolescent girls in the United States continually diet, but that only 16% are actually overweight. Most girls dream and wish for beautiful, lean, and trim bodies, and many of them tend not to be satisfied with their own bodies. More recently, adolescent boys have begun to develop eating disorders (Harris & Cumella, 2006).

Two common eating disorders that lead to serious medical complications, and even death, if not treated correctly or at all are **anorexia nervosa** and **bulimia.** The tragedy is that most adolescents who experience these two disorders are skilled at hiding them until medical problems become severe. Nurses who work closely with adolescents need to be highly skilled in assessing and monitoring adolescents who are at risk for these eating disorders. Refer to Box 6.5 for warning signs and symptoms for which nurses need to monitor. Other than weight loss, some signs that may alert the nurse to these disorders include the need to be "perfect" or a high achiever, low self-esteem, open displays of intense guilt, signs of depression, or signs of obsession with food, calories, fat grams, or weight.

For many adolescents, **obesity** has become a disturbing problem. Adolescents who are obese tend to be very self-conscious of how they look to others, which may lead to a lifelong cycle of anxiety, depression, and overeating. Chronic overeating and obesity lead to severe health problems, such as heart disease, hypertension, type 2 diabetes, and respiratory problems.

The fact that these eating disorders exist in many adolescents is a warning that severe emotional hurting is present. In turn, if left undetected or untreated, the emotional distress may progress to more disturbing behavior, such as complete withdrawal, being friendless, expressions of anger and aggression, and self-harm. Psychotherapy is the treatment of choice, and nurses need to monitor for warning

BOX 6.5 ETHICAL FORMATIONS: WARNING SIGNS OF EATING DISORDERS: ANOREXIA NERVOSA AND BULIMIA

- Sudden and dramatic weight loss
- Relentless exercising
- Ritual eating—tiny bites, rearranging food on the plate
- Obsession with counting calories
- High achiever or a need to be perfect
- Frequent weighing on scales
- Common use of laxatives, diuretics, and diet suppressants
- Binge eating or purging
- Avoiding meals altogether or often eating alone
- Self-image of being and looking fat even though weight loss continues
- Interpersonal relationship problems
- Sense of helplessness that is curbed with controlling eating

Source: Harris, M., & Cumella, E. J. (2006). Eating disorders across the life span. *Journal of Psychosocial Nursing, 44*(4), 20–26.

signs of all of these disorders and talk with the adolescent and parents so that the nurse can make the appropriate referrals to a primary care provider and a psychotherapist.

Facing Death

Losing a Loved One

Losing a loved one is a catastrophic tragedy for an adolescent. Healing strategies include simple activities for the nurse, such as being present, conducting attentive listening, and allowing adolescents to express themselves as long as they need to do so. It is important for nurses to realize that some adolescents do not want to disclose information about their feelings of losing someone, and they need to be alone. Many adolescents turn to prayer, hope, and a belief in absoluteness, or a higher being. Some adolescents heal through self-talk, memories, and dreams. It is a difficult thing for an adolescent to lose a parent. Robert, a 16-year-old boy, expressed his thoughts about the memory of his mother 3 years after her death (Markowitz & McPhee, 2002) in Box 6.6. He was only 13 years old when his mother died.

Although people can expect death at some point in life, most of the time people are not prepared for it, especially adolescents. In 2000, more than 20,000 school-aged children or teens, ranging in age between 5 and 18 years, died in the United States (Lazenby, 2006). When a student dies, often the teacher and school nurse will hold off on their grief and focus on the children left behind in the school. Lazenby conducted qualitative research to explore how teachers deal with the death of a student. When the researchers asked the teachers about their perception of received support, one of the informants stated: "They never acknowledged to us [teachers] that maybe we needed to do something too and we were not allowed time to sit down and gather all our thoughts or listen to the counselors" (p. 56). Refer to Box 6.7 regarding two teachers' experiences with the death of a student.

BOX 6.6 ETHICAL FORMATIONS: SOMETIMES I DREAM ABOUT HER

Words of an adolescent boy about the loss of his mother:

Every day I miss her, but it is just something that I've accepted that I have to deal with and can't change. One time I followed someone [in the car] until she turned, because she had the same color hair as my mom. Even though I knew it wasn't her, there was the fascination of, "What if it was . . . ?" Sometimes I dream about her, but then I wake up . . . and it knocks me back down to earth. It isn't a sad thing, because it is nice to see her again. . . . The thing that stops me in my tracks is seeing her handwriting. I still have a list of chores she'd written out—there was so much personality in her voice and in her writing, that even though it was just a chore list it is something that is so beautiful to me.

Source: Quoted from Robert, age 16. Markowitz, A., & McPhee, S. (2002). Adolescent grief: "It never really hit me . . . until it actually happened." *Journal of the American Medical Association, 288*(21), 2741.

If allowed to grieve appropriately, however, in most cases adolescents will heal without permanent scarring. When death is unexpected, such as in violence or an accident, screams and loud bursts of "Oh God, why?" and "No!" from adolescents are often voiced. The death of a fellow student may shock others to a state of numbness and disbelief. When adolescents unexpectedly or expectedly lose someone they love, be it friend or family member, how do they say goodbye, progress through the hurting and pain, and move on?

Adolescents realize that death is a final and irreversible act. When grieving has not progressed appropriately, however, dysfunctional grieving may occur. It is normal for adolescents to live in the present and often not think in terms of consequences. Grief is a complex process for anyone, but especially for adolescents. During the grieving process, they may take more risks than usual and harm themselves. They may even seek thrills that are potentially life-threatening events.

Ethically, the nurse or school nurse must try to promote beneficence and nonmaleficence by helping adolescents through the 10 stages of grief when they lose a loved one (see Box 6.8). If a long-term nurse–adolescent relationship exists, the nurse must try to help the adolescent overcome barriers to development tasks.

BOX 6.7 ETHICAL FORMATIONS: TEACHERS AND STUDENT DEATHS

One Teacher's Experience with the Death of Billy

It was a sunny Friday morning as the teacher stood before her fourth-grade class calling roll. She was struck by Billy's absence as he had not missed a day of school the entire year. Making comments to the effect that he was probably sick, she proceeded with the day as usual. Upon her arrival home, she received a phone call informing her that Billy had been murdered by a family member earlier that day. Her first thoughts were of denial and guilt. It was possible that she had been talking about the child at the exact moment that life left his body.

How will this teacher face her fourth-grade class on Monday after one of their beloved friends has lost his life? How will she have the strength to clear all of the items from his desk or remove his name from the roll? How many other teachers will experience the death of a student during the school year? What emotions will those teachers experience? (p. 50)

One Teacher's Irony of a Student's Final Day at School

[One teacher] recalled the irony of his student's final day of school. While sharing with his class about the statistics and dangers of drinking and driving, the student was engaged in conversation with another student. The teacher's perception was that the student was intending to do the very thing he was telling the students to avoid: drinking and driving. The teacher vividly remembered thinking, "I wish he would listen to me." That was on Friday. The student was buried on Monday as the result of a motor vehicle accident involving alcohol. (p. 54)

Source: Lazenby, R. B. (2006). Teachers dealing with the death of students: A qualitative analysis. *Journal of Hospice and Palliative Nursing, 8*(1), 50–56.

Nurses and teachers need to be aware of dysfunctional grieving signs other than adolescents taking abnormal risks, such as (1) symptoms of chronic depression, sleeping problems, and low self-esteem issues; (2) low academic performance or an indifference to school-related activities; and (3) relationship problems with family members and old friends. School nurses are in an ideal situation to provide support to grieving adolescents and to educate teachers on how to cope with death and dying in school settings. Lazenby (2006) emphasized that there is considerable research that has revealed a deficit of knowledge and "know-how" for teachers working with adolescents coping with death and dying of their peers and family members.

Adolescents Facing Their Own Deaths

Adolescents facing their own deaths may have a terminal illness. In this case, they also may take life-threatening risks to impress their peers or others. Stillion and Papadatou (2002) poignantly stated: "Terminally-ill young people find themselves struggling with major issues of identity in the face of a foreclosed future" (p. 302).

BOX 6.8 ETHICAL FORMATIONS: STAGES OF GRIEF

General Stages of Grief for Those Who Are Experiencing Dying

Stage 1 Denial
Stage 2 Anger
Stage 3 Bargaining
Stage 4 Depression
Stage 5 Acceptance

Stages of Grief for Loss of a Loved One

Stage 1 Shock
Stage 2 Expression of emotion
Stage 3 Depression and loneliness
Stage 4 Physical symptoms of distress
Stage 5 Panic
Stage 6 Guilt
Stage 7 Anger and resentment
Stage 8 Resistance
Stage 9 Hope
Stage 10 Affirmation of reality

Source: Adapted From National Education Association. (2000). *Book 4: Hands on assistance—Tools for educators: Crisis communications guide and toolkit. Tool 32—Children's concept of death.* Retrieved from http://www.preventionweb.net/files/3949_Toolsforeducators.pdf

They ask questions such as "Who am I now?", "Who was I?", "Who would I like to become?", "Who will I be?", and "How will I be remembered by my friends?" (p. 303). The stages of grief that people go through when they know they are dying are different from when a person is grieving for another person. In this case, grieving consists of five stages that have been widely recognized: Stage 1—Denial; Stage 2—Anger; Stage 3—Bargaining; Stage 4—Depression; and Stage 5—Acceptance (Kübler-Ross, 1970; see Box 6.8).

While struggling with whether to engage in intimate relationships and searching for purpose and meaning to their time-limited lives, adolescents with a terminal illness may live almost aimlessly from day to day. They may fear that they will hurt others if they die. "They [adolescents] must learn to live in two worlds—the medical world with the threat of painful treatment, relapse, and death; and the normal world of home, school, and community, with all the challenges that healthy children face" (Stillion & Papadatou, 2002, p. 303).

The central ethical principles involved in this type of nurse–adolescent relationship are beneficence, nonmaleficence, and autonomy. The same grief stages that apply to the death of a loved one are at work here as well, and nurses who are involved with dying adolescents need to first explain the stages to the adolescent. Then, nurses and family members need to be alert to problems that may arise. Extreme behaviors and risk-taking are signs that can alert nurses and family members to take measures to prevent harm (nonmaleficence). Benefiting or doing good for terminally ill adolescents includes maintaining or improving their quality of life as much as possible. Ways to improve quality of life are to allow expressions of their fears and concerns, to be sensitive to meeting cultural and spiritual needs, to have compassion and show benevolence (kindness), and to remember that they experience most of the same challenges that healthy adolescents experience. Nurses must encourage sick adolescents to engage in autonomous decision making, as appropriate, as they progress through these developmental challenges.

Nursing Care

In this chapter, there has already been considerable discussion about the ethical management of adolescents concerning consent, confidentiality, prevention, and illness. In addition to these issues are fundamental moral virtues that nurses need to understand and practice consistently in all areas with adolescents. The ANA *Code of Ethics for Nurses with Interpretive Statements* (2001) has essential aspects that relate to the moral integrity of nurses and their practice (see Box 6.9). Nurses who base their practice on a moral framework that includes the following virtues are more likely to be successful in developing a respectful relationship between themselves and the adolescents with whom they work.

BOX 6.9 ETHICAL FORMATIONS: ESSENTIAL ASPECTS FROM THE *CODE OF ETHICS FOR NURSES WITH INTERPRETIVE STATEMENTS* FOR CULTIVATING CARE FOR ADOLESCENTS

- Only information pertinent to a patient's treatment and welfare is disclosed, and only to those directly involved with the patient's care. Duties of confidentiality, however, are not absolute and may need to be modified in order to protect the patient, other innocent parties, and in circumstances of mandatory disclosure for public health reasons. (3.2, p. 12)
- Nurses have a duty to remain consistent with both their personal and professional values and to accept compromise only to the degree that it remains an integrity-preserving compromise. An integrity-preserving compromise does not jeopardize the dignity or well-being of the nurse or others. (5.4, p. 19)
- Virtues are habits of character that predispose persons to meet their moral obligations; that is, to do what is right. Excellences are habits of character that predispose a person to do a particular job or task well. (6.1, p. 20).
- Virtues such as wisdom, honesty, and courage are habits or attributes of the morally good person. Excellences such as compassion, patience, and skill are habits of character of the morally good nurse. For the nurse, virtues and excellences are those habits that affirm and promote the values of human dignity, well-being, respect, health, independence, and other values central to nurses. (6.1, p. 20)

Trustworthiness

Trustworthiness, as already defined, means that nurses are dependable and authentic because they take responsibility for their own behavior and commit to their obligations (Gullotta et al., 2000). For example, a teen girl trusts that a school nurse is going to follow through with an appointment to discuss a sensitive issue, such as the possibility of the girl being pregnant and the choices that are available to her.

Genuineness

Adolescents are more perceptive to how genuine a person is than any other population (Gullotta et al., 2000). **Genuineness** is how credible or real the nurse is. For example, if the nurse puts on a facade that there is genuineness in a relationship with an adolescent because of not desiring a genuine relationship, the adolescent will perceive the disingenuousness. The pretense may be more damaging to the adolescent than the nurse admitting the desire not to have a genuine relationship.

Compassion

Compassion means for the nurse to have an understanding of the adolescent's suffering and a desire to take action to alleviate that suffering. The display of compassion is uncommon but is a human quality that nurses need to possess. In the ANA *Code of Ethics for Nurses with Interpretive Statements* (2001) and the International

Council of Nurses *ICN Code of Ethics for Nurses* (2006), compassion and alleviation of suffering are common themes.

An example of a compassionate action by a nurse is to intervene on behalf of an adolescent who has a hidden hurt. A hidden hurt is one that causes a great degree of mental stress, such as when family members or peers tease, make fun of, or bully a person because of a weight problem, poor grades in school, freckles, a big nose, other facial distortions, or other perceived shortcomings (Urban Programs Resource Network, 2011). The victimized person feels emotionally abused and belittled and, over time, a lowered sense of self-worth will occur, with a display of extremes in behaviors such as aggression, violence, passiveness, or becoming withdrawn. An example of a compassionate school nurse is one who takes immediate measures to stop the aggressive behavior and compassionately acts by attempting to establish a trusting relationship with an adolescent who is being bullied or teased continuously. Notifying the school counselor or the principal and talking with the adolescent's parents are important considerations.

Honesty

The old cliché of "honesty is the best policy" has proved to be a good one for nurse relationships. **Honesty** means being forthright, truthful, and not deceptive. According to Gullotta et al. (2000), "without honesty there can be no relationship" (p. 281). Nurses should express their feelings and emotions in relationships. For example, expressing sadness, dissatisfaction, pleasure, or displeasure about an adolescent's behavior is better than trying to cover up feelings. Hiding one's feelings can cause a barrier in the relationship—and irreparable damage.

If nurses practice the virtues of trustworthiness, genuineness, compassion, and honesty with adolescent care, a healthy and respectful relationship between the nurse and adolescent is more likely to develop. However, the adolescent must be able to perceive that the virtues are evident in the nurse's practice, otherwise a trusting relationship between the two may never evolve.

Spiritual Considerations

One of the most important things we can do to nurture the spiritual growth of our youth is listen to their stories and share with them ours. We have a spiritual emptiness in our society, even in the face of spirituality as an essential part of being human. If adolescents believe in a higher being, or what some may call absoluteness, they usually voice comfort in living with this belief. For adolescents, spirituality can provide a type of healthy, nonpunitive socialization and acceptance. Nurses can facilitate an adolescent's spiritual growth by remembering the little actions that help adolescents' spirituality, such as attentive listening, being present, or keeping commitments to them. Spirituality transcends all religious beliefs; therefore, nurses could better help teens by being familiar with different religious beliefs.

CASE STUDY: AN ADOLESCENT COUPLE WITH HIV

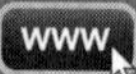

Alexa was a 17-year-old senior in high school and had been an "A" student in school her whole life. Her goal was to earn a bachelor's degree in science and to one day become a physician. She had gone steady with Robert for 3 years, but he was 2 years older and was already at the local university. Robert was going to be an accountant. They were planning on marriage at some point in time. They were having unprotected sex on a regular basis, but to prevent pregnancy she was on oral contraceptives. She did not worry. However, Alexa began to get sick often, such as having no appetite, losing weight, and having nausea, diarrhea, cramping, and other mysterious symptoms. She finally went to her physician. She received a diagnosis of HIV. She was shocked! She had never had sex with anyone but Robert and she never doubted Robert's faithfulness to her. After confronting him, she found out that Robert had been getting high on drugs and having unprotected group sex with college friends of both genders since he began his studies. Although he too had been having symptoms, he was unaware that he had HIV on the night when Alexa confronted him. He later received a diagnosis of HIV.

Case Study Questions

- You are the nurse who is working the day that Alexa finds out that she has HIV. She is in the clinic for more than one hour with you while you try to counsel and console her. You have had formal HIV counseling training, so you go through the official guidelines with her. Several weeks later, after Alexa is more composed and has had time to think more about her situation, she drops by the clinic and wants to talk with you on a more personal basis. She needs comforting. What approaches are you going to take with Alexa? Please explore how to use and apply the virtues to help Alexa. Be specific with your approaches.
- You know that spiritual promotion for adolescents is an important consideration. What are methods that you would use with Alexa to promote her spirituality? Be very specific. In doing so, consider her life goals with or without her boyfriend, what might happen to her relationship with Robert, her medical future, and her future in general. Imagine what you might actually say to her and do for her. Imagine a conversation that would take place between the two of you. An option to try is role-play with your peers.

Nurses can do several things to help adolescents with spiritual growth. It should be emphasized that if nurses help promote adolescents' spirituality, nurses may consciously or unconsciously begin developing their own spiritual growth. Small actions that may help to deliver huge positive consequences are showing love and showing compassion.

Love is difficult to define, but many people know it when they feel it. Showing love to patients from a nursing perspective is necessary and it takes a certain degree of willingness to accomplish showing love. Nurses need to maintain a perceptive eye in differentiating this type of nurturing from unethical and illegal sexual advances.

Compassion is one of the virtues already mentioned in the *Nursing Care* section of this chapter. For a nurse to promote spiritual growth by practicing compassion, several related virtues emerge:

- **Forgiveness**: Always being open to others' situations and reasons for the circumstances
- **Patience and tolerance**: Detaching from one's own agenda and outcomes and waiting on and being open to another's agenda
- **Equanimity**: Being engaged in a situation with a patient and working toward a patient's well-being without the unhealthy attachment that may cause harm to the relationship
- **Sense of responsibility**: Knowing that people are interconnected and that responsibility grows from the interconnectedness
- **Sense of harmony**: Remaining in contact with the reality of a situation and with others
- **Contentment**: An intermittent feeling of comfort that comes to a person as a result of practicing and following a spiritual direction (Ingersoll, 2000)

Many Americans have taken a renewed interest in spirituality and would prefer the label of "spiritual" rather than "religious." One reason for this interest is that most people believe that spirituality is at the core of human life experience. If nurses talk with adolescents and truly listen to them, spiritual growth may occur for both adolescents and nurses. Please refer to Box 6.9 for essential aspects from the ANA *Code of Ethics for Nurses with Interpretive Statements* in caring for adolescents.

KEY POINTS

- The adolescent three-phase developmental process includes early adolescence, middle adolescence, and late adolescence. Risk-taking behaviors are at the highest rate in middle adolescence.
- When implementing any type of prevention intervention program for adolescents, nurses need to incorporate theory-based health risk messages along with behavioral interventions that are beneficial and nonharmful.
- Nurses are faced with the dilemma of choosing a program that is appropriate and healthy for a particular group. There are a variety of standardized and evidence-based programs for adolescents. Misleading, age- or content-inappropriate information, or non-theory-based information can cause more harm than good and may be a factor in an increase of unhealthy risky behaviors.
- An increasingly difficult challenge exists for nurses to provide ethical and acceptable sexual education to adolescents, and ensure that the information

KEY POINTS (continued)

taught is actually heard as intended. Nurses need to know where along the sexual abstinence–comprehensive sexual education continuum that information becomes unethical, nonbeneficial, or even harmful.

- There are three major ethical concerns for nurses teaching along this continuum: (1) there is no clear definition of sexual abstinence today; (2) adolescent sexual intimacy is alive and well, and long-term abstinence has the potential to damage a young person's capacity to love with greater depth and integrity; and (3) there continues to be controversy as to whether abstinence-only programs are working.
- Nurses must gain trust by relentlessly proving themselves to adolescents by being consistent, giving correct information, keeping commitments, and showing concern and caring. These strategies are tried and true ways to gain trust with others, especially with adolescents. A trust-privacy-confidentiality dilemma emerges when the nurse is entrusted with an adolescent's confidential health and social information. In fact, research has revealed that the likelihood that adolescents will seek health services for sensitive issues depends on how well their confidential issues will be maintained. There are limits to confidentiality when potential harm to others or self is at stake. Limits of confidentiality generally include suicidal ideation, homicidal ideation, physical abuse, sexual abuse, and other behaviors that place the adolescent at risk of physical harm.
- If adolescents ever really have autonomous decision-making capacity for consenting to or refusing treatments, it is closely linked to their moral self-development characteristics and how self-directed they are. Information that is gathered in a nurse–adolescent relationship must be kept private and confidential by the nurse, with the exception limits of confidentiality.
- Adolescents cope differently and sometimes worse than do adults. When a peer at school dies suddenly, reactions are usually widespread throughout the community and school. Shock and disbelief will emotionally paralyze the adolescents. Teachers and school nurses must hold off on their grief to focus on supporting and helping the grieving adolescents. The school nurse or community nurse must try to promote beneficence and nonmaleficence by helping adolescents through the 10 stages of grief when they lose a loved one or classmate. Adolescents facing their own death will experience the 5 stages of grief that were labeled by Kübler-Ross. It is likely that adolescents grieving for self or the death of classmates will engage in high-risk behaviors intermittently.
- Nurses need to base their practice with adolescents on a moral framework of virtues that includes trustworthiness, genuineness, compassion, and honesty. The ANA *Code of Ethics for Nurses with Interpretive Statements* (2001) and

KEY POINTS (continued)

the *ICN Code of Ethics for Nurses* (2006) emphasize moral integrity in practice. Spiritual considerations are important to adolescents in all aspects of tribulations experienced. Nurses should practice the virtues of spirituality as well as teach these virtues to adolescents.

- Listen to adolescents, their stories, and their problems.
- Remember the little things that nurses can do in times of stress and need.
- Be compassionate.
- Be forgiving and remain open to others.
- Stay engaged in a situation with adolescents as needed.
- Maintain a sense of responsibility.
- Develop a sense of harmony.
- Be content.

References

American Academy of Child & Adolescent Psychiatry. (2008). *Facts for families, No. 10*: Teen suicide. Retrieved from http://www.aacap.org/cs/root/facts_for_families/teen_suicide

American Nurses Association. (2001). *Code of ethics for nurses with interpretive statements.* Silver Spring, MD: Author.

Bandura, A. (1977). *Social learning theory.* New York, NY: General Learning Press.

Banks, S. (1999). *Ethical issues in youth work.* New York, NY: Routledge.

Blustein, J., & Moreno, J. D. (1999). Valid consent to treatment and the unsupervised adolescent. In J. Blustein, C. Levine, & N. N. Dubler (Eds.), *The adolescent alone: Decision making in health care in the United States* (pp. 100–110). New York, NY: Cambridge University Press.

Bowman, D. H. (2004). Cover story: Abstinence-only debate heating up. *Education Week, 23*(22), 1–2.

Butts, J. B., & Hartman, S. (2002). Project BART: Effectiveness of a behavioral intervention to reduce HIV risk in adolescents. *Journal of Maternal Child Nursing, 27*(3), 163–169.

Centers for Disease Control and Prevention. (2010). Youth risk behavior surveillance—United States, 2009. *Morbidity and Morality Weekly Report, 59*(SS-5), 1–148. Retrieved from http://www.cdc.gov/mmwr/pdf/ss/ss5905.pdf

Cook, R. J., Dickens, B. M., & Fathalla, M. F. (2003). *Reproductive health and human rights: Integrating medicine, ethics, and law.* New York, NY: Oxford University Press/Clarendon.

DiClemente, R. J., Hansen, W. B., & Ponton, L. E. (1996). *Handbook of adolescent health risk behavior.* New York, NY: Plenum.

Dryfoos, J. G., & Barkin, C. (2006). *Adolescence: Growing up in America today.* New York, NY: Oxford University Press.

Erikson, E. (1963). *Childhood and society* (2nd ed.). New York, NY: Norton.

Feliz, J. (2011, January 12). *Survey: Exposure to anti-drug messages among teens drops dramatically by two-thirds as drug use goes up.* The Partnership at Drugfree.org—Newsroom. Retrieved from http://www.drugfree.org/newsroom/survey-exposure-to-anti-drug-messages-among-teens-drops-dramatically-by-two-thirds-as-drug-use-goes-up

Fisher, J. D., & Fisher, W. A. (1992). Changing AIDS risk behavior. *Psychological Bulletin, 111*, 455–474.

Gullotta, T. P., Adams, G. R., & Markstrom, C. A. (2000). *The adolescent experience* (4th ed.). San Diego, CA: Academic.

Guttmacher Institute. (2011a). *Facts on American teens' sources of information about sex: Sex, pregnancy, and abortion.* Retrieved from http://www.guttmacher.org/pubs/FB-Teen-Sex-Ed.html

Guttmacher Institute. (2011b, August 1). *State policies in brief: Parental involvement in minors' abortions.* Retrieved from http://www.guttmacher.org/statecenter/spibs/spib_PIMA.pdf

Harris, M., & Cumella, E. J. (2006). Eating disorders across the life span. *Journal of Psychosocial Nursing, 44*(4), 20–26.

Hartwig, M. J. (2000). *The poetics of intimacy and the problem of sexual abstinence.* New York, NY: Peter Lang.

Ingersoll, R. E. (2000, May). Spirituality as a counseling resource for adolescents: Reality is complex, complexity is our friend. MetroHealth presentation. Retrieved from http://www. csuohio.edu/casal/spirsyl.htm

International Council of Nurses. (2006). *ICN Code of ethics for nurses.* Geneva, Switzerland: Author. Retrieved from http://www.icn.ch/icncode.pdf

Jessor, R., Van Den Bos, J., Vanderryn, J., Costa, F., & Turbin, M. (1995). Protective factors in adolescent problem behavior: Moderator effects and developmental change. *Developmental Psychology, 31*, 923–933.

Kübler-Ross, E. (1970). *On death and dying.* New York, NY: Macmillan.

Lazenby, R. B. (2006). CE education: Teachers dealing with the death of students: A qualitative analysis. *Journal of Hospice and Palliative Nursing, 8*(1), 50–56.

Leffert, N., & Petersen, A. C. (1999). Adolescent development: Implications for the adolescents alone. In J. Blustein, C. Levine, & N. N. Dubler (Eds.), *The adolescent alone: Decision making in health care in the United States* (pp. 31–49). New York, NY: Cambridge University Press.

Lindberg, L. D., Boggess, S., & Williams, S. (2000). *Multiple threats: The co-occurrence of teen health risk behaviors.* Office of the Assistant Secretary for Planning & Evaluation [Contract No. HHS-100-95-0021]. Retrieved from http://www.urban.org/publications/410248.html

Markowitz, A. J., & McPhee, S. J. (2002). Adolescent grief: "It never really hit me until it actually happened." *Journal of the American Medical Association, 288*(21), 2741.

McGuinness, T. M. (2006). Nothing to sniff at: Inhalant abuse & youth. *Journal of Psychosocial Nursing, 44*(8), 15–18.

McIntosh, J. L. (for the American Association of Suicidology). (2010). *U.S.A. suicide 2007: Official final data.* Washington, DC: American Association of Suicidology. Dated May 23, 2010. Retrieved from http://www.suicidology.org/c/document_library/get_file?folderId=228&name=DLFE-227.pdf

McKay, S. (2003). Adolescent risk behaviors and communication research: Current directions. *Journal of Language and Social Psychology, 22*(1), 74–82.

National Education Association. (2000). *Book 4: Hands on assistance—Tools for educators: Crisis communications guide and toolkit. Tool 32—Children's concept of death.* Retrieved from http://www.preventionweb.net/files/3949_Toolsforeducators.pdf

National Institute on Alcohol Abuse and Alcoholism. (2010). *Underage drinking research initiative.* Retrieved from http://www.niaaa.nih.gov/AboutNIAAA/NIAAASponsoredPrograms/underage.htm

Planned Parenthood Action Fund. (2010). *Title X: America's family planning program.* Retrieved from http://www.plannedparenthoodaction.org/positions/title-x-americas-family-planning-program-855.htm

Population Reference Bureau. (2011). *United States—Demographic highlights*. Retrieved from http://www.prb.org/Datafinder/Geography/Summary.aspx?region=72®ion_type=2

ProCon.org. (2011). *16 legal medical marijuana states and DC*. Retrieved from http://medicalmarijuana.procon.org/view.resource.php?resourceID=000881

Remez, L. (2000). Oral sex among adolescents: Is it sex or is it abstinence? *Family Planning Perspectives, 32*(6), 298–304.

St. Lawrence, J. S. (1994). *Becoming a responsible teen [BART]: An HIV risk program for adolescents*. Jackson, MS: Jackson State University.

St. Lawrence, J. S., Brasfield T., Jefferson, K. W., Alleyne, E., O'Bannon, R. E., & Shirley, A. (1995). Cognitive-behavioral intervention to reduce African-American adolescents' risk for HIV infection. *Journal of Consulting and Clinical Psychology, 63*(2), 221–237.

Stillion, J. M., & Papadatou, D. (2002). Suffer the children: An examination of psychosocial issues in children and adolescents with terminal illness. *American Behavioral Scientist, 46*(2), 299–315.

Turnbull, C. M. (1983). *The human cycle*. New York, NY: Simon and Schuster.

UNAIDS—The Joint United Nations Programme for HIV/AIDS. (2010). *UNAIDS report on the global AIDS epidemic* (Chapter 1). Retrieved from http://www.unaids.org/documents/20101123_GlobalReport_Chap1_em.pdf

Underage drinking debate: Zero tolerance vs. teaching responsibility. (2006). *The Brown University Child and Adolescent Behavior Letter, 22*(3), 1, 6, 7.

United Nations Population Fund. (2011). *Adolescents and youth—Giving young people top priority*. Retrieved from http://www.unfpa.org/public/adolescents/dhs_adolescent_guides.html

University of Chicago, Pritzker School of Medicine. (2005). *Approach to assessing adolescents on serious or sensitive issues and confidentiality*. Retrieved from http://pedclerk.bsd.uchicago.edu/confidentiality.html

Urban Programs Resource Network. (2011). *Family works: Respect and hidden hurts*. Retrieved from http://urbanext.illinois.edu/familyworks/respect-03.html

Whitlock, E. P., Williams, S. B., Gold, R., Smith, P. R., & Shipman, S. A. (2005). Screening and interventions for childhood overweight: A summary of evidence for the U.S. Preventive Services Task Force. *Pediatrics, 116*, e125–e144.

Wiseman, R. (2001). *Queenbees and wannabees: Helping your daughter survive cliques, gossip, boyfriends, and other realities of adolescence*. New York, NY: Three Rivers.

Witte, K., Meyer, G., & Martell, D. (2001). *Effective health risk messages: A step-by-step guide*. Thousand Oaks, CA: Sage.

Wolfe, D. A., Jaffe, P. G., & Crooks, C. V. (2006). *Adolescent risk behaviors: Why teens experiment and strategies to keep them safe*. New Haven, CT: Yale University Press.

For a full suite of assignments and additional learning activities, use the access code located in the front of your book to visit this exclusive website: http://go.jblearning.com/butts. If you do not have an access code, you can obtain one at the site.

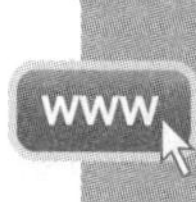

Adult Health Nursing Ethics

Janie B. Butts

The depth and strength of a human character are defined by its moral reserves. People reveal themselves completely only when they are thrown out of the customary conditions of their life, for only then do they have to fall back on their reserves.

—LEONARDO DA VINCI

OBJECTIVES

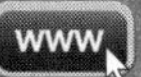

After reading this chapter, the reader should be able to:

1. Explore medicalization in terms of the changes in physician predominance and health care that have taken place since the 1970s.
2. Differentiate between the following terms: compliance, noncompliance, adherence, nonadherence, and concordance.
3. Examine cultural views related to self-determination, decision making, and American healthcare professionals' values of medicalization and therapeutic regimens.
4. Construct nursing care interventions in accordance with the nine themes that emerged from the interviews between the Chronic Illness Alliance researchers and patients with chronic illness and disease.
5. Delineate strategies that nurses can practice to create an ethical environment for chronically ill and suffering patients.
6. Contrast the organ procurement methods of presumed consent, mandated choice, donor cards, and required response in terms of a utilitarian framework, a virtue ethics approach, and a deontology framework.

7. Evaluate the three current ethical debates regarding retrieval of a person's organs as related to the dead donor rule.
8. Imagine ways in which nursing care would change from the perspective of an expanded legal definition of death to include patients with higher brain functioning, but no lower brain functioning.
9. Recommend nursing care strategies for families of brain-dead donors during the period of uncertainty and shock, during the life-sustaining mechanical ventilation period, and during the harvesting process.

Medicalization

Medicalization developed from a process whereby medical professionals diagnose human social problems, disorders, and syndromes as medical conditions. **Medicalization** is "a problem [that] is defined in medical terms, described using medical language, understood through the adoption of a medical framework, or 'treated' with a medical intervention" (Conrad, 2007, p. 5). Cure over care is emphasized in this medical model. A key point for understanding the definition of medicalization is that an illness, disorder, or disease "is not ipso facto a medical problem, rather, it needs to become defined as one" for the problem to become medicalized (Conrad, 2007, p. 6).

Medicalization has been scrutinized widely in the literature since the 1970s, but its meaning has evolved over time because of the changes in the medical process and the healthcare system (Conrad, 2007). Some critics say that medicalization has transformed nonmedical, social, or personal problems into medical conditions and has narrowed the range of what is acceptable for everyday living (e.g., Illich, 1975/2010). According to Conrad (2007), medical professionals classify and label the symptoms and decide who is sick. What some individuals or groups perceive as advantages to medicalization may be perceived as disadvantages by others, and vice versa. By labeling social conditions as a medical problem, medicalization has allowed for the extension of the sick role, has reduced individual blame for the problem, and has led to a focus on the individual rather than the social context. Many people have been helped by medications and treatment for their problems, such as alcoholism, erectile dysfunction, baldness, and many more human conditions.

Even though physicians remain the gatekeepers for medical treatment and continue to treat most of the disorders, three market-driven interests continue to expand the medicalization of society: (1) managed care, (2) biotechnology—such as genetic possibilities and pharmaceutical treatments, and (3) consumers. The trend for labeling human social conditions as medical problems has been increasing and there are no signs of waning (Conrad, 2007).

As the shift to managed care emerged, patients began to think like consumers when it came to the medical care they receive, the physicians they want, and the types of health insurance policies they can purchase. Consumer-patients have become more vocal and active in their own care and are demanding more services. During this same time period, pharmaceutical companies made enormous profits, and continue to do so, on new drug treatments; by the 1990s, the Human Genome Project shifted society's focus to new possibilities in diagnoses and treatments. As the 1990s ended, medical professional dominance in health care and treatments diminished somewhat, although physicians continue to practice with a high degree of control. Even though the market has shifted some of the traditional power away from physicians, many consumers are still experiencing the hegemonic practices of the medical profession in regard to their health care. Conrad (2007) emphasized that medicalization will continue to be a dominant force for a wide range of human problems.

Compliance, Adherence, and Concordance

The terms *compliance*, *adherence*, and *concordance* fall under the umbrella of medicalization. In a healthcare context, **compliance** refers to a patient's written or nonwritten approval of a physician's medical treatment or nurse's healthcare regimen, which represents the patient's intentions of obeying the wishes of the provider and following the suggested course of treatment. Compliance could border on coerciveness or indicate a paternalistic approach by physicians and nurses to make or force a patient to behave in a manner that reveals a submission to provider regimens.

In the last few decades, there has been a decline in the use of the term compliance because of the negative connotations in terms of the lack of patient involvement and autonomy in the physician–patient relationship. Within this negative connotation, **noncompliance** could be perceived as patient incompetence and deviance because the patient exhibits behaviors that do not conform to the physician and nurse's regimens. However, noncompliance remains a persistent concern for nursing practice; Russell, Daly, Hughes, and Hoog (2003) believe that "nurses can play an important role in providing a broader approach to compliance [and] nurses integrating an understanding of patient contexts with current nursing practice will result in more effective inventions" (p. 286).

Barofsky (1978; as cited in Berg, Evangelista, & Dunbar-Jacob, 2002) emphasized three levels on a self-care continuum of patient responses to treatments outlined by physicians and nurses: (1) compliance, (2) adherence, and (3) therapeutic alliance. In Barofsky's continuum, compliance means coercion, adherence means conformity, and self-care is a therapeutic alliance between the providers of care and the patient.

There are other ways that adherence has been defined. Adherence began to be used as a substitute for compliance in an attempt to deemphasize provider control and to emphasize patient self-determination and freedom to choose the extent of adhering to the medical regimen. **Adherence** is defined as the degree to which patients' behaviors match the recommendations agreed upon by the physician or nurse and the patient (Horne, Weinman, Barber, Elliott, & Morgan, 2005). The use of the term *adherence* is a clear indication that there should be an emphasis on the need for agreement between the physician or nurse and the patient.

Providers sometimes define **nonadherence** as an all-or-nothing patient approach (patients follow either all or none of a treatment plan), but a more therapeutic definition of nonadherence is the extent to which the desired treatment or therapeutic result is unlikely to be realized. There are unintentional and intentional reasons for patients not adhering to the therapeutic regimen: unintentional reasons include resource limitations or patients' constraints of memory or dexterity, while intentional nonadherence could be caused by constraints of patient or family beliefs, attitudes, or expectations. Patients' adherence or nonadherence should not be characterized as good or bad; more acceptable are the terms high and low adherence. In practice, physicians and nurses often find that determining adherence is difficult because the patient's degree of adherence often is not verbalized or mentioned during a clinical encounter.

Similar to Barofsky's (1978) term *therapeutic alliance* is the term ***concordance***, which is defined as an approach to the prescribing and taking of medicines. A patient and physician agreement is reached after negotiation that includes the beliefs and wishes of the patient in determining whether, when, and how medicines need to be taken (Horne et al., 2005). Concordance has been practiced more in the United Kingdom than any other country. The practice of concordance has many advantages, but Horne et al. believe that the term needs more conceptualization and understanding for its increased use in practice. Those providers who practice concordance have encountered frequent issues when it comes to discriminating concordance from compliance and adherence.

In the healthcare system today, the issue of doing more with less, with a focus on cost containment, is critical to providers promoting strategies that have the potential to improve a person's health. The ethical issue of promoting healthy behaviors and prescribing therapeutic regimens, yet trying to respect one's rights to self-determination, is a catch-22 situation. An ethical question to answer is: How far should providers of care go in terms of respecting the autonomy of patients when some of the patient behaviors burden society with enormous costs, both in terms of money and nonmonetary resources? For physicians and nurses to practice ethically, they must be attuned to patients' freedom to self-determination and attempt to be nonpaternalistic and less coercive in teaching patients strategies to promote healthy behaviors (Berg et al., 2002). At the same time, variables that must be considered include efficient cost containment of treatments, patient and provider risks and benefits of proposed treatments, the costs to society for patients to maintain unhealthy behaviors, and the responsibility that patients have regarding their self-care.

Cultural Views on Medicalization and Therapeutic Regimens

In this complex mix of therapeutic regimens and medicalization, providers of care must take into consideration the cultural values regarding autonomy, independence, self-care, and authoritative figures of the family. In the United States, healthcare professionals value and depend on their ability to teach patients self-care strategies to reduce illness and disease; they value efficiency; and they value self-control (Galanti, 2004). In so doing, some patients and families view the eagerness of providers to teach them self-care as more of a coercive tactic. Patients of various cultures do not necessarily appreciate the upfront way that American providers of care practice, and can have trouble with such tactics as giving warnings of consequences if unhealthy behaviors are continued or getting caught up in a procedure while not paying attention to the patient's modesty. The patient's values often conflict with the values of American providers of care.

Another cultural consideration is the manner in which the decision is made. Generally speaking, all human beings want to know how to care for themselves, but sometimes patients will value input from their families and will not make decisions without direction from them. The decisions will come from a group "think and do" approach, rather than unilateral patient decisions. Some cultures, such as those from Asia, have the head of the family make the decisions, whereas Native Americans would prefer that grandparents make the healthcare decisions. Beliefs such as these can be in conflict with the traditional view in the United States, where healthcare providers emphasize self-control, self-care, autonomy, money, and cure over care. The focus on curing, no matter how much the cure costs, is demonstrated by practices such as the extensive use of life support, fetal monitoring, organ transplants, and many other life-controlling and life-sustaining methods.

Many people have learned how to adapt their cultural traditions to the broader environment so that they can function without much difficulty. Galanti (2004) emphasized, "When cultural conflicts occur, it is often because what is successful under one set of environmental circumstances may be less so under others" (p. 17). Galanti proposed the **adaptation theory** to reduce cultural conflicts—that is, people adapting to the physical and social environment where they live. Nurses specifically can promote adaptation to a point of individual comfort so that social isolation and anonymity do not occur (see Box 7.1). In the *Code of Ethics for Nurses with Interpretive Statements*, the ANA (2001) emphasized that nurses are to care for patients in a respectful and an unbiased way (see Appendix A for the ANA code of

BOX 7.1 ETHICAL FORMATIONS: EXPERIENCE WITH MEDICALIZATION

Discuss one situation where you have experienced the effects of medicalization and a patient's adherence to a therapeutic regimen in your nursing practice, either as a nurse or nursing student.

Describe these effects as either positive or negative and think about the influences by the healthcare system, nurses and other providers of care, the hospital or agency, and the family. How did these influences affect patient outcomes with regard to the whole person?
Do you recall the context of the care? Were human dignity, privacy, respect, and other ethical concepts a consideration? Please give your rationale for your answers.
Were there cultural variances that needed attention and sensitivity? Please explain.
What ethical frameworks or principles would guide the practice of providers (nurses and physicians) in a healthcare facility with a major concern of "doing more with less"? What conflicts might you encounter if you practiced according to your moral conscience derived from the *Code of Ethics for Nurses*?

ethics). In the Preamble of the International Council of Nurses (ICN) *ICN Code of Ethics for Nurses* (2006; see Appendix B for the ICN code of ethics), the ICN stated:

> Inherent in nursing is respect for human rights, including cultural rights, the right to life and choice, to dignity and to be treated with respect. Nursing care is respectful of and unrestricted by considerations of age, colour, creed, culture, disability or illness, gender, sexual orientation, nationality, politics, race or social status. (p. 3)

Chronic Illness

> *Life is full of misery, loneliness, and suffering—and it's all over much too soon.*
>
> —Woody Allen

As advances in medical technology and treatment increase exponentially, the length of life of those people who have chronic illnesses also continues to increase. A powerful statement by Booth, Gordon, Carlson, and Hamilton (2000) conveys the global problem of chronicity: "Our society is at war. Although it may not be commonly publicized in this manner, make no mistake, our society, and even the world's population in general, is truly at war against a common enemy. That enemy is modern chronic disease" (p. 775). The Chronic Illness Alliance (CIA, 2011) defined **chronic illness** as "an illness that is permanent or lasts a long time. It may get slowly worse over time. It may lead to death, or it may finally go away. It may cause permanent changes to the body. It will certainly affect the person's quality of life" (para. 2). Many CIA members, who are located largely in Australia, convened in 2002 in an attempt to define chronic illness as a result of their qualitative interviews. In the final research report by the CIA, the team could not agree on a definition, so the definition on the alliance's website remains unchanged. What *is* interesting in this research are the comments made by the informants about their chronic illness and how it has affected their lives. Most informants saw chronic illness as a negative term and state of being that robbed them of any hope of recovery. Box 7.2 provides a summation of the informants' comments on chronic illness.

This Australian research has significant implications globally for those who care for patients with chronic illness. Erlen (2002) proposed three fundamental ethical concerns related to chronically ill persons: "lack of control, suffering, and access to services" (p. 416). These three concerns link closely to the concept of medicalization discussed in the previous section.

Patients with chronic illnesses frequently feel as if their illnesses are controlling them, rather than feeling that they are in control of their own lives. As indicated in the CIA (2002) report, the reality of power imbalances between vulnerable-feeling patients and the persuasion of healthcare providers magnify negative feelings of lack of control. Unless patients are inclined to cause harm to themselves or others, healthcare professionals need to honor patients' desires to be in control of their own lives.

Catherine Garrett's (2005) work on chronic illness and suffering was based on her own chronic illness experience with irritable bowel syndrome, a cluster of symptoms that include gastric pain, intestinal pain and spasms, and malfunctioning digestion. Garrett has lived with this pain and suffering for more than 40 years, and her desire in writing the book titled *Gut Feelings: Chronic Illness and the Search for Healing* was to recount and share her story and scholarly research on sickness, disability, violence, grief, loss, confusion, and despair. These symptoms make up what she called her suffering. Garrett explained that the suffering related to chronic illness is just one kind of suffering, but that people suffer in many ways.

Garrett (2005) stated that her work was a quest for the physical, emotional, intellectual, and spiritual components that connect to chronic illness and suffering. The excellent quotation by Woody Allen at the beginning of this section reflects these broad perspectives on suffering. Suffering related to chronic illness is similar to the tormenting symptoms of suffering so familiar in dying patients and their families.

Chronic illness results in a relentless, ongoing, and unhealing suffering, and if any inseparable part is suffering, the whole person will suffer. Garrett (2005) highlighted the extent of suffering to Aristotle's four inseparable parts—appetitive, vegetative, deliberative, and contemplative. Chronic conditions produce enormous demands and conflicts to which the ill person must respond. Patient suffering related to chronic illness can be a result of many entities such as unrelieved pain,

BOX 7.2 ETHICAL FORMATIONS: RESEARCH BRIEF ON CHRONIC ILLNESS: INFORMANTS' VIEWS

The 43 informants of this Australian study reported 27 different chronic illnesses. Arthritis or musculoskeletal diseases topped the list, followed by mental depression, multiple sclerosis, breast cancer, chronic pain, asthma, epilepsy, stroke, thyroid problems, and hypertension. Other diseases were less frequent. The researchers extrapolated 9 major themes from the 43 interviewees. The themes were:

The social impact of living with a chronic illness: Included not being able to work; living with an illness that they know will lead to their dependency on someone or even lead to death, poverty, isolation, and loneliness; and requiring many types of support in the home.

The relationship between the patient with a chronic illness and the medical providers: Patients' feelings that healthcare providers were frustrated by their patients' chronicity, healthcare staff not properly trained to care for them, the medical model dominance in terms of the many treatments and medications that did not seem to help, poor medical management, and inconsistent treatments.

The stigma associated with chronic illness: Patients' feelings of discrimination and stigmatization, friends and family telling the loved one to try harder, patients labeled as noncompliant by medical and nursing providers of care if they did not or could not follow the regimen, and patients labeled as difficult if they verbalized that the regimen was not working well.

The way that they were labeled or classified: Patients' feelings of being labeled or classified in a certain medical language brought about negativity from the wider global perception, and terms such as *chronic*, *long-standing*, and *long-term* were labels that brought about discrimination against them.

The need for a new definition of chronic illness: Patients' desire for a new definition with a broader perspective on chronic illness and patients' feelings for including the complexity of one's experience in chronic illness.

The essential features of chronic illness for patients: Patients' beliefs that their chronic illness had the following features:

- Ongoing and problematic
- Quality of work compromised
- Relationships compromised
- Lifelong and substantial commitment by caregiver
- Elements of uncertainty
- Expensive treatments and visits to providers
- Incurable
- Untreatable
- Requires complex and ongoing management
- Life threatening
- Unresolved
- Complex
- Permeates the whole of life
- Fatigue

BOX 7.2 ETHICAL FORMATIONS: RESEARCH BRIEF ON CHRONIC ILLNESS: INFORMANTS' VIEWS (continued)

The need for a "health-promoting" definition of chronic illness: Patients' desire for a new "health-promoting" definition to help others understand their difficulties and needs.

Consumers' views that policies should account for chronic illness: Patients' fears that society and the government punished them for their chronic illness.

Chronic illness and activism: Patients' commitment to fight for rights.

Source: From Chronic Illness Alliance. (2002). *Developing a shared definition of chronic illness: The implications and benefits for general practice* (GPEP 843: Final Report). Retrieved from http://www.chronicillness.org.au/reports.htm#shareddefinition

the stigma of chronic illness, and disparities between extending life and the potential consequences to quality of life that results from the ability to extend it.

Patients with chronic illness feel alone and miserable, as Woody Allen so stated about the misery of life, or put another way, the self is suffering and the signs of suffering become evident. Many chronically ill patients often struggle with trying to attach meaning to their suffering through searching their soul, through spirituality, or by just trying to find out why they are the ones having to suffer so much, no matter whether the illness is depression, alcoholism, arthritis, diabetes mellitus, or multiple other conditions.

People suffering with chronic illness have feelings of fear, anxiety, shame, guilt, anger, and depression, all of which may bring them to a belief that they often cause their own suffering (Garrett, 2005). In Box 7.3, the writers of the lyrics of the song "Questions Make Me Free" were conveying the struggle and suffering that conforming to a conventional lifestyle (rite) can bring to people who chronically suffer. These song lyrics are exemplary in revealing how people will hide from themselves and push their own feelings away to avoid the pain and suffering of seeing the reality of themselves.

Ethical Nursing Care for Chronically Ill Patients

How can nurses intervene or help chronically ill patients who are suffering and struggling? Erlen (2002) discussed several ways in which nurses can create an ethical environment for giving care: (1) nurses need to increase their understanding of ethics, (2) nurses need to be advocates for their chronically ill patients, and (3) nurses need to communicate effectively with their patients and with other members of the healthcare team.

The first intervention, increasing their knowledge of ethics, requires that nurses understand the substance and depth of human dignity, respect, autonomy (patient self-determination), beneficence (doing good for the patient), nonmaleficence (doing no harm), and justice (fair treatment). Ways that nurses can increase their

BOX 7.3 ETHICAL FORMATIONS: A SCENARIO OF SUFFERING: "QUESTIONS MAKE ME FREE"

Questions Make Me Free

Lying in bed
Cried to sleep.
Tried to do rite–
It failed ME!

This round world
Looks flat to ME
If U come inside
I know how to hide from ME!
Prayn' it makes sense
Struggling deep inside!
I can't give up now,
But my dreams are running dry!

The answer's all around
But I still can't see.
Loved U so much
Pushed U away
Didn't want U to hurt
The Hurt that's been Killing Me!

Not much time
Gone through hell.
No answers?
But the QUESTION:
Can't U see,
Look in the mirror.
If U find yourself,
You can just be free!
All along it's been RIGHT IN FRONT OF ME!

Source: Lyrics by David and Annie Butts. Copyright 2007.

knowledge and understanding of ethics are by attending ethics conferences, reading, participating in journal ethics clubs in a live or online classroom, completing live or online classroom courses on ethics, and identifying a mentor who has expertise in ethics.

The second intervention involves nurses being advocates for their chronically ill patients. In the Australian research by the Chronic Illness Alliance group

(2002), the predominant echo that infiltrated all of the nine major themes was the need for a clear health-promoting definition of chronic illness so that labeling and stereotyping are avoided. Another strong theme that emerged was that people with chronic illnesses require special attention and understanding at a level that other patients may not require. Building a therapeutic partnership with chronically ill patients serves as an avenue for advocacy. Relationships need to be ongoing and long term in the sense that nurses and patients develop a long, trustworthy relationship. Even though medical management is a concern and sometimes a requirement, patients with chronic illness need emotional support, gentle prodding or teaching, and most of all, the security of knowing that the nurse will be there for them. As Erlen (2002) emphasized, advocacy requires that nurses take a risk in the relationship, a risk in speaking out for their chronically ill patients, and a risk of being caught in the middle of a conflict between the patient and others.

Instead of nurses building a wall of self-protection to avoid personal injury, they need to see the possibilities of "what could be" in the nurse–patient relationship by sensitizing themselves toward the human side of chronically ill person. Experiencing a patients' pain and suffering can sometimes be emotionally and physically draining for a nurse, which brings the advocacy intervention back to nurses and their self-care practices. Rituals of self-care are vital for replenishing physical and emotional energy that is needed in ethical relationships and when being an advocate for chronically ill patients. Garrett (2005) performed ritualistic behaviors to promote self-healing, such as yoga, spiritual meditations, stress-relieving activities, reiki, storytelling, writing, and some other mystical experiences. Nurses can choose their healing ritual for their own soul, but equally important is that nurses need to encourage chronically ill and suffering patients to create some type of ritualistic behaviors for their ongoing healing process.

Communicating effectively, Erlen's (2002) third intervention, relates to nurses being an advocate by conveying the issues and concerns of chronically ill patients to ethics committees, political action groups, professional organizations, and the media. Nurses must speak out about the concerns and issues of chronically ill patients. One such example would be speaking out for improved access to healthcare services and individualized care instead of the band-aid type of care that many patients experience (see Box 7.4).

Organ Transplantation

Every day in the United States, approximately 75 people receive an organ transplant, and another 20 people die while waiting on an organ (U.S. Department of Health and Human Services, 2011). In 1954, a surgeon named Joseph Murray performed the first successful kidney transplant in Boston (President's Council on Bioethics, 2003); in 1990, Murray received a Nobel Prize for Medicine. The first

BOX 7.4 ETHICAL FORMATIONS: A CHRONICALLY ILL MIDDLE-AGED PATIENT

You have a middle-aged female patient, Ms. S., with a 23-year history of crippling rheumatoid arthritis. Ms. S. has returned to the hospital with an injury to her head because she fell. She has no complaints of pain regarding the bump on her head; however, she is suffering with extreme and relentless arthritic pain and has a long history of bilateral swelling of her hands and feet, severe fatigue, intermittent fever, and general aching and pain all over her body. Her hands and feet are crippled from years of inflammation and the erosion of the joints and bones, and therefore she must rely on others for care and support. As her nurse, you see that Ms. S. is suffering to the point that her whole existence seems weakened and compromised. The suffering experience has robbed Ms. S. of joy, contentment, and enthusiasm. In your conversations with her, she related to you that her passion for living is gone and she wants to be free from her burden of suffering.

Explore the feelings that Ms. S. conveyed as one who is chronically ill and experiencing suffering. What are the ethical issues that nurses encounter when they care for chronically ill and suffering patients who are experiencing a predominance of medicalization and medical regimens?

Discuss the moral imperatives that are critical for nurses to practice in the care of chronically ill and suffering patients.

Integrate an ethic of care approach in your plan of care. Discuss ways that you could care for Ms. S. based on your ethical plan.

Explore ways that you could offer support to Ms. S. in terms of nursing and a multidisciplinary approach.

BOX 7.5 ETHICAL FORMATIONS: WOULD YOU CHOOSE THE LION OR SWIM FROM THE CROCODILES?

The First Human Heart Transplant

A heart surgeon named Christiaan Barnard and his 19 team members pushed the medical and scientific limits in 1967 to perform the first human heart transplant. Barnard stated: "On Saturday, I was a surgeon in South Africa, very little known. . . . On Monday, I was world renowned" (para. 4).

Barnard transplanted the heart of a 25-year-old female auto-crash victim into a 55-year-old South African man named Louis Washkansky who at the time was dying of heart disease. For Louis Washkansky, the choice was to live a little longer with the donated heart or die very soon with his diseased heart. Barnard stated:

> For a dying man it is not a difficult decision...because he knows he is at the end. If a lion chases you to the bank of a river filled with crocodiles, you will leap into the water convinced you have a chance to swim to the other side. But you would not accept such odds if there were no lion. (para. 18)

There was success with the surgery. The heart began beating during surgery. Louis Washkansky's prescribed medication for preventing rejection of his "new" heart caused failure of his immune system. He died 18 days after his surgery.

Source: Pioneer heart surgeon Barnard dies. (2001, September 3). *TVNZ.* Retrieved from http://tvnz.co.nz/content/55309/425826/article.html

human heart transplant was performed in 1967 by a surgeon named Christiaan Barnard from Cape Town, South Africa (see Box 7.5).

Organ transplantation is more accepted in the 21st century than it was in the 1950s. The ethical questions regarding removing organs from dead donors then were just as intense and angst-provoking as the ethical questions faced today regarding human cloning. One issue in the 1950s was that, for the first time in history, surgeons were forced to decide criteria for organ recipients in light of a severely sparse supply of organs; in other words, for the first time ever, surgeons were literally choosing who would live and who would die. Another major issue was that many people were dying from organ rejection because of inadequate and harmful antirejection medications. It was not until 1978 that the effective immunosuppressive medication cyclosporin was available for use.

More than 50 years after the first kidney transplant, ethical issues regarding organ donation and transplantation are still debated; however, the issues in the 21st century have shifted to a more diverse set of problems. One major issue is the societal pressure for organ harvesting, resulting from a global demand for organs that far outweighs the supply. Another major issue involves individuals questioning their own moral beliefs about death and the legal definition of death as it relates to organ donation.

Organ Procurement

As of October 2011, there were 112,294 candidates on the waiting list for organs in the United States (United Network for Organ Sharing [UNOS], 2011). There is evidence that people are increasingly refusing to donate their organs, which is one of the reasons for the severe imbalance in supply and demand (Kerridge, Saul, Lowe, McPhee, & Williams, 2002). **Organ procurement** is defined as the obtaining, transferring, and processing of organs for transplantation through systems, organizations, or programs. Organ donation is a delicate subject for most people. The very thought of donating an organ could lead to individuals having disturbing thoughts about their own death or loss of a body part.

To counterbalance the supply–demand crisis, the U.S. Department of Health and Human Services has implemented new programs to increase organ supply. Meanwhile, people continue to die in the United States while on the waiting list for an organ. A societal ethical conflict exists between the national officials' proposals and the values of potential donors. Many program coordinators want to use a utilitarian ethical framework as a basis for setting and accomplishing the goals of increasing organ supply, whereas potential donors, especially in the Western world, value and presently abide by a deontological ethical framework of respect for autonomy and human dignity. With autonomy and decision making as a focus for individuals, utilitarian-based programs find it a challenge to increase the number of organ donors. For a utilitarian approach, some countries use a **presumed consent** approach, meaning that individuals automatically consent to donating their organs unless they specifically indicate otherwise (Brannigan & Boss, 2001). Another approach is **mandated choice**, which means that competent individuals would be required to make a choice as to whether they wanted to become an organ donor on license applications, tax returns, and other official state identification records. Once they decide to become a donor, this mandated choice binds them by way of the cards they signed; however, an advance directive or a written change of mind can reverse that decision.

In the United States, donor cards are a legal, but rarely the sole, document used in the organ donation process. **Donor cards** that are carried by people give permission for the use of their bodily organs in the event of death. Advance directives also are legal documents that are used to express one's desires about organ donation. The UNOS ethics committee has requested that U.S. citizens use a method named **required response**, which means that all adults are required to express their wishes regarding organ donation. At that time, they will be able to object or willingly agree to donate their organs, in addition to having an opportunity to allow a relative to be their designated surrogate.

Death and the Dead Donor Rule

According to the **1981 Uniform Determination of Death Act** (UDDA), **death** is an irreversible cessation of circulatory and respiratory functions or irreversible cessation of all functions of the brain (President's Commission for the Study of Ethical Problems in Medicine and Biomedical and Behavioral Research, 1981). Rubenstein, Cohen, and Jackson (2006) posed the following questions: (1) "Why does having a sound definition of death matter at all?" (2) "What are the human goods at stake in getting this question right?" and (3) "What are the moral hazards in getting it wrong?" (Introduction, para. 5). The medical community has adopted two guiding moral principles, known as the dead donor rule, as the norm for managing potential organ donors. The principles of the **dead donor rule** are: (1) the donor must first be dead before the retrieval of organs, and (2) a person's life and care "must never be compromised in favor of potential organ recipients" (DeGrazia & Mappes, 2001, p. 325).

There are three unresolved ethical debates regarding the retrieval of a person's organs in accordance with the legal definition of death. The issues are: (1) the issue of properly caring for the dying person until death is pronounced, (2) the issue of the well-being of the loved ones who must say goodbye to the dying one, and (3) the issue of the good of the organ donation itself (Rubenstein et al., 2006). The first issue is the assurance of uncompromised and competent care until the person is dead. The dead donor rule, if followed, applies here. Nurses and physicians must first tend to the care of this dying patient, which could mean administering aggressive treatment or affirming that this person's treatment is medically futile.

The second ethical issue is the well-being of families, and an additional concern is the issue of the well-being of healthcare professionals. When the potential donor is declared brain dead, the dead patient continues to remain on a mechanical ventilator as if "still living"—having warm skin and up and down chest movement—and receiving intravenous fluids. Families see this pronounced-dead patient's chest moving up and down and see their still-living loved one. This picture leaves healthcare professionals and families with feelings of ambiguity.

Nurses experience moral distress when they see these types of moral uncertainties. Normally, once a person is declared dead, medical treatment and ventilation support are suspended. Following a declaration of death for potential organ donors, however, providers of care maintain the physical body by way of ventilation and circulatory support until the organ procurement team can harvest the organs. The procurement teams, well trained in their field, tread on morally shaky ground with families of a newly pronounced-dead loved one. Approaching the grieving family at this time is difficult, even when the team just needs to confirm the patient's or family's wish of wanting to donate the organs. Sometimes the person's death will have occurred suddenly, such as in car accidents or other injuries, and families must have time to sort out or come to terms with the death of their loved one.

A point that Rubenstein et al. (2006) made was, "these final moments of life and first moments of death *belong* to the grieving at least as much as to the departed person" (Introduction, para. 7), yet this same window of time also belongs to the procurement team and surgeons. The procurement team needs to act quickly to remove the organs and deliver them to the unknown beneficiary. The ethical issue involved here is the risk of causing harm to the families when there has not been sufficient time given for them to grieve and process the information versus the risk of not having viable organs if the families wait too long to come to terms with the death.

The third issue involves the good of organ donation itself. From one perspective, the donation of organs can give death a certain degree of meaning, allowing a last act of benevolence and selflessness. An example could be the parents' wish to donate their newly brain-dead child's organs as an imagined way to carry on that child's life. From another perspective, patients who preregister their desires to be a donor have autonomy and self-determination. The procurement team often views itself as an advocate for carrying out the patient's wish after death, which actually goes beyond the principle of autonomy in health care; however, this view of autonomy and beneficence for the recipient, or the releasing of the dead person's organs for the good of another person, is a widely accepted utilitarianism paradigm in society.

There is an intensely debated ethical issue surrounding the dead donor rule and its legitimacy in today's society: Is the dead donor rule outdated? Alan Shewmon (2004; as cited in Rubenstein et al., 2006) clarified his latest thoughts on death as an unreal and unknowing ontological (study of being or existence) event that is without significant meaning, especially when society defines a person as dead by the legal standard that humans created in the last 26 years. Shewmon stated:

> "Is the patient dead?" is not only the wrong question to ask on the practical, physical level; it is not even a meaningful one when asked on a microscopic time-scale in the transition between life and death. This would be like zooming in on the prismatic spectrum midway between green and blue, and demanding that someone not only identify that point unequivocally as either "green" or "blue" but also have a convincing, logical rationale for doing so. (p. 292)

Many bioethicists are attempting to define death as an event versus death as a process as they grapple with expanding the utilitarianism perspective to overturn the dead donor rule so that organs can be retrieved from patients who have no higher brain function. Examples include patients with only lower brain (and no higher brain) function, such as those in a persistent vegetative state (PVS) like Terri Schiavo and babies born with anencephaly. Patients with no higher brain function, such as patients in a PVS, have an intact brain stem and usually breathe without the assistance of mechanical ventilation.

Pronouncing dead those patients with a functioning brain stem but without higher brain functioning would be a complete ontological shift in how society views death. Overturning the dead donor rule and retrieving organs from patients who are still alive by the UDDA definition of death would be a utilitarian ethical framework when viewed from the perspective of longer-term quality of life and the number of people that could be saved—for example, one person's organs may save three or four people. For patients in a PVS, higher brain functioning does not exist. For anencephalic babies, there is usually very little, if any, higher brain function. Society must answer these questions:

1. If the dead donor rule changes so that organ teams can harvest organs from patients without higher brain function—only lower brain function—how will the definition of death change to include these patients?
2. Do patients without higher brain function, but who are not dead by the current legal definition of death, have full moral standing?
3. If persons can breathe on their own, such as those in a PVS, could they ever be dead as defined by a new legal definition of death?

Society must also reckon with the utilitarian morality of a dead person's organs being good for several people versus being good for only one family. Finally, society needs to search for what death really means in terms of the moral imperative of doing good for others versus acting within moral limits and respecting *primum non nocere* (first do no harm).

Non-Heart-Beating Organ Donors

Organ donation was originally based on the principle of procuring organs from cadavers. A **non-heart-beating donor (NHBD)** is one whose heart has ceased at the time that the organ is retrieved. There are two types. **Controlled NHBDs** are donors who are maintained on mechanical ventilation until their organs are harvested; many times, these donors have advance directives. **Uncontrolled NHBDs** are donors who have a cardiorespiratory arrest outside the hospital and cannot be resuscitated but have a declaration of death prior to retrieval of their organs. There are two critical NHBD protocols that physicians must follow: there can be no discussion with family members about organ donation or the consent process before the decision has been made by everyone concerned to withdraw life support, and the physician who declares death cannot be linked with any organ recovery agency, transplant team, or recovery team (UNOS, 2011). Nurses must adhere to the first protocol.

Social Justice and Organ Transplantation

Social justice is a consideration that cannot be overlooked in the face of scarce healthcare resources and an especially scarce supply of organs (Gillett, 2000). The ethical question is twofold: How are people chosen for the organ "wait list," and how are they chosen to receive the organ? Gillett stated:

> Our ability to act for the benefit of any given individual must be tempered by the requirements of justice. If there is one kidney and more than one possible recipient, some basis has to be found to make the choice between recipients. It is tempting to believe that there must be some ethical way of regulating such choices....The obvious way is to accept the principle of first-come first-served. (p. 249)

First-come, first-served may not be an adequate guideline for many people because this method would not address the sickest people first; rather, it is based on a fairness principle. Organ coordinators face complex decisions regarding the allocation of organs, deciding who gets the organ, and then justifying that decision. The sickest patients have many more complications and suffer more; however, if they are chosen first, as they often have been in the past, their success rate with the new organ may not be as good as that of a recipient chosen based on other criteria. The approach of using the sickest patients first is a medical entitlement method, similar to that of medical emergency department triage.

Trying to select organ recipients based on social worth, self-destructive behavior, and a potential for rehabilitation is difficult to justify from an ethical perspective. One example of a self-destructive behavior is chronic smoking. Suppose there is a chronic smoker who needs a lung transplant. Would the organ team determine that this smoker is not as worthy to live or to receive an organ as another potential recipient because the person smokes? Is this not a value judgment?

If potential recipients were chosen from a utilitarian–consequential perspective, they would receive an organ based on their potential for longer-term survival with a higher quality of life. Gillett (2000) stated about utilitarianism: "Every individual should count for one and nobody for more than one....The more one debates the issue, the more it seems the only fair way to determine how to distribute scarce resources" (p. 249).

Nurses and Organ Donors

Nurses coordinate and give care to potential organ donors, recipients, and their families, and the organ procurement teams consist of nurses, surgeons, and other healthcare professionals. According to the *Code of Ethics for Nurses*, nurses work within a moral framework of good personal character to promote the principle of beneficence. Refer to Box 7.6 for essential aspects of the ANA *Code of Ethics for*

BOX 7.6 ETHICAL FORMATIONS: ESSENTIAL ASPECTS FROM THE *CODE OF ETHICS FOR NURSES WITH INTERPRETIVE STATEMENTS FOR CARE OF ADULT PATIENTS*

An individual's lifestyle, value system, and religious beliefs should be considered in planning care with and for each patient. (1.2, p. 7)

Nurses actively participate in assessing and ensuring the responsible and appropriate use of interventions in order to minimize unwarranted or unwanted treatment and patient suffering. (1.3, p. 8)

Support of autonomy in the broadest sense also includes recognition that people of some cultures place less weight on individualism and more value in deferring decisions to family members. (1.4, p. 9)

Respect not just for the specific decision, but also for the patient's method of decision making, is consistent with the principle of autonomy. (1.4, p. 9)

Nursing holds a fundamental commitment to the uniqueness of the individual patient; therefore, any plan of care must reflect that uniqueness. (2.1, p. 9)

Moral respect accords moral worth and dignity to all human beings irrespective of their personal attributes or life situation. Such respect extends to oneself as well; the same duties that we owe to others we owe to ourselves. (5.1, p. 18)

For the nurse, virtues and excellences are those habits that affirm and promote the values of human dignity, well-being, respect, health, independence, and other values central to nursing. (6.1, p. 20)

All nurses, regardless of role, have a responsibility to create, maintain, and contribute to environments of practice that support nurses in fulfilling their ethical obligations. (6.2, p. 21)

The nurse should affirm human dignity and show respect for the values and practices associated with different cultures and use approaches to care that reflect awareness and sensitivity. (8.2, p. 24)

Nurses that apply to the care of adult patients. Most of the time, nurses want to have a sense of satisfaction based on their belief that they promote human good, preserve their patients' dignity as much as possible, and maintain a caring environment. Nurses in intensive care units and on transplant teams coordinate organ donations and transplants on a daily basis. The psychosocial impact and outcome of the organ transplantation process for donors, donor families, and recipients are unique.

Pearson, Robertson-Malt, Walsh, and Fitzgerald (2001) conducted a study of the attitudes of intensive care nurses toward brain-dead organ donors. Two major themes of caring that emerged from the study were the family and the nurse.

The Family

Of central importance to the nurses in the study was meeting the needs of their patients' families. Some important considerations for nursing care of donor family members are:

Prioritizing the family's needs
Empathizing with the family's tragedy
Supporting the family's decisions
Realizing that caring for the patient shows care for the family
Encouraging space and privacy for the family to grieve, say their goodbyes, and, hopefully, accept the situation
Not intruding on the family's grief (Pearson et al., 2001, p. 135)

The Nurse

A challenge for intensive care nurses is finding meaning in the case of each brain-dead patient, including the potential donors (Pearson et al., 2001). In this study, nurses stated that brain-dead patients should be treated as if they were alive because this action shows respect for the patients and their families, and they were adamant that family members must be shown respect and kindness. A compassionate way to show ultimate kindness is to give excellent care to the families' loved ones.

In the midst of giving competent care, tending to family needs, and providing much-needed emotional support, nurses tend to become emotionally drained from feeling a need to clarify the definition of brain death and other medical terms to the families. Nurses also feel emotional strain in regard to their own ambiguities about the definition of brain death. With the ever-increasing organ procurement system, nurses find themselves experiencing moral suffering because of internal moral conflicts regarding the uncertainties of life and death. If nurses take advantage of extra education on organ transplantation nursing care and grieving families, they may be better prepared for managing their own personal emotions and those of families in crisis.

CASE STUDY: WHO WILL RECEIVE THE LIVER?

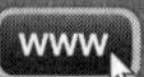

Mr. Mann, 50 years old, has been a heavy drinker since high school and has end-stage liver disease (ESLD) due to alcoholic cirrhosis. He will soon die if he does not receive a liver. He has been unemployed for years, even before his illness, and has received state financial assistance. Mr. Mann has stated that once he receives his new liver he will try to quit drinking on a long-term basis, but will make no promises. He is not drinking now because he is in the hospital and knows he must remain abstinent for a period of time before the actual organ transplant and during the recovery process. Mr. Mann is divorced, lives alone, and has two sons who are married and working. Mr. Mann and his two sons are not on good terms.

Mrs. Bay, 37 years old, has ESLD due to hepatitis B. Mrs. Bay is a wife and a mother of two children, one who is 16 years old and the other 12. The family is well known and active in the community. The family members have a great relationship. The children have stated that they do not want to lose their mother but Mrs. Bay is very sick, though not in the hospital. At this time, Mrs. Bay experiences days when she feels critically sick and cannot move from the bed. Other days are a little better. Her prognosis is grave while she waits for a liver. She is ahead of Mr. Mann on the "wait list."

Based on your knowledge of the two diseases, you know that alcoholic cirrhosis patients with new livers may have a better success rate and longer life than do those suffering from hepatitis B, despite the fact that recovering alcoholics may have a high recidivism (relapsing to old behavior) rate. Giving hepatitis B patients new livers is controversial, and the success rate is varied. Mr. Mann is at the maximum end of the age range for organ recipients (usually age 50 or more).

Case Study Questions

Explore all situations between the two organ candidates. Whom do you choose? Give a full justification for choosing your candidate for the liver. You could briefly search the Internet regarding qualification criteria for organ recipients. Then you could search for these two diseases—alcoholic cirrhosis and hepatitis B—on past success rates of organ transplantation in similar patients. Think about the following ranking criteria for allocating organs, some of which are discussed in this chapter:

The sickest patients: Medical entitlement method

First-come, first-served: Fairness principle

Social worth principle: A method of placing more value on some people and not on others because of certain individual characteristics

Best success rate and long-term outcome: Utilitarian-consequential perspective

Proximity: Location in relation to the area of the hospital where the organ will be transplanted (immediate area, county, region). What about the United States versus another country?

KEY POINTS

- The traditional concept of medicalization from the 1970s, in what was known as the "golden age of doctoring," and three market-driven forces have caused the physician's role to shift from one of dominance (in the 1970s) to one of more deference that borders on subordinate.
- The three forces that contributed to this medical paradigm shift were managed care, biotechnology, and consumers. With the shift, patients now think like consumers as they cleverly choose types of medical services and physicians and select the types of insurance policies they want.
- The ethical issue of promoting healthy behaviors, yet trying to respect one's rights to self-determination, is a catch-22 situation. An ethical question to consider is: How far should providers of care go in terms of respecting the self-determination of patients when some noncompliant behaviors can cost society a great deal of money and resources?
- Under the umbrella of medicalization are the concepts of compliance, adherence, and concordance.
- Chronic illness includes concepts such as suffering, labeling, isolation, and loneliness associated with long-standing disease.
- The Chronic Illness Alliance research in 2002 began developing a newly expanded definition of chronic illness, one that would include health-promoting concepts.
- Ethical nursing care for chronically ill patients involves themes from Erlen's (2002) thoughts on creating an ethical environment: (1) nurses need to increase their understanding of ethics, (2) nurses need to be advocates for their chronically ill patients, and (3) nurses need to communicate effectively with their patients and with other members of the healthcare team.
- There is a supply-and-demand crisis for organ donation. Utilitarian-based programs to increase the number of organs remain challenged.
- Expert bioethicists continue to debate the pros and cons of altering the dead donor rule so that patients who have lower brain function, but no higher brain function, can be considered potential organ donors.
- To provide ethical care regarding organ procurement and transplantation, nurses need to consider the methods of organ procurement, the dead donor rule, and the three unresolved ethical debates regarding the retrieval of a person's organs: the legal definition of death, non-heart-beating organ donors, and social justice regarding organ transplantation.

References

American Nurses Association. (2001). *Code of ethics for nurses with interpretive statements.* Silver Spring, MD: Author.

Barofsky, L. (1978). Compliance, adherence, and the therapeutic alliance: Steps in the development of self-care. *Social Science and Medicine, 12*, 369–376.

Berg, J., Evangelista, L. S., & Dunbar-Jacob, J. M. (2002). Compliance. In I. M. Lubkin & P. D. Larsen (Eds.), *Chronic illness: Impact and interventions* (5th ed.) (pp. 203–232). Sudbury, MA: Jones and Bartlett.

Booth, F. W., Gordon, S. E., Carlson, C. J., & Hamilton, M. T. (2000). Waging war on modern chronic diseases: Primary prevention through exercise biology. *Journal of Applied Physiology, 88*, 774–787.

Brannigan, M. C., & Boss, J. A. (2001). *Healthcare ethics in a diverse society.* Mountain View, CA: Mayfield.

Butts, D., & Butts, A. (2007). Song lyrics: Questions make me free. Personal collection. Hattiesburg, Mississippi.

Chronic Illness Alliance. (2002). *Developing a shared definition of chronic illness: The implications and benefits for general practice* (GPEP 843: Final Report). Retrieved from http://www.chronicillness.org.au/reports.htm#shareddefinition

Chronic Illness Alliance. (2011). *Chronic illness.* Retrieved from http://www.chronicillness.org.au/

Conrad, P. (2007). *The medicalization of society: On the transformation of human conditions into treatable disorders.* Baltimore, MD: The Johns Hopkins University Press.

DeGrazia, D., & Mappes, T. A. (2001). *Biomedical ethics* (5th ed.) Boston, MA: McGraw-Hill.

Erlen, J. A. (2002). Ethics in chronic illness. In I. M. Lubkin & P. D. Larsen (Eds.), *Chronic illness: Impact and interventions* (5th ed.) (pp. 407–430). Sudbury, MA: Jones and Bartlett.

Galanti, G. A. (2004). *Caring for patients from different cultures* (3rd ed.). Philadelphia, PA: University of Pennsylvania Press.

Garrett, C. (2005). *Gut feelings: Chronic illness and the search for healing* (At the Interface/Probing the Boundaries series, Vol. 16). Amsterdam, Netherlands: Rodopi.

Gillett, G. (2000). Ethics and images in organ transplantation. In P. T. Trzepacz & A. F. DiMartini (Eds.), *The transplant patient: Biological, psychiatric, and ethical issues in organ transplantation* (pp. 239–254). Cambridge, UK: Cambridge University Press.

Horne, R., Weinman, J., Barber, N., Elliott, R., & Morgan, M. (2005, December). Concordance, adherence and compliance in medicine taking. *Report for the national co-ordinating centre for NHS service delivery and organisation R & D (NCCSDO).* Retrieved from http://www.medslearning.leeds.ac.uk/pages/documents/useful_docs/76-final-report%5B1%5D.pdf

Illich, I. (1975/2010). The medicalization of life. *Limits to medicine—Medical nemesis: The exploration of health* (Chap. 2, pp. 39–125). London, UK: Marion Boyars.

International Council of Nurses. (2006). *ICN code of ethics for nurses.* Geneva, Switzerland: Author.

Kerridge, I. H., Saul, P., Lowe, M., McPhee, J., & Williams, D. (2002). Death, dying and donation: Organ transplantation and the diagnosis of death. *Journal of Medical Ethics, 28*, 89–94.

Pearson, A., Robertson-Malt, S., Walsh, K., & Fitzgerald, M. (2001). Intensive care nurses' experiences of caring for brain dead organ donor patients. *Journal of Clinical Nursing, 10*, 132–139.

Pioneer heart surgeon Barnard dies. TVNZ. (2001, September 3). *TVNZ*. Retrieved from http://tvnz.co.nz/content/55309/425826/article.html

President's Commission for the Study of Ethical Problems in Medicine and Biomedical and Behavioral Research. (1981). *Defining death*. Washington, DC: Government Printing Office.

President's Council on Bioethics. (2003, January). *Organ transplantation: Ethical dilemmas and policies*. Retrieved from http://ia410331.us.archive.org/peth04/20041015170807/http://bioethics.gov/background/org_transplant.html

Rubenstein, A., Cohen, E., & Jackson, E. (2006, September). *PCBE: The definition of death and the ethics of organ procurement from the deceased*. Washington, DC: PCBE. Retrieved from http://permanent.access.gpo.gov/lps92742/rubenstein.html

Russell, S., Daly, J., Hughes, E., & Hoog, C. (2003). Nurses and "difficult" patients: Negotiating non-compliance. *Journal of Advanced Nursing, 43*(3), 281–287.

Shewmon, D. A. (2004). The dead donor rule: Lessons from linguistics. *Kennedy Institute of Ethics Journal, 14*(3), 277–300.

United Network for Organ Sharing. (2011). *Organ donation and transplantation*. Retrieved from http://www.unos.org

U.S. Department of Health and Human Services. (2011). *The need is real data: Data*. Retrieved from http://www.organdonor.gov/aboutStatsFacts.asp

For a full suite of assignments and additional learning activities, use the access code located in the front of your book to visit this exclusive website: http://go.jblearning.com/butts. If you do not have an access code, you can obtain one at the site.

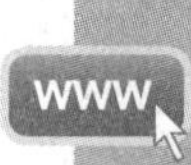

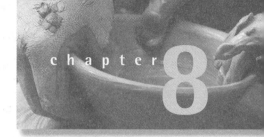

chapter 8

Ethics and the Nursing Care of Elders

Karen L. Rich

At first, people wanted to help the old ones in any way they could, but the women would not allow too much assistance, for they enjoyed their newly found independence. So the people showed respect for the two women by listening to what they had to say.

—*Velma Wallis*, Two Old Women: An Alaska Legend of Betrayal, Courage, and Survival, *1993, p. 135*

OBJECTIVES

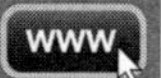

After reading this chapter, the reader should be able to:

1. Define ageism.
2. Identify factors that influence elders' experiences of living meaningful lives.
3. Discuss the principle of autonomy as it relates to the ethical care of elders.
4. Assess the range of paternalism as it relates to ethical nursing practice.
5. Discriminate between different levels of moral agency.
6. Discuss different perspectives about quality-of-life assessments.
7. Identify the signs of elder abuse and appropriate nursing interventions.
8. Discuss the ANA's *Code of Ethics for Nurses* in relation to the nursing care of elders.

Aging in America

The President's Council on Bioethics (2005) proposed that "we are on the threshold of a 'mass geriatric society,' a society of more long-lived individuals than ever before in human history" (p. xvii). People are living longer and healthier lives due to the technological advances that have occurred in medicine and public health during the last century. According to the U.S. Census Bureau (2011), there were approximately 50 million Americans over the age of 62 in 2010, which represents an increase of 21.1% since 2000. The number of people 100 years of age and over increased 5.8% between 2000 and 2010. Although the quantity of human life years has been extended, questions remain about how the quality of those years is threatened by chronic debilitating conditions, ageism, and limited support and resources for elders and their caregivers.

Often, chronic conditions such as cerebrovascular disease and Alzheimer's disease cause elders to lose their most crucial link with others: their voice within society. A loss of voice to express their individual feelings, desires, and needs is arguably one of the most profound causes of isolation for elders (Smith, Kotthoff-Burrell, & Post, 2002). Considerations about the loss of the voice of elderly persons and diminished societal recognition of the meaningfulness of their lives underlie many of the ethical issues discussed in this chapter. A large portion of elder-focused ethics is based on the relationships that elders have with other people in society, including their families and healthcare professionals. Often, the lives of elders are "set aside" from the lives of other adults in communities. It is this overall view of separateness among generations that makes it necessary to study elder-focused ethics.

Ageism, a way of thinking that was originally described by Butler (1975), has influenced some people within society to view elders as fundamentally different from others; consequently, some people cease to identify elders as normal human beings (Agich, 2003). Just as racism and sexism describe the stereotyping of and discrimination against people because of their skin color or gender, **ageism** involves the same type of negative perceptions toward older adults based on age. Ageism perpetuates the idea that elders as a population are cognitively impaired, "set in their ways," and "old-fashioned" in regard to their morals and abilities (Agich, 2003; Butler, 1975).

It probably is disquieting to elders when they realize how youth oriented Western society is today. One can see that the media's target audience is most often young adults and the financially affluent, young, middle-aged population. Media emphasis is placed on having beautiful bodies even if expensive elective surgery is needed to do so. Pictures of beautiful and famous young people and couples are prominently displayed on magazine covers, and young athletes are revered in Western society. Older actors, and particularly actresses, lament the lack of "good roles" for them in the movie industry. It is not surprising that as people age, they often become despondent about the losses that they experience in regard to their appearance and physical abilities. The seemingly vital, active, and glamorous lives of the young people portrayed in the media serve as a stark contrast to what many elderly persons may be experiencing. Agich (2003) proposed that "a society that values productivity and material wealth above other values is understandably youth oriented; a natural consequence is that the old come to be seen, and to see themselves, as obsolete and redundant" (p. 54).

So, who are the elders in today's society? Savishinsky (1991) stated:

> The class of the elderly includes both the rich and poor, sick and well, sane and insane; it also embraces the relatively healthy so-called young old between 60 and 75 and the more vulnerable old old who are living beyond their eighth decade. Some are intimately connected with family and community, whereas others are cut off from their kin. Some are active and ardent; others are disengaged and hopeless. (p. 2)

In the late 1700s and early 1800s, old people were encouraged to view their lives as a pilgrimage and to prepare for death while still participating in service to family and community. However, starting around the 1850s, societies began to instill the belief that thoughts about death should be avoided. The emphasis changed to a focus on valuing "the virtues of youth rather than age, the new rather than the old, self-reliance and autonomy rather than community" (Callahan, 1995, p. 39).

These views formed the foundation of the beginning of ageism in the 20th century. The realities of old age were not consistent with the new world view of the morality of self-control and autonomy; rather, the decay inherent in aging was associated with dependence and failure. Though ageism began to be a general social theme after World War II, today it may be focused more on elderly persons who are disabled (Cohen, 1988).

The lives of people of all ages are overshadowed by an awareness of their eventual aging and death, and it is during one's later years that these issues can no longer be ignored. When one actually does confront the facts of unavoidable aging and death, the mysteries involved can be startling. The feminist philosopher Simone de Beauvoir (1972) proposed that "the old are invisible because we see death with a clearer eye than old age itself" (p. 4). Agich (2003) interpreted this statement to mean that old people are set apart from the rest of society because people tend to look beyond the elderly persons themselves, who they perceive as close to death, and instead see the prospects of their own death.

Moody (1992) proposed that the modern advances in biomedical technology that have facilitated longer lives for many elderly persons have made it necessary to confront critical ethical questions that society may want to ignore. These questions involve dilemmas about death and dying, the perception of what is meant by quality of life, and judgments about the mental and physical functional capacity of old adults. Moody questioned whether the typical models and approaches to bioethics based on rights and duties fit well with considerations of ethics and aging. He asked the question, "What ethical ideals are appropriate for an aging society?" (p. 243).

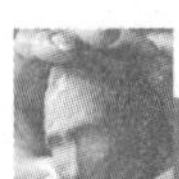

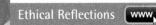

Ethical Reflections www

- Can an ethicist or nurse simply apply the bioethical principles of autonomy, beneficence, nonmaleficence, and justice to situations involving elderly patients? Why or why not? What is a good approach to elder-focused ethics?
- How can nurses combat ageism in their local, state, and national communities?
- Do you believe that ageism is based solely on age or on the degree of an elderly person's disability? On socioeconomic level? Explain the rationale for your beliefs.

According to Moody, focusing on individual autonomy and justice between generations will not provide people with the desired ethical model for engaging in relationships with elders. Elder-focused ethics includes negotiation and a foundation in the virtues. Principles and rules also must be included, but principles and rules can thwart desired ends if the practical wisdom and good character of caregivers are not emphasized as a part of the overall scheme of ethics.

Life Meaning and Significance

Once, while Mahatma Gandhi's train was pulling slowly out of the station, a European reporter ran up to his compartment window. "Do you have a message I can take back to my people?" he asked. It was Gandhi's day of silence, a vital respite from his demanding speaking schedule, so he didn't reply. Instead, he scrawled a few words on a scrap of paper and passed it to the reporter: "My life is my message."

—*E.* EASWARAN, YOUR LIFE IS YOUR MESSAGE, *1992,* P. *1*

The issues of autonomy, vulnerability, dependency, and good relationships are important when considering ethics and elders. However, there is another issue that is important to the moral world of elders and those with whom they relate: elderly persons' own feelings about the significance and meaning of their lives. According to Callahan (1995), underlying the strong desire by society and scientists to abolish the biology of aging is "a profound failure of meaning" (p. 39).

As people age, often they begin to realize the truth of Gandhi's words—that their life is their message—but does Western society support elders reflecting on the meaning and significance of their lives? In earlier times, tradition was highly valued by society, and the meaning and significance of elderly persons' lives were viewed differently than they are today in our culturally and morally diverse society (Callahan, 1995). In the past, elders had an elevated status in communities because their wisdom was prized for its own sake and because their wisdom placed them in a special position of being called on to perpetuate and interpret societal moral traditions.

The diverse moral views of current Western culture sometimes undermine the community-wide role of elderly persons in passing on moral traditions; therefore, one of the traditional societal purposes for elders has diminished. Today, elderly persons are important to businesses if they are financially well off, to families if they are willing and able to provide care for grandchildren and financial support, to politicians as a voting block, and to nonprofit agencies as volunteers (Callahan,

1995). Some people believe that these roles for elders make older persons valuable within society. However, upon closer inspection, one can determine that it is not age that is held in high regard, but the accidental features of old age such as disposable income and free time.

According to Cole (1986), meaning is "an intuitive expression of one's overall appraisal of living. Existentially, meaning refers to lived perceptions of coherence, sense, or significance, in experiences" (p. 4). Callahan (1995) described meaning as an inner feeling supported by "some specifiable traditions, beliefs, concepts or ideas, that one's life" has purpose and is well structured in "relating the inner self and the outer world—and that even in the face of aging and death, it is a life which makes sense to oneself; that is, one can give a plausible, relatively satisfying account" (p. 33). Callahan described significance as "the social attribution of value to old age, that it has a sturdy and cherished place in the structure of society and politics, and provides a coherence among the generations that is understood to be important if not indispensable" (p. 33).

Nurses may question why it is relevant to nursing ethics for them to consider elderly persons' pursuit of life meaning and significance. The answer is that nursing ethics is first and foremost about relationships, alleviating patients' suffering, and facilitating patients' well-being. In relation to elders, nursing ethics also is focused on helping elderly persons find and keep their voice or means of expressing their values and feelings. Finding meaning and significance alleviates suffering and promotes well-being for many elderly persons (see Box 8.1).

The Search for Meaning

The Viennese neurologist and psychiatrist, Viktor Frankl (1905–1997), wrote the influential book *Man's Search for Meaning*, which was originally published in 1959. Over 10 million copies of this book have been sold, and it was rated as one of the 10 most influential books read by respondents in a survey conducted by the Library of Congress (Greening, 1998). The book is about how Frankl found meaning in his

BOX 8.1 ETHICAL FORMATIONS: DISCOVERING MEANING

In the story *The Fall of Freddie the Leaf*, a leaf named Freddie questioned a wise older leaf, Daniel, about life and its meaning. When Daniel told Freddie that all of the leaves on their tree and even the tree itself would eventually die, Freddie asked, "Then what has been the reason for all of this? Why were we here at all if we only have to fall and die?"

Daniel answered, "It's been about the sun and the moon. It's been about happy times together. It's been about the shade and the old people and the children [that sat and played beneath the tree]. It's been about colors in Fall. It's been about seasons. Isn't that enough?"

Source: Buscaglia, L. (1982). *The fall of Freddie the leaf: A story of life for all ages.* Thorofare, NJ: Charles B. Slack, pp. 19–20.

experiences in Auschwitz and other concentration camps during World War II. In the preface to the third edition of the book, Allport (1984) stated that Frankl proposed that "to live is to suffer, to survive is to find meaning in the suffering. If there is a purpose in life at all, there must be a purpose in suffering and in dying" (p. 9).

Frankl (1959/1984) suggested that meaning is the primary motivation in the lives of humans. He determined that the last of his human freedoms in the concentration camp was to choose his attitude toward his suffering. Being in a concentration camp was an unchangeable situation for Frankl, as are the facts that aging will happen to all people who do not die young and that all people will eventually die. It is in continuing to choose to find meaning in the circumstances that people encounter as their life stories are created and unfold that will eventually form the fabric of a meaningful life when people are old.

Frankl (1959/1984) believed that the transitoriness, or fleeting nature, of life, similar to what Buddhists call impermanence, must not be denied by persons who are interested in putting the search for meaning at the center of their lives. Rather, even suffering and dying can be actualizing experiences. Though no one can supply another person's life meaning, nurses can help elderly people on their journey through life by helping them to discover meaning in their lives and to feel that they are significant members of communities.

Updating the Eriksonian Life Cycle

In exploring the moral treatment of elderly persons, Callahan (1995) proposed that the search for common meaning in aging requires a consideration of the updated theory of the life cycle as elaborated by Erik Erikson. Erikson's book, *The Life Cycle Completed*, first published in 1982, emphasized that all eight stages of the Eriksonian life cycle cannot be distinctly separated, but are interrelated. After Erikson's death at age 91, his wife Joan used her own ideas and notes written by her husband to update the book. She proposed a ninth stage of development and addressed other issues related to old-old people. Joan Erikson was in her 90s when she wrote this updated book, and she used her voice to speak for many old-old people about their experiences.

The ninth stage of the life cycle is an extension of the eighth stage, which is a time that elders develop to some degree either despair and disgust or integrity. Wisdom is the strength or virtue that some elders depend on to successfully navigate both the eighth and ninth stages of development. The ninth stage is the stage of the lived experiences of persons in their eighth or ninth decade of life. The following are some of the difficulties that occur in the ninth stage that make wisdom and integrity hard for elders to achieve (Erikson & Erikson, 1997):

- Wisdom requires the senses of sight and hearing to see, hear, and remember. Integrity is compared with tact (as in the word *intact*), which is related to touch. In their 90s, elderly persons often lose or have impaired senses of sight, hearing, and touch.

- When persons reach the age of late 80s or enter the decade of their 90s, despair may occur because people realize that life is too short now to try to make up for missed opportunities.
- Despair may occur because the old-old person is just trying to "get through the day" because of their physical limitations, even without the added burdens of regrets about one's earlier life. When persons believe that their lives are not what they wished them to be, the despair is deepened.
- Persons in their 80s and 90s are likely to have experienced losses of relationships to a greater degree than at any other age. In addition to the suffering directly related to these losses, suffering is generated when the person realizes that "death's door is open and not so far away." (p. 113)

Like virtue ethicists who have drawn connections between the "good life" and being a vital member of a community (Blum, 1994; MacIntyre, 1984), Joan Erikson (1997) said that her husband, Erik, often proposed that the life cycle cannot be appropriately understood if it is not viewed within a social context or in terms of the community in which it is actually lived. The Eriksons' belief that individuals and society are interrelated and that people are constantly involved with the give and take of a dynamic community is a key position of communitarian ethicists today. When society lacks a sound ideal of old age, a holistic view of life is not well integrated into communities. If elders are excluded from the valued members of a community, they are often viewed as the embodiment of shame instead of the embodiment of wisdom.

Joan Erikson was convinced that if persons in their 80s and 90s had developed hope and trust in earlier life stages, they would be able to move further down the path to gerotranscendence, a concept she borrowed from the work of Lars Tornstam. Transcendence means "to rise above or go beyond a limit, [to] exceed, [to] excel" (Erikson & Erikson, 1997, p. 124). Erikson described the experiences of gerotranscendent individuals as:

- Feeling a cosmic union with the universal spirit
- Perceiving time as being limited to now or maybe only next week; otherwise the future is misty
- Feeling that the dimensions of space have been decreased to the perimeter of what the person's physical capabilities allow
- Feeling that death is a sustaining presence for the person and viewing death as being "the way of all living things" (p. 124)
- Having an expanded sense of self that includes "a wider range of interrelated others" (p. 124)

Erikson then activated the word transcendence into the word transcen*dance* to associate its meaning with the arts and specifically "the dance of life [that] can

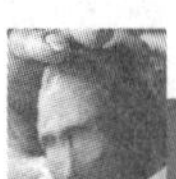

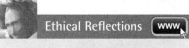

Ethical Reflections www

- In what ways does society perpetuate elders being viewed as the embodiment of shame?
- Joan Erikson said "to grow old is a great privilege" (Erikson & Erikson, 1997, p. 128). How can nurses help elderly persons realize this privilege?

transport us into all realms of making and doing with every item of body, mind, and spirit involved" (p. 127).

Moral Agency

It is generally believed that elders are a vulnerable population because of the natural progression toward frailty that occurs with aging. Because of this vulnerability, moral agency is a key consideration in relationships with elders. The ability to make deliberate choices and to act deliberately in regard to important life experiences that affect the suffering and well-being of sentient beings, including oneself, refers to a person's moral agency. **Moral agency** implies that people are responsible for their beliefs and actions. Arguments about moral agency generally result from debates about a person's mental capacity in regard to decision making. Referring to whether the person is or is not autonomous usually is at the heart of the debate.

Decisional Capacity

Decisional capacity or incapacity is the ability or inability to come to what most adults would consider to be reasonable conclusions or resolutions. Decisional capacity can generally be equated with the concept of competence, though competence has more of a legal connotation, as it is closely tied to formal situations that legally require informed consent. Questions of decisional capacity and competence are associated most often with the three populations of "(a) mentally disabled persons, (b) cognitively impaired elderly persons, and (c) children" (Stanley, Sieber, & Melton, 2003, p. 398). Decisional capacity in regard to minor children and mentally disabled persons is discussed in Chapters 10 and 5, respectively.

There is no one set of published criteria to be used in all assessments of decisional capacity and competence. A method cited by Beauchamp and Childress (2009) is unique because it includes a range of the inabilities that someone who is incompetent would exhibit as opposed to being based on the person's actual abilities. The standards begin by describing the behaviors that persons with the least competence exhibit and moves toward those standards that require higher ability. The standards are:

- Inability to express or communicate a preference or choice
- Inability to understand one's situation and its consequences
- Inability to understand relevant information
- Inability to give a reason
- Inability to give a rational reason (although some supporting reasons may be given)

- Inability to give risk- or benefit-related reasons (although some rational supporting reasons may be given)
- Inability to reach a reasonable decision (as judged, for example, by a reasonable person's standard) (pp. 114–115)

Nurses must be sensitive to the fact that vulnerable and dependent elderly patients often are assumed to be mentally incapacitated or incompetent based on faulty impressions and ageism. When ungrounded assumptions are made based on a person's frail appearance, for example, elderly patients can be left out of the process of decision making that is important to their well-being. Elders who are physically frail may not be included in making decisions ranging from deciding when they want to take their bath in a long-term care facility to healthcare professionals aiding family members in legally taking away the older person's decisional capacity for treatment options and the management of their financial affairs.

Though in most cases family members have ethical motives when caring for elderly family members, this is not always the case. Occasionally, family members and caregivers are more interested in their own self-serving desires than the well-being of an elder when the family or caregivers want to deem the elder as incompetent. Biased decisions, which are intentional or unintentional, may be based on a desire to gain or maintain access to an elder's money or on feelings of disgust or exasperation. Nurses must be cautiously and wisely alert when assessing patients and situations that affect determinations of elders' decisional capacity. As directed in the *Code of Ethics for Nurses* (American Nurses Association [ANA], 2001), a nurse's primary commitment is to the patient.

Autonomy and Paternalism

Autonomy in bioethics means that persons are rational and allowed to direct their own health-related and life decisions. **Paternalism** occurs when a healthcare professional makes choices for a patient based on the healthcare professional's beliefs about "the best interest of the patient" or "the patient's own good." Physicians and nurses sometimes believe that patients are unable to understand the full extent of their care needs; a less-justifiable reason for paternalistic behavior is based on healthcare professionals' belief that their profession accords them a warranted place of power over patients.

Although the practice of paternalism was once an expected behavior among healthcare professionals and was encouraged by educators, it is not as readily accepted today by professionals or the recipients of their care. However, elders are still at a high risk for having their autonomy violated by healthcare professionals. This often results from incorrect assumptions about elders' decisional capacities because of their frail appearance and the influences of societal ageism. Even when elders are confused regarding the minor details of a situation, they may retain decisional capacity. In fact, elderly persons may be disoriented regarding time and the names and roles of other persons and still retain the capacity to make reasonable decisions regarding their lives and treatment. For example, if an elderly patient does not remember the name of an emergency department physician when the physician comes and goes in and out of the room, this does not necessarily mean that the patient is not competent to make treatment decisions. A more important assessment would be whether the patient knows that she is in a hospital emergency department. However, even this determination may not be sufficient to determine decisional capacity in regard to treatment decisions.

When elders are confused about some of the details regarding their current situation, healthcare professionals may be tempted to act paternalistically. Even if an elder does not know that she is in a hospital emergency department, healthcare professionals should not automatically overrule the patient's refusal of treatment. Instead, the whole context of the elder's life must be evaluated in terms of the ability to understand the benefits, risks, and consequences of decisions as well as the overall consistency of the elder's conversations and expressions of wishes over time. Healthcare professionals need to assess whether the elder's current wishes are consistent with previously expressed desires and ways of being. People sometimes want to quickly overrule elders' decisions and requests when their autonomy should rightfully be honored.

Some ethicists believe that the excessive paternalistic behavior exhibited by physicians and nurses in the past has caused a backlash, currently resulting in an elevated and imbalanced interest in respecting a patient's autonomy. According to some ethicists, the pendulum has now swung too far in the direction of an overinflated interest in preserving autonomy, and this stance minimizes the importance of the give and take needed for good human relationships, a desire to cultivate a strong sense of community, and the usefulness of virtues (Agich, 2003; Callahan, 1995; Hester, 2001; MacIntyre, 1984, 1999; Moody, 1992). Therefore, behavior exhibited toward elderly patients may fall somewhere along a wide continuum from a point of unjustified paternalism to a point of rigid adherence to respecting autonomy. Hester, a communitarian ethicist, has argued that healing requires communal involvement, not an overdeveloped interest in autonomy; when autonomy becomes the consuming focus in health care, the involvement of communities and personal relationships may be sidelined.

Elderly patients often need the care of nurses not because they need someone to respect their capacity for autonomy but because they have lost mental and/or physical abilities. Rather than focusing on the use of rules and principles such as autonomy, a humanistic focus on facilitating the well-being and alleviating the suffering of elders may be the more important focal point of care. Respect for autonomy remains extremely important in bioethics and nursing ethics, but a humanistic approach that puts the patient's humanity and well-being at the center of care is needed, rather than an unquestioned allegiance to rule-oriented behavior.

Also, nurses may believe that they should minimize family involvement in order to support an elderly patient's autonomy. Although healthcare providers need to support elders in maintaining self-direction, family caregivers usually should not be excluded from decision making regarding elders' care. Autonomous elderly patients are not necessarily bound by their family's decisions or recommendations, and often elders appreciate the caring concern of their family and even the appropriate decisional support provided by trusted nurses. Caregivers, including nurses who are well-known by elderly patients through repeated contacts over time, are intimates to the patient, not strangers. It is unreasonable to believe that nurses who care about the well-being of their patients would be objectively detached from actively interacting with patients regarding the patients' healthcare decisions. When providing decisional support to elders, nurses need to use practical wisdom in evaluating whether capricious assumptions, ageism, and prejudices are influencing the support and direction that they are providing to patients. Ultimately, wise and compassionate decisional support is a critically important part of nursing care and patient advocacy.

Vulnerability and Dependence

In addition to autonomy, vulnerability and dependence are integrally related to moral agency. In order to facilitate communities working toward the common good of their members, MacIntyre (1999) emphasized that people need to acknowledge their animal nature. When realizing that human nature is also animal nature, vulnerability and dependence are accepted as natural human conditions. Vulnerability and dependence are inherent human conditions as people move from childhood to adulthood; barring complicating circumstances, people progress from vulnerability and dependence in childhood to being capable of independent practical reasoning as adults.

As adults, however, humans may reexperience vulnerability and dependence due to the effects of physical and cognitive changes during aging. According to MacIntyre (1999), ethicists frequently talk in terms of stronger, independent persons benevolently bestowing their virtues on people who are vulnerable and dependent. Nurses would do well to keep in mind that all people are subject to vulnerabilities and dependence, even nurses themselves. There is a vast amount of knowledge to learn from vulnerable and dependent elders if nurses are open to hearing and relating to their patients' life stories (Butts & Rich, 2004).

Dementia

Nurses, particularly nurses working in home care and long-term care settings, often provide care to patients with dementia. Kitwood (1997) suggested that our evolving culture has supported society and healthcare communities treating persons with dementia as the "new outcasts of society" (p. 44). According to Jenkins and Price (1996), the loss experienced by persons with dementia can be likened to a loss of personhood. Examples of personal tendencies that depersonalize other people are listed in Box 8.2.

When people become adjusted to the dwindling capacities of persons with dementia, they often begin reacting to these people as if they are less than persons (Moody, 1992). People with dementia can still be aware of their feelings even when the person they once seemed to be appears to be withering away. It is reasonable to assume that an extreme sense of vulnerability can occur as a person enters the early and middle stages of a progressive dementia. This occurs when a remainder of cognitive ability may still exist in the awareness of personhood and connectedness to the environment and to others.

Kitwood's (1997) reference to persons with dementia becoming the outcasts of society becomes very relevant when these people lose their dignity in terms of how

BOX 8.2 ETHICAL FORMATIONS: DEPERSONALIZING TENDENCIES TO AVOID

1. Treachery: Using deception to distract or manipulate
2. Disempowerment: Not allowing persons to use their abilities
3. Infantalization: Patronizing; acting as an insensitive parent would act toward a child
4. Intimidation: Inducing fear through physical power or threats
5. Labeling: Using a category, such as dementia, as the basis for interactions and explanations
6. Stigmatization: Treating someone as an outcast or a diseased object
7. Outpacing: Pressuring others to act faster than they are able; presenting information too rapidly
8. Invalidation: Failing to acknowledge others' subjective experiences and feelings
9. Banishment: Physical or psychological exclusion
10. Objectification: Treating others as a "lump of matter" rather than as sentient beings
11. Ignoring: Talking or interacting with others in the presence of a person as if he or she is not there
12. Imposition: Forcing a person to do something; overriding or denying the possibility of choice
13. Withholding: Refusing to provide asked-for attention or to meet evident needs
14. Accusation: Blaming for actions or failures that arise from lack of ability or misunderstanding
15. Disruption: Crudely intruding into a person's actions or reflections
16. Mockery: Humiliating; making jokes at another's expense
17. Disparagement: Damaging another person's self-esteem; conveying messages that someone is useless, worthless, [or] incompetent

Source: Kitwood, T. (1997). *Dementia reconsidered.* Buckingham, UK: Open University Press, pp. 46–47.

other people perceive them. Dignity is acknowledged or denied in the relatedness of daily interactions between people with dementia and their significant others and healthcare professionals. Though families and nurses may not recognize the subtle risks involved, dignity may be jeopardized when caregivers are so focused on making ethical decisions regarding the care of persons with dementia that they forget to actually relate to the persons themselves (Moody, 1992).

Family and paid caregivers of people with dementia often become frustrated and anxious. Nurses can serve as mentors to other caregivers by exhibiting the virtues of compassion and equanimity when interacting with patients with dementia and their families. Gentle communication used by nurses helps to support the overall sense of dignity surrounding the care of patients with dementia. Environmental calm is created with gentle words as opposed to an environment of fear and anxiousness that can be created when loud and harsh words are used. Inexperienced caregivers learn by observing nurses. Nurses always must be aware of their potential to ultimately help or harm patients by the example they set for others.

Virtues Needed by Elders

May (1986) asserted that aging is a mystery rather than a problem, and as a society, people must focus on how they behave toward aging rather than on how to fix it. Doctors and nurses' position of power as compared to the seemingly passive beneficiary position of vulnerable patients is an important topic in bioethics. The behavior of healthcare professionals directed toward aged individuals is significant because elderly persons sometimes perceive that the treatment they receive from healthcare professionals is symbolic of what they can expect from the larger community.

May (1986) proposed that even when they are seemingly powerless, elderly persons remain moral agents who are personally responsible for the quality of their lives. An ethic of caregiving that is one sided on the part of nurses and physicians is not the answer to power imbalances between healthcare professionals and patients. Elders may experience more meaning in their lives if they remain dynamically involved in creating their own sense of well-being. Life is not static; it can be vital into old age.

The following are virtues that May (1986) proposed that elders need to cultivate in order to enhance the quality of their moral lives. These virtues articulated by May were considered valuable enough to be included by the President's Council on Bioethics (2005) in their report *Taking Care: Ethical Caregiving in Our Aging Society*. Nurses who are aware of the continued moral development that occurs in old age can support elderly patients in cultivating these virtues as elders continue their journey of moral progress.

Courage: Courage is consistent with St. Thomas Aquinas's definition of courage as "a firmness of soul in the face of adversity" (May, 1986, p. 51).

Elderly persons need courage when facing the certainty of death and loss in their lives.

Humility: Elderly people need humility when their dignity is assaulted through seeing and feeling their bodily decay, when they interpret the looks that they receive from young people as a sign that their frailty is noticeable and possibly repugnant to others, and when they progressively lose more people and things of value in their lives. Humility is a virtue also needed by caregivers to counteract the arrogance that may arise because of their position of power in their relationships with elders. Nurses need to be receivers as well as givers in patient–professional relationships; nurses can receive the gifts of insight and practical wisdom when they actively listen to the narratives of their elderly patients who have lived many years and experienced many joys and sufferings.

Patience: Although old age sometimes stimulates the emotions of bitterness and anger, a positive conception of the virtue of patience can help combat these reactive emotions. "Patience is purposive waiting, receiving, willing . . . it requires taking control of one's spirit precisely when all else goes out of control" (May, 1986, p. 52). Patience is the virtue that can help elders bear the frustrations of their frail bodies, rather than "cursing their fate" and becoming frustrated with issues such as being short of breath when trying to walk short distances.

Simplicity: Simplicity is a virtue referred to by Benedictine monks as a moral mark of old age. Simplicity becomes the virtue of a pilgrim who "has at long last learned how to travel light" (May, 1986, p. 53). Simplicity is exhibited when elderly persons experience great joy in the small pleasures of life, such as a meal with friends, rather than in accumulating material possessions.

Benignity: Benignity is another moral mark of old age, according to the Benedictines. Benignity is defined "as a kind of purified benevolence" (May, 1986, p. 53). It is opposed to the vice of grasping and avarice (greed) that has been associated with some elders' attempts to hold onto life in the face of death. Benevolence provides an answer to the tightfistedness of avarice "not with the empty-handedness of death, but the openhandedness of love" (p. 53). Elders who exhibit the virtue of benignity usually have realized the meaning of their lives as well as the meaning that can be found in their deaths. They have learned to find joy in serving others.

Integrity: The virtue of integrity represents "an inclusive unity of character" (May, 1986, p. 53) that summarizes all of the other virtues of character in old age. Character is a moral structure and requires an overriding virtue when character is "at one with itself" (p. 53). Integrity, or an intactness of character, is the foundation that helps elders remain kind and optimistic in

BOX 8.3 ETHICAL FORMATIONS: FLEXIBILITY AND LIFE

"When a man is living, he is soft and supple; when he is dead he becomes hard and rigid. When a plant is living, it is soft and tender; when it is dead, it becomes withered and dry. Hence, the hard and rigid belongs to the company of the dead. The soft and supple belongs to the company of the living."

Source: Tzu, L. (1989). *Tao teh ching* (J.C.H. Wu, Trans.). Boston, MA: Shambhala, p. 155. (Original work published 1961)

terms of their transcendent connection with the universe, even when loss and impermanence could easily pull them in a more negative direction.

Wisdom (prudence): Wisdom or prudence makes integrity possible through the lessons learned from the experiences of one's past. Prudence was defined by medieval moralists as consisting of three parts: memoria, docilitus, and solertia. Memoria "characterizes the person who remains open to his or her past, without retouching, falsifying, or glorifying it" (May, 1986, p. 57). Docilitus does not represent the passiveness of one who is merely docile, but rather is "a capacity to take in the present—an alertness, an attentiveness in the moment" (p. 58). It implies a contrasting state from the need to talk excessively that sometimes serves to separate elders from others. Solertia is "a readiness for the unexpected" (p. 58). It provides a contrast to being inflexible with routines (see Box 8.3); however, it should be noted that some amount of ritual helps elders develop strength of character.

Detachment and nonchalance: Detachment and nonchalance are similar virtues. May (1986) proposed that detachment is a virtue linked with wisdom and is consistent with what Erikson defined as "an attitude that depends in part upon a store of experience" (May, p. 58). People who are experienced weigh and react to situations wisely, calmly, and with love; people who are inexperienced overreact and become engulfed by catastrophe. May based nonchalance on a Biblical virtue that allows one the "capacity to take in one's stride life's gifts and blows" (p. 59). For example, the virtue of detachment or nonchalance might allow elderly persons who have serious medical problems to enjoy the gifts in their lives, such as being with their great-grandchildren, while calmly accepting the realistic assessment that they may not live to see their great-grandchildren graduate from college.

Courtesy: Courtesy, too, is based on a Biblical link to wisdom. Courtesy is the "capacity to deal honorably with all that is urgent, jarring, and rancorous on the social scene" (May, 1986, p. 59). (See Box 8.4.)

Hilarity: A final virtue outlined by May (1986) is another virtue of old age identified by Benedictine monks. Though the risk for depression is more common in elders than at other ages because of conditions such as naturally

BOX 8.4 ETHICAL FORMATIONS: LAST ACTS OF COURTESY

Ida was a 79-year-old Alzheimer's patient seen by Dr. Muller, a psychiatrist, in the emergency room (ER) because she became agitated at her foster home. Ida looked younger than her years and "still had some of the light that usually leaves the face of the demented. Her score was 7 out of 30 on the Mini Mental Status Exam. "Ida gave little information during the interview, though she showed every sign of wanting to cooperate." Plans were made for Ida to be discharged back to the foster home on Haldol. When Dr. Muller went to say good-bye to Ida he found her "straightening the sheet and flattening out the pillow on the gurney where she had been placed prior to the interview. She was trying to put [styrofoam cups and food wrappers] into a trash container" but was having difficulty in doing so. Dr. Muller stated "I was struck by what was still left of this sweet lady's demented brain and mind—which did not know the year, season, month, or day—that made her want to attempt these last acts of courtesy before leaving the ER." Muller quoted the neurologist, Oliver Sacks, who stated "style, neurologically, is the deepest part of one's being, and may be preserved, almost to the last, in a dementia."

Source: Muller, R. (2003). *Psych ER.* Hillsdale, NJ: The Analytic Press, pp. 63–65.

lowered serotonin levels; anxiety over fixed incomes; physical, personal, and material losses; and disturbed sleep patterns, the monks wisely believed that hilarity is a realistic virtue of old age. Hilaritas is "a kind of celestial gaiety in those who have seen a lot, done a lot, grieved a lot, but now acquire that humored detachment of the fly on the ceiling looking down on the human scene" (p. 60). It involves not taking oneself too seriously.

Ethical Reflections www

- How important is elders' personal responsibility for the moral nature of their lives and relationships? As a nurse, how can you positively affect an elder's personal views regarding this responsibility?
- How can nurses help elderly persons cultivate the virtues identified by May?
- Discuss your experiences with elders. Provide examples of situations in which you have observed elders displaying May's virtues. Provide examples of situations in which elders seemed to need the virtues but lacked them.

Quality of Life

What do people mean when they discuss the issue of quality of life? Often, people, including healthcare professionals, talk about quality of life as if it is a concept that is self-evident. But is it? According to Jonsen, Siegler, and Winslade (2010), determinations of quality of life are value judgments, and value judgments imply variations among the people who are determining value. If it is determined that a patient's quality of life is seriously diminished, justifications often are proposed to refrain from life-prolonging medical treatments. Some people find this position problematic because of their views about the sanctity of life—these people believe that because all human life is sacred, life must be preserved no matter what the quality of that life might be.

Many people do believe that treatment can be withheld or withdrawn based on quality-of-life determinations while still preserving a reverence for the sanctity of life. Scales have been developed and measures of physical and psychological functions have been suggested to objectify quality-of-life determinations. However, people differ significantly in how they respond to scales and measurements that are supposed to quantify the quality of their own or others' lives. Studies have shown that at least one group of healthcare professionals—physicians—frequently rate the quality of a patient's life lower than the patient rates it (Jonsen et al., 2010).

Determination of the quality of a life can be divided into categories of personal evaluations and observer evaluations. According to Jonsen et al. (2010), a **personal evaluation** is "the personal satisfaction expressed or experienced by individuals in their own physical, mental, and social situation" (p. 113). **Observer evaluations** refer to quality-of-life judgments made by someone other than the person "living the life." Observers tend to base their evaluations on some standard below which they believe that life is not desirable. It is observer evaluations that generate most ethical problems in regard to quality-of-life determinations, because observer evaluations can reflect incorrect assumptions, biases, prejudices, or beliefs about conditions that are not necessarily permanent, such as homelessness or family conditions.

Problems with quality-of-life determinations that are specifically related to elderly patients can arise due to discrimination against patients by healthcare professionals based on the patient's chronological age, a perception of a patient's social worth, a patient's dementia, or differences between the professional's and the patient's life goals and values (Faden & German, 1994; Jonsen et al., 2010). Decisions regarding treatment must always be made based on honest determinations of medical need and patients' current or previously communicated preferences. If a patient's wishes were not previously communicated, decisions should be based on projections of what loved ones believe that the patient would want done. Problems can easily arise when professionals try to project what a "reasonable person" would want in a particular situation, and it is at this point that prejudices and biased discriminations based on ageism can enter into observer evaluations.

When acting in regard to elderly patients, special attention needs to be focused on an assumption that values and goals are different among people of different age groups (Faden & German, 1994; Jonsen et al., 2010). The values that might be consistent among young healthcare professionals could be expected to be different from the values held by old-old adults. Automatic projections of values by nurses and other healthcare professionals are not consistent with the moral care of elderly persons. Elders may view their lives as having quality when younger persons, still in the prime of their lives, do not readily see the same quality. In addition to nurses using moral imagination in simply stopping to reflect about the dangers of forming automatic assumptions, conducting a values history with elderly patients when

BOX 8.5 ETHICAL FORMATIONS: CONDUCTING A VALUES HISTORY

Sample questions for conducting a values history with elders:

1. What would you like to say to someone reading [a] document about your overall attitude toward life?
2. What, for you, makes life worth living?
3. How do you feel about your health problems or disabilities? What would you like others (family, friends, doctors, nurses) to know about these feelings?
4. How do you expect friends, family, and others to support your decisions regarding medical treatment you may need now or in the future?
5. If your current physical or mental health gets worse, how would you feel?
6. How does independence or dependence affect your life?
7. What will be important to you when you are dying (e.g., physical comfort, no pain, family members present)?
8. Where would you prefer to die?
9. What general comments would you like to make about medical treatment?
10. How do your religious background or beliefs affect your feelings toward serious, chronic, or terminal illness?

Source: Institute for Ethics, University of New Mexico. (n.d.). *Values history.* Retrieved from http://hsc.unm.edu/ethics/docs/Values_History.pdf

they enter a new healthcare system can be invaluable in trying to ensure the ethical treatment of elders. This history must be reevaluated as appropriate (see Box 8.5).

As previously discussed, Frankl (1959/1984) maintained that "man's search for meaning is the primary motivation in his life" (p. 105). Humans embark on the search for meaning in order to alleviate and understand suffering and to move toward well-being. Frankl proposed that inner tension, rather than inner equilibrium, may result from the search for meaning, and he believed that inner tension is a prerequisite for mental health. Valuing the need to strive toward equilibrium and homeostasis (a tensionless state) is a dangerous misconception, according to Frankl. This way of thinking can be especially true when interacting with elderly persons whose whole being does not generally remain in a state of equilibrium.

An acceptance of the belief that equilibrium is not necessarily the healthiest state supports the belief that suffering should not be attacked as if it is something to eliminate at all costs. Rather, well-being often involves the relief of suffering through the acceptance of suffering. In discussing the often misguided goals of a modernist society, Callahan (1995) proposed that the novelist George Eliot had captured this philosophy with the word *meliorism*. The concept of meliorism describes "an ethic of action oriented toward the relief, not the acceptance, of pain and suffering" (p. 30).

An emphasis on holistic care has helped to eliminate some of the beliefs from the Enlightenment period that the human body can be compared with a machine (sometimes referred to as reductionism). Mechanics fix machines, but the healthcare professional–patient relationship should not be viewed in a similar way. However, the healthcare system and healthcare professionals today often still perpetuate the meliorism described by Eliot. Meliorism causes doctors and nurses to work toward curing disease and relieving suffering at all costs. In working with patients of all ages, but especially in patients' later years, attempts must be made to alleviate suffering while realizing that completely relieving suffering and curing diseases is not always possible. In these instances, the nurse's goal is to help patients accept the pain and suffering that cannot be changed and find meaning in their suffering. Amid the chaos and pain of patients' suffering, nurses can be compared to the calm person described by the Buddhist monk Thich Nhat Hanh (see Box 8.6). Patients' suffering can lead to a profound, transforming life experience for both patients and nurses.

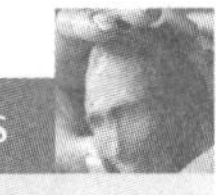

www Ethical Reflections

- A decision not to attempt to resuscitate an unconscious, frail, elderly person in an emergency department should not be made based solely on chronological age. What factors must be considered in such a decision?
- How might ageism affect end-of-life decisions and the elderly? What can nurses do to combat end-of-life care and decisions based solely on ageism?

Assessing the Capacity to Remain at Home

Assessing elders' capacity to safely continue to live alone in their own homes is a problem often faced by nurses working in the community and nurses helping to plan discharges of patients from acute care to home care. These determinations become particularly difficult when frail elders adamantly want to remain in or return to their homes and caregivers disagree with an elder's decisions. Caregivers must consider the real and perceived capacities and incapacities of elders and question the safety of their living situation. Ways to assess cognitive capacity have been covered earlier in this chapter and will also be addressed in Chapter 10. If it is believed that an elder is incapacitated, a consideration of respecting elders' autonomy versus supporting caregivers' beneficence may be needed. The ethical issue becomes a matter of deciding whether to act in a way that Beauchamp and Childress (2009) called **weak** or **soft paternalism**, which is a concept that was originally suggested by Feinberg.

BOX 8.6 ETHICAL FORMATIONS: CALM WITHIN THE STORM

In Vietnam there are many people, called boat people, who leave the country in small boats. Often the boats are caught in rough seas or storms, the people may panic, and boats can sink. But if even one person aboard can remain calm, lucid, knowing what to do and what not to do, he or she can help the boat survive. His or her expression—face, voice—communicates clarity and calmness, and people have trust in that person. They will listen to what he or she says. One such person can save the lives of many.

Source: Thich Nhat Hanh. (2001). *Thich Nhat Hanh: Essential writings* (R. Ellsberg, Ed.). New York, NY: Orbis Books, p. 162.

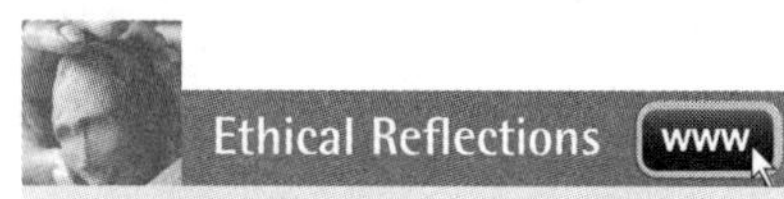

- Healthcare professionals' beliefs about the proper treatment of elders falls along a continuum from discounting elders' personal quality-of-life judgments to believing that only curing disease and being successful in eliminating physical suffering are worthwhile goals. Provide examples of nurses' opportunities to act as patient advocates in relation to this continuum.

"In soft paternalism, an agent intervenes in the life of another person on grounds of beneficence or nonmaleficence with the goal of preventing substantially-*nonvoluntary* conduct" (Beauchamp & Childress, 2009, p. 209). Nonvoluntary or nonautonomous actions are actions that are not based on rational decision making. Persons who are the receivers of soft paternalistic actions must have some form of compromised ability for this form of weak paternalism to be justified. It is debatable as to whether soft paternalism actually qualifies to be labeled as paternalism, as acting in a person's best interest is not usually disputed when people must be protected from harm resulting from circumstances that are beyond their control, including a personal desire based on faulty information when a person is incapacitated. However, issues of self-harm often constitute dilemmas when elders with intact decisional capacity want to remain at home when it is not safe to do so because of the elder's physical limitations. Family caregivers and healthcare providers must carefully weigh when and the degree to which weak paternalism is justified in preventing self-harm.

Long-Term Care

Issues regarding moral relationships between nurses and patients in long-term care facilities are similar to other issues discussed in this chapter; that is, the relationships often are focused on issues of autonomy. However, as previously proposed, focusing too narrowly on respecting autonomy can cause nurses to miss the real day-to-day complexities that make up moral relationships with elders. In many instances, elders are in long-term care facilities because they no longer are able to exercise self-direction in safely caring for themselves. This fact sometimes makes attempts at trying to respect and preserve autonomy, in a comprehensive sense, a futile undertaking. When unrealistic goals are not acknowledged in long-term care, it often frustrates nurses and aides who work in long-term care facilities; unfortunately, these frustrations can ultimately be directed against long-term care residents.

Pullman (1998) proposed that an ethic of dignity be used, as opposed to an ethic of autonomy, in long-term care. With an ethic of dignity, the moral character of caregivers is the focus, rather than the autonomy of the recipients of care. Of course, autonomy must be respected when it is realistic to do so, but when working with long-term care residents who are no longer able to exercise their full autonomy, a communal ethic of dignity can provide a compassionate means of care. Even when elders are able to fully exercise their autonomous choices, an ethic of dignity provides an appropriate grounding framework from which to work.

Pullman (1998) divided dignity into **basic dignity**, which is the dignity inherent in all humans, and **personal dignity**, which is an evaluative type of dignity decided upon by communities that does not have to be solely tied to a person's autonomy. Personal dignity can be viewed as a community's valuing of the interrelationship of members of the community. Acknowledging elders' basic and personal dignity, through the adoption of an ethic of dignity, includes the "confidence that caregivers will strive to serve the on-going interests of their patients to the best of their abilities" (Pullman, 1998, p. 37). If there is a belief that elderly residents of long-term care facilities need to be independent because being dependent is bad, and if the goal is to minimize the elders' need for care rather than to provide more care, then the relationships between nurses and elderly residents of long-term care facilities are in trouble from their outset.

Pullman (1998) suggested that long-term care often requires paternalistic interventions from the beginning of patient–healthcare provider relationships. He defined a rule of **justified paternalism** as a guide for these paternalistic interventions; that rule is: "the degree of paternalistic intervention justified or required, is inversely proportional to the degree of autonomy present" (p. 37). Nurses must be extremely sensitive and aware in ensuring that they cultivate the intellectual virtue of practical wisdom so that errors in judgments are not made about respecting patients' autonomy versus practicing justified or weak paternalism in patient care.

When elders have the capacity to make choices regarding treatments and daily living activities, they must have the freedom to make personal decisions. Those options include such things as choosing to refuse medications and refusing physical therapy treatments. However, respecting elders' autonomy does not mean that compassionate nurses should not take considerable time, if needed, to calmly discuss the potential consequences of controversial choices made by elderly persons. Nurses who work from an ethic of dignity are not emotionally detached from their patients but, instead, are willing to risk feeling a personal sense of failure or loss when their elderly patients make choices that a nurse believes are not in the elder's best interest.

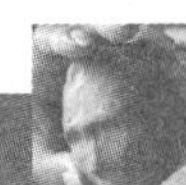

www Ethical Reflections

- Cohen (1988) said that elders often focus all of their energy toward avoiding "the ultimate defeat, which is not death but institutionalization and which is regarded as a living death" (p. 25). How can nurses help to change the experience of residence in a long-term care facility being like a "living death"?
- When caring for elders, both chemical and physical restrictions and restraints should be limited to the least amount possible to maintain the safety of patients and caregivers. Imagine that you are working as an RN in a large, long-term care facility. You are asked to help with something on your colleague's wing of the facility. As you are walking down the hall of her wing, you hear a resident crying out very loudly. You enter the resident's room and notice that the resident is tightly restrained to the bed. What would you do?
- Do you believe that nurses who work in long-term care facilities are stigmatized in any way? If so, what do you believe is the underlying cause of this stigmatization? How can this perception be changed?

Elder Abuse

Nurses are frequently the first people to recognize that patients are the victims of violence or abuse; this is especially true in regard to emergency department and home care nurses. Moral care of elders requires nurses to be interested in recognizing the signs of abuse and in taking appropriate actions. Elder abuse includes physical abuse, sexual abuse, emotional or psychological abuse, neglect, abandonment, financial or material exploitation, and self-neglect (National Center on Elder Abuse [NCEA], 2011b).

A survey report regarding abuse of adults 60 years of age and older, which was prepared for the National Center on Elder Abuse and conducted and coauthored by the National Committee for the Prevention of Elder Abuse in conjunction with the National Adult Protective Services Association (2006), revealed that there has been a significant increase in reports of elder abuse, neglect, and exploitation since the 2000 survey. Between 2000 and 2004, the reports of abuse of adults of all ages increased by 19%. The alleged abuse usually occurred in a home (89.3%), and women were much more likely to be victims of abuse than men. Perpetrators of elder abuse and neglect were women in 52.7% of cases reviewed in the survey. Adult children accounted for 32.6% of the total number of perpetrators, and other family members accounted for 21.5%.

Clues that abuse may be occurring include explanations about injuries that seem inconsistent with what the nurse actually sees; delays in seeking treatment for conditions and injuries; and unusual behaviors, such as caregivers giving extensive details about the elder's injuries, refusing to allow the elder to be interviewed or treated by the nurse without the caregiver being present, and showing an unreasonable interest in the cost of treatment (Ramsey, 2006). The conditions of elder abuse are often different from abuse involving other adults or children (Bergeron, 2000). Older males are more prone to abuse than younger males, and generally there are limited resources in terms of safe houses for males. Elderly persons who are abused tend to be less accepting of help from police and the court system than younger victims of abuse; this reluctance is particularly prevalent when the abuser is the elder's child. When an abuser is a spouse, elderly persons are more resistant to seeking a divorce or separation from the spouse than happens with younger persons. Because of limited financial resources, elderly persons usually feel more constrained by their housing and living situations and are reluctant to disrupt the *status quo* even when they are being abused.

The NCEA (2005) recommended that accurate elder abuse data need to be continuously collected at both the state and national levels. Trends need to be tracked, studied, and addressed through appropriate interventions, and education about identifying and reporting elder abuse needs to be increased. Nurses can have a key role in regard to all of these recommendations. It is morally imperative that nurses be active in recognizing the abuse of elders and knowing state statutes regarding the

BOX 8.7 ETHICAL REFLECTIONS: WAYS TO RAISE AWARENESS ABOUT ELDER ABUSE

- Organize a candlelight vigil or a march down Main Street in recognition of World Elder Abuse Awareness Day.
- Host a rally on World Elder Abuse Awareness Day and invite seniors, advocates, spokespersons, and government officials to talk about the issues and the ways that citizens can become involved in prevention. Don't forget to invite the local press!
- Distribute elder abuse public awareness materials at a local sporting event, concert, or fair.
- Ask local banks or utility companies to include small elder abuse awareness inserts (that your organization supplies) with the May or June statements. You can find fact sheets on the NCEA website to use or modify for the inserts, and don't forget to mention any other "Join Us" activities your community is holding.
- Purple is the color designated for elder abuse awareness. Distribute purple ribbons to your staff, nursing home professionals, Adult Protective Service [APS] staff, law enforcement, and other community organizations and members in recognition of World Elder Abuse Awareness Day.
- Partner with a local nursing home for a World Elder Abuse Awareness Day barbeque or picnic. Include activities and food for residents and their families, staff, and the community. Ask volunteers to bring food and games to play and coordinate the activities with nursing home staff. Invite the press for added exposure and increased elder abuse awareness.
- Start an elder abuse awareness group on a social networking site, such as "Facebook," and encourage "friends" to join the group. Start a campaign to get "X" number of "friends" to join by World Elder Abuse Awareness Day.
- Hold a community yard sale at a central location such as a senior center or church/synagogue with proceeds going to an elder abuse support group or community outreach efforts to help elderly in crisis.
- Organize a "Letter to the Editor" writing campaign to raise awareness not only of elder abuse but of the local resources that are available through APS, area agency on aging offices, and other organizations. Be sure to include contact information and hotline/helpline phone numbers, as well as web addresses for relevant organizations.

Source: National Center on Elder Abuse. (2011). *How your organization can generate awareness & foster action in the fight against elder abuse.* Retrieved from http://ncea.aoa.gov/Ncearoot/Main_Site/pdf/publication/Join_Us_Campaign_tipsheet_org_final.pdf

handling of elder abuse. Nurses also have a key role in teaching other healthcare professionals and the community about recognizing and reporting elder abuse. The following list provides a guideline for meeting moral responsibility in reporting abuse.

Report to:

- Adult Protective Services
- Long-term care ombudsman (usually when an agency or healthcare provider is involved)
- State licensing board (when a healthcare provider is involved)
- Law enforcement (if required under statute)

When:

- Written or verbal report within 24 hours of incident (Ramsey, 2006, p. 58)

In conjunction with the 2011 annual World Elder Abuse Awareness Day, the National Center on Elder Abuse (2011a) encouraged people to volunteer to help raise awareness about elder abuse and to sponsor World Day activities (see Box 8.7). State and local resources often are lacking to help elders who are abused or are at high risk for abuse. The bottom line in the moral care of abused elders is that nurses must be persistent in their efforts to obtain help for these vulnerable adults.

Age-Based Distribution of Healthcare Resources

There has been substantial debate among bioethicists and philosophers about the need for a plan to fairly distribute healthcare resources among different generations (Callahan, 1995; Daniels, 1988; Moody, 1992). The Alliance for Aging Research, a nonprofit group focused on improving the well-being of elders, published a report in 2003 that outlined five ways that the U.S. healthcare system has failed elders (see Box 8.8). According to the Alliance, the reason underlying these failures is a fundamental ageist bias in U.S. society.

Even if one concedes that there is an ageist bias among the American public, it is known that a large percentage of all U.S. healthcare dollars is spent on the care of elders during their last year of life. Because of the expensive health care that they often receive, it is the very young (neonates) and the very old who are the focus of debates about the distribution of healthcare resources. Currently, no plan for fairly distributing healthcare dollars among different generations has received widespread acceptance in the United States.

Social justice in distributing healthcare resources according to age has been described as a type of rationing. Moody (1992) defined rationing as a system that

BOX 8.8 ETHICAL FORMATIONS: FIVE DIMENSIONS OF AGEIST BIAS

1. Healthcare professionals do not receive enough training in geriatrics to properly care for many older patients.
2. Older patients are less likely than younger people to receive preventive care.
3. Older patients are less likely to be tested or screened for diseases and other health problems.
4. Proven medical interventions for older patients are often ignored, leading to inappropriate or incomplete treatment.
5. Older people are consistently excluded from clinical trials, even though they are the largest users of approved drugs.

Source: Alliance for Aging Research. (2003). *Ageism: How healthcare fails the elderly.* Retrieved from http://www.agingresearch.org/content/article/detail/694/

is associated with crisis situations, like the rationing of gasoline during oil embargoes and butter during World War II. Rationing is used when there is a scarcity of resources, but it is often only a temporary solution. Rationing usually is not a method that is appropriate to use in making decisions about the distribution of healthcare resources, especially in nonemergency situations. American healthcare practices that can be compared to acts of rationing include: "the distribution of organs for transplantation, the practice of triage in admission to hospital emergency rooms, [and] extensive queuing for healthcare services provided through the Veterans Administration" (Moody, 1992, p. 199).

In fact, Moody (1992) said that the United States already has an allocation scheme for making decisions regarding health care for elders in the form of the Medicare program, which was established in 1965. The Medicare program has limits in regard to the care and treatment that can be provided under the program, but these limits usually are not referred to as rationing. However, the limits of the Medicare program, unfortunately, may contribute to the ineffective system of distributing resources; for example, restrictions on payments for home care may contribute to the number of elders living in long-term care facilities.

Callahan (1995) proposed that the idea of the "natural life span" and a "tolerable death" might need to be included in considerations about distributing healthcare resources to elders. Callahan defined these terms as "a fitting life span followed by a death that is relatively acceptable in its timeliness within that life span" (p. 64) (see Box 8.9). Moody (1992) agreed that using considerations of a natural life span can be helpful in the rationing/allocation debate, but he added that in the real world, bringing theory and practice together is very difficult and requires prudent political judgment. The debate regarding allocating healthcare resources among different generations is a heated one, and seems to have no immediate end in sight.

BOX 8.9 ETHICAL FORMATIONS: IS THERE A DUTY TO DIE?

Hardwig (2000) proposed that "death does not always come at the right time" and that death does not happen to hermits, that is, "death is a death in the family" (p. 81). In regard to his own life, Hardwig stated that he may "one day have a duty to die" because of his connections with his family. He suggested that in some situations "preserving my life can only devastate the lives of those who care about me" (p. 86).

1. Do you believe that people ever have a "duty to die"? If so, under what circumstances?
2. Defend your position.

Source: Hardwig, J. (2000). *Is there a duty to die? and other essays in medical ethics.* New York, NY: Routledge.

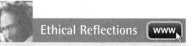

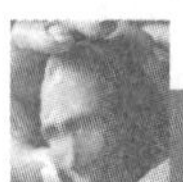

Ethical Reflections 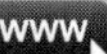

In the United States, approximately $8,160 is spent per capita annually on health care. This figure is more than the money spent on health care per capita in any other country. However, health indicators and outcomes in the United States do not reflect this great expenditure–for example, life expectancy in the United States is below the level of other industrialized countries, and infant mortality rates in the United States are high.

- Discuss the ethics of how money is allocated for the health care provided to different-aged populations in the United States. Is the allocation system justice based? Why or why not?
- Is too much money allocated to caring for people at both ends of the spectrum of life, the very young and the very old? What is the rationale for your answer to this question?
- Do you believe that the U.S. public would spend less on health care during the last year of an elder's life if more preventive care was provided to the population of elders? Explain and include examples.
- Why is the intergenerational distribution of healthcare resources an ethical issue of concern for nurses?

Ethics and the Humanistic Nursing Care of Elders

Travelbee (1971) described the human-to-human relationship between a nurse and the recipient of care as a "mutually significant experience" (p. 123). According to Travelbee, "each participant in the relationship perceives and responds to the human-ness of the other; that is, the 'patient' is perceived and responded to as a unique human being—not as 'an illness,' 'a room number,' or as a 'task to be performed'" (p. 124). Unfortunately, elders often feel dehumanized when interacting with healthcare professionals, which further compounds the dehumanization that they encounter in society. Travelbee made a profound statement: if just 1 healthcare professional would treat a recipient of care as a human being, this gesture might give the person the strength to cope with 10 other healthcare professionals who perceive that same person as merely a patient.

Nurses who are compassionate dedicate themselves to helping patients transcend or accept unavoidable suffering. It is a challenge to relate to others compassionately, to really communicate to the heart, according to Chodron (1997). "Compassion is not a relationship between the healer and the wounded. It is a relationship between equals" (Chodron, 2001, p. 50).

For many elders, the world is a lonely place. Nurses who have a sincere desire to take action to alleviate or facilitate acceptance of the suffering of this vulnerable group are widening the circle of compassion in the world. Solomon (2001) stated that research has revealed that elders have a higher response to placebo treatment than is normally expected, which has been attributed to the attention that elderly persons receive when they participate in research studies. He proposed that elders must be very lonely for this slight attention to provide them with such a lift.

Compassion and healing can be thought of as paired needs of elders. Capra (1982) described healing as a "complex interplay among the physical, psychological, social, and environmental aspects of the human condition" (p. 124). Capra postulated that healing has been excluded from medical science because it cannot be understood in terms of reductionism. Healing suggests moving toward a wholeness that goes

CASE STUDY: WHOSE WISHES SHOULD BE HONORED?

Mrs. R., a frail, 85-year-old woman who lives alone, was admitted to a gero-psychiatric unit because of irritability, confusion, and increasing incontinence. Mrs. R.'s family stated that she was continually refusing assistance from her home health aides and became angry when her family and home care nurses tried to reason with her about these refusals. During her hospital admission, Mrs. R. was hydrated with intravenous fluids and a couple of her medications were adjusted. She subsequently became calm and cooperative with the care that she received while in the hospital. When the RN and social worker talked with Mrs. R. about the safety risks of her living in her home alone, the patient stated, "I am 85 years old and think that I should be able to decide how I want to live the rest of my life. I'm willing to take my chances. I will die if I go to a nursing home." Mrs. R. was often unsure about the correct day of the week when questioned, yet she knew the name of the hospital and the reason that she was admitted for treatment. She was often confused about the names of the hospital staff but was able to state her own name and the names of her children. Though Mrs. R. agreed to cooperate with home care providers, her family continued to insist that Mrs. R. be admitted to a long-term care facility. Her family requested that the psychiatrist complete the paperwork so that a judge could have the patient declared incompetent. The psychiatrist did not usually seem sincerely interested in his patients, and he had spent little time with Mrs. R. This psychiatrist was usually willing to comply with most families' wishes. The RN and social worker disagreed with the decision to declare Mrs. R. to be incompetent and were in favor of allowing her to return home as she wished.

Case Study Questions

1. Based on the information provided, does it seem that Mrs. R. has decision-making capacity? What criteria can be used as a basis for your decision? What needs to be included in a complete assessment of Mrs. R.'s decision-making capacity?
2. Does safety at home for Mrs. R. seem feasible? If so, how might this be accomplished? If not, why not?
3. What could the RN and social worker do to try to resolve the disagreement among the patient, her family, the doctor, and themselves?
4. Is a form of paternalism being used by any of the people involved in this case? If so, is it a form of weak or justified paternalism? Does the approach seem to be ethical? Why or why not?
5. What type of quality-of-life evaluation is most appropriate in this situation? Explain.
6. How is the issue of Mrs. R.'s dignity involved in this case?
7. How might the RN and social worker enter into a discussion of life meaning with Mrs. R.? With her family? With the physician?

beyond a single human being; it is consistent with a belief in the interconnection of all beings and the universe. Healing does not imply curing; it is a realization that not all things can be fixed. This idea of healing encompasses the recognition of the nature of impermanence and accepts unpredictability and the inability to strictly control events.

BOX 8.10 **ETHICAL FORMATIONS: *CODE OF ETHICS FOR NURSES***

- The worth of an individual is not affected by disease, disability, functional status, or proximity to death (1.3, p. 7).
- Nursing care aims to maximize the values that the patient has treasured in life and extends supportive care to the family and significant others (1.3, p. 7).
- The nurse preserves, protects, and supports [patients' self-determination] by assessing the patient's comprehension of both the information presented and the implications of decisions (1.4, p. 8).
- Nurses may not delegate responsibilities such as assessment and evaluation; they may delegate tasks. The nurse must not knowingly assign or delegate to any member of the nursing team a task for which that person is not prepared or qualified (4.4, p. 17).

Source: American Nurses Association. (2001). *Code of ethics for nurses with interpretive statements.* Silver Spring, MD: Author.

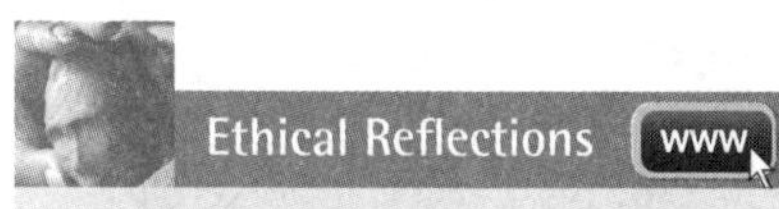

- Box 8.10 contains examples from the ANA's (2001) *Code of Ethics for Nurses with Interpretive Statements.* How are these examples relevant to the nursing care of elders?
- What other provisions and statements in the ANA's *Code of Ethics for Nurses* are particularly pertinent to the nursing care of elders (see Appendix A)? Discuss these provisions and provide examples of how they apply to nursing practice.

Nurses must establish human-to-human relationships with elderly patients and recognize the interplay of many factors that may affect the older person's state of well-being. Many factors that affect elders cannot be changed; they must be peacefully accepted and used in achieving integrity. However, there are active healing interventions that nurses can employ.

The need for physical touch is heightened at a time when elders are already experiencing significant losses in their lives—loved ones, belongings, and sensory abilities. Touch is one form of healing communication that nurses can use to convey compassion to elders. Many elders perceive the nurse's touch as a comforting touch. In her experimental study, Butts (1998, 2001) found that in long-term care facilities, the nurse's comforting touch significantly improved female elderly residents' perceptions of five factors—self-esteem, well-being and social status, health status, life satisfaction and self-actualization, and faith and belief—as compared to those female elders in long-term care facilities who were not touched.

Caring for elders requires dynamic interventions blending art and science. Suffering and loss are inherent in the daily lives of elders, and the reality of impermanence forms a glaring presence that is difficult for the aged to ignore. Although there are many approaches in the ethical care of elderly patients, nurses might adopt an approach to care similar to a way of being suggested by Thich Nhat Hanh (1998), based on the Buddhist Lotus Sutra. Thich Nhat Hanh stated that the sutra advises one "to look and listen with the eyes of compassion." He further stated that "compassionate listening brings about healing" (p. 86). Compassionate listening by nurses gives individual elders their voice in an often uncompassionate world.

KEY POINTS

- Ageism, or discrimination based on chronological age, underlies many ethical issues related to elders.
- Society often neglects to notice the meaning of elders' lives as scientists work to abolish the biology of aging.
- Determinations of decisional capacity in regard to elders are sometimes made based upon prejudiced assumptions rather than facts.
- Elders may perceive the quality of their lives to be higher than healthcare professionals perceive it based on observational judgments.
- Weak or justified paternalism is sometimes a compassionate approach to caring for elderly persons.
- Focusing on an ethic of dignity rather than a strict ethic of autonomy may be more realistic in caring for some elders, especially in long-term care facilities, when elderly persons are not completely able to exercise their autonomy.

References

Agich, G. J. (2003). *Dependence and autonomy in old age: An ethical framework for long-term care* (2nd ed.). Cambridge, UK: Cambridge University Press.

Alliance for Aging Research. (2003). *Ageism: How healthcare fails the elderly*. Retrieved from http://www.agingresearch.org/content/article/detail/694/

Allport, G. W. (1984). Preface. In V. E. Frankl, *Man's search for meaning: An introduction to logotherapy* (3rd ed., pp. 7–10). New York, NY: Simon and Schuster.

American Nurses Association. (2001). *Code of ethics for nurses with interpretive statements*. Silver Spring, MD: Author.

Beauchamp, T. L., & Childress, J. F. (2009). *Principles of biomedical ethics* (6th ed.). New York, NY: Oxford University Press.

Bergeron, R. (2000, September). Servicing the needs of elder abuse victims. *Policy & Practice*, 40–45.

Blum, L. A. (1994). *Moral perception and particularity*. Cambridge, UK: Cambridge University Press.

Buscaglia, L. (1982). *The fall of Freddie the leaf: A story of life for all ages*. Thorofare, NJ: Charles B. Slack.

Butler, R. (1975). *Why survive? Being old in America*. New York, NY: Harper & Row.

Butts, J. B. (1998). *Outcomes of comfort touch in institutionalized elderly female residents*. Unpublished doctoral dissertation, University of Alabama at Birmingham.

Butts, J. B. (2001). Outcomes of comfort touch in institutionalized elderly female residents. *Geriatric Nursing, 22*(4), 180–184.

Butts, J. B., & Rich, K. L. (2004). Acknowledging dependence: A MacIntyrean perspective on relationships involving Alzheimer's disease. *Nursing Ethics, 11*(4), 400–410.

Callahan, D. (1995). *Setting limits: Medical goals in an aging society with "a response to my critics."* Washington, DC: Georgetown University Press.

Capra, F. (1982). *The turning point: Science, society, and the rising culture*. New York, NY: Bantam Books.

Chodron, P. (1997). *When things fall apart: Heart advice for difficult times.* Boston, MA: Shambhala.

Chodron, P. (2001). *The places that scare you: A guide to fearlessness in difficult times.* Boston, MA: Shambhala.

Cohen, E. S. (1988). The elderly mystique: Constraints on the autonomy of the elderly with disabilities. *Gerontologist, 28*(Suppl.), 24–31.

Cole, T. R. (1986). The tattered web of cultural meanings. In T. R. Cole & S. Gadow (Eds.), *What does it mean to grow old? Reflections from the humanities* (pp. 3–7). Durham, NC: Duke University Press.

Daniels, N. (1988). *Am I my parents' keeper?* New York, NY: Oxford University Press.

de Beauvoir, S. (1972). *The coming of age* (P. O'Brien, Trans.). New York, NY: Putnam.

Easwaran, E. (1992). *Your life is your message: Finding harmony with yourself, others, and the earth.* New York, NY: Hyperion.

Erikson, E. H., & Erikson, J. M. (1997). *The life cycle completed* (extended version). New York, NY: W.W. Norton & Company.

Faden, R., & German, P. S. (1994). Quality of life: Considerations in geriatrics. *Clinics in Geriatric Medicine, 19*(3), 541–551.

Frankl, V. E. (1984). *Man's search for meaning: An introduction to logotherapy* (3rd ed.). New York, NY: Simon and Schuster. (Original work published 1959)

Greening, T. (1998). Viktor Frankl, 1905–1997. *Journal of Humanistic Psychology, 38*(1), 10–11.

Hardwig, J. (2000). *Is there a duty to die? and other essays in medical ethics.* New York, NY: Routledge.

Hester, D. M. (2001). *Community as healing: Pragmatist ethics in medical encounters.* Lanham, MD: Rowman & Littlefield.

Institute for Ethics, University of New Mexico. (n.d.). *Values history.* Retrieved from http://hsc.unm.edu/ethics/docs/Values_History.pdf

Jenkins, D., & Price, B. (1996). Dementia and personhood: A focus for care? *Journal of Advanced Nursing, 24*(1), 84–90.

Jonsen, A. R., Siegler, M., & Winslade, W. J. (2010). *Clinical ethics: A practical approach to ethical decisions in clinical medicine* (7th ed.). New York, NY: McGraw-Hill.

Kitwood, T. (1997). *Dementia reconsidered: The person comes first.* Buckingham, UK: Open University Press.

MacIntyre, A. (1984). *After virtue.* Notre Dame, IN: University of Notre Dame Press.

MacIntyre, A. (1999). *Dependent rational animals: Why human beings need the virtues.* Chicago, IL: Open Court.

May, W. F. (1986). The virtues and vices of the elderly. In T. R. Cole & S. Gadow (Eds.), *What does it mean to grow old? Reflections from the humanities* (pp. 43–61). Durham, NC: Duke University Press.

Moody, H. R. (1992). *Ethics in an aging society.* Baltimore, MD: The Johns Hopkins University Press.

Muller, R. J. (2003). *Psych ER.* Hillsdale, NJ: The Analytic Press.

National Center on Elder Abuse. (2005). *Fact sheet: Abuse of adults aged 60+, 2004 survey of adult protective services.* Retrieved from http://www.ncea.aoa.gov/ncearoot/Main_Site/pdf/publication/FinalStatistics050331.pdf

National Center on Elder Abuse. (2011a). *How your organization can generate awareness & foster action in the fight against elder abuse.* Retrieved from http://ncea.aoa.gov/ncearoot/Main_Site/pdf/publication/Join_Us_Campaign_tipsheet_org_final.pdf

National Center on Elder Abuse. (2011b). *The basics: Major types of elder abuse.* Retrieved from http://www.ncea.aoa.gov/ncearoot/Main_Site/FAQ/Basics/Types_Of_Abuse.aspx

National Committee for the Prevention of Elder Abuse and National Adult Protective Services Association. (2006). *The 2004 survey of state adult protective services: Abuse of adults 60 years of age and older.* Retrieved from http://www.ncea.aoa.gov/ncearoot/main_site/pdf/2-14-06%20final%2060+report.pdf

President's Council on Bioethics. (2005). *Taking care: Ethical caregiving in our aging society.* Washington, DC: Author.

Pullman, D. (1998). The ethics of autonomy and dignity in long-term care. *Canadian Journal on Aging, 18*(1), 26–46.

Ramsey, S. B. (2006). Abusive situations. In S. W. Killion & K. Dempski (Eds.), *Quick look nursing: Legal and ethical issues* (pp. 58–59). Sudbury, MA: Jones and Bartlett.

Savishinsky, J. S. (1991). *The ends of time: Life and work in a nursing home.* New York, NY: Bergin & Garvey.

Smith, N. L., Kotthoff-Burrell, E., & Post, L. F. (2002). Protecting the patient's voice on team. In M. D. Mezey, C. K. Cassel, M. M. Bottrell, K. Hyer, J. L. Howe, & T. T. Fulmer (Eds.), *Ethical patient care: A casebook for geriatric health care teams* (pp. 83–101). Baltimore, MD: The Johns Hopkins University Press.

Solomon, A. (2001). *The noonday demon: An atlas of depression.* New York, NY: Scribner.

Stanley, B., Sieber, J. E., & Melton, G. B. (2003). Empirical studies of ethical issues in research: A research agenda. In D. N. Bersoff (Ed.), *Ethical conflicts in psychology* (3rd ed., pp. 398–402). Washington, DC: American Psychological Association.

Thich Nhat Hanh. (1998). *The heart of the Buddha's teaching: Transforming suffering into peace, joy and liberation.* New York, NY: Broadway.

Thich Nhat Hanh. (2001). *Thich Nhat Hanh: Essential writings* (R. Ellsberg, Ed.). New York, NY: Orbis.

Travelbee, J. (1971). *Interpersonal aspects of nursing* (2nd ed.). Philadelphia, PA: F. A. Davis.

Tzu, L. (1989). *Tao teh ching* (J. C. H. Wu, Trans.). Boston, MA: Shambhala. (This edition originally published 1961)

U.S. Census Bureau. (2011). *2010 census briefs: Age and sex composition: 2010.* Retrieved from http://www.census.gov/prod/cen2010/briefs/c2010br-03.pdf

Wallis, V. (1993). *Two old women: An Alaska legend of betrayal, courage, and survival* (10th anniversary ed.). New York, NY: Perennial.

For a full suite of assignments and additional learning activities, use the access code located in the front of your book to visit this exclusive website: http://go.jblearning.com/butts. If you do not have an access code, you can obtain one at the site.

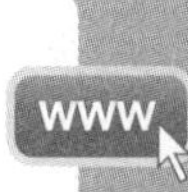

Ethical Issues in End-of-Life Nursing Care

Janie B. Butts

A place to stay untouched by death does not exist. It does not exist in space, it does not exist in the ocean, nor if you stay in the middle of a mountain.

—THE BUDDHA

OBJECTIVES

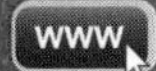

After reading this chapter, the reader should be able to:

1. Discuss the issues and forces surrounding death anxiety and the ideal death.
2. Explore the meaning of imaginative dramatic rehearsal in terms of one's own death.
3. Explain the nursing care of suffering patients as it relates to suffering from the perspective of Aristotle's four inseparable parts of the human soul, the American Nurses Association (ANA) *Code of Ethics for Nurses*, and the International Council of Nurses (ICN) *Code of Ethics for Nurses*.
4. Compare and contrast the different types of euthanasia: active, passive, voluntary, nonvoluntary, and involuntary.
5. Identify the historical death practices and issues that led to the President's Commission *Uniform Determination of Death Act* in 1981.
6. Define the three standards of death that have emerged since the President's Commission report in 1981.
7. Contrast the criteria for whole-brain death and higher-brain death.
8. Discuss the strengths and weaknesses of each type of advance directive.

9. Explore the nurse's role in communicating information about the types of advance directives to dying patients and their families, patients who are not necessarily dying, and the public.
10. Explain the types of decision-making standards in which surrogate decision makers may participate.
11. Discuss the seven principles regarding surrogate decisions for incompetent patients as they relate to the Terri Schiavo case.
12. Discuss the standard used by the surrogate in the Terri Schiavo case.
13. Analyze the issues that will arise in the decision-making process for patients, families, and healthcare team members for a patient whose treatment has been evaluated as medically futile.
14. Describe types of cases or illnesses that a nurse may see in a palliative care situation.
15. Analyze the substantive moral differences between the three highlighted legal cases of Quinlan, Cruzan, and Schiavo: withholding life-sustaining treatment vs. withdrawing life-sustaining treatment; withholding artificial nutrition and hydration vs. withdrawing artificial nutrition and hydration; and letting go vs. an intentional inducement of death.
16. Delineate the nurse's role, according to the ANA *Code of Ethics for Nurses with Interpretive Statements*, Provision 1, regarding the three conditions of the rule of double effect when caring for a dying patient.
17. Contrast terminal sedation, physician-assisted suicide, and relieving pain and suffering with opiates or opiate-synthetic drugs.
18. Discuss the nurse's moral distress and conflicts when caring for dying patients and their families.
19. Delineate the World Health Organization's pain ladder for patients receiving palliative care.
20. Identify the core principles for end-of-life care and relate them to a previous experience with a dying patient or a would-be dying patient.
21. Explore ways in which nurses could give and manage the spiritual care of dying patients and their families.

What Is Death?

Contemporary ethical discussions about death and dying relate to philosophers attempting to answer captivating questions such as, "What is a good death?" and "How will we all die?" In recent years, the focus has been on the challenging issues of readiness to die, acceptance of death, and knowing the right time to die (Battin, 1994; Connelly, 2003; Hester, 2003). Many questions about death are unanswerable, but individuals can develop a subjective notion about the meaning of death. For people to face death more peacefully, they need to come to their own understanding of death and beyond (and if a "beyond" exists), as well as develop a personal knowing of death's connection. Nietzsche, a German philosopher, proposed that everyone needs a philosophy of life in relation to death. Victor Frankl has credited Nietzsche with saying: "He who has a *why* to live can bear almost any *how*" (Wackernagel & Rieger, 1878, as cited in Frank & Anselmi, 2011, p. 15).

The Ideal Death

Philosopher Andrew Lustig (2003) stated that he has been amazed at how bioethicists are engaging in passionate conversations about the meaning of death, and yet personalizing the truth of our own mortality is difficult. As the title character in the nonfiction bestseller *Tuesdays with Morrie* puts it, "Everyone knows they're going to die, but nobody believes it" (Albom, 1997, p. 81). People "talk death" and romanticize death as if it was something ideal rather than a confrontation with mortality.

People use phrases such as "he passed away" to keep from saying the words "he died" or to avoid facing the reality of death (Spiegel, 1993). Yalom (1980) defined **death anxiety** as a "dread of death that resides in the unconscious, a dread that is formed early in life at a time prior to the development of precise conceptual formation, a dread that is terrible and inchoate and exists outside of language and image" (p. 189). Existential philosophers such as Kierkegaard, Heidegger, and Sartre emphasized that it is in facing death and the possibility of nonbeing that a person comes to know oneself best; in other words, a person first has to put death in perspective to understand any portion of life.

Yalom (1980) stated that individuals avoid facing their own mortality in two ways, or defenses. The first defense against death is through immortality projects, where people throw themselves into commendable projects, their work, or raising children. People thoroughly and completely engage in these activities and, by doing so, they insulate themselves from death. The second defense is through dependence on a rescuer, believing that another person can provide a sense of safety or protection from death. Almost all people want to feel some sense of insulation from elements of threat; death is one of those elements, and dying is a fearful process. Many times patients look to nurses, physicians, and other healthcare professionals to fulfill a rescuer role.

In his studies about death and dying, Spiegel (1993) consulted several hundred people regarding what they fear most about death. Spiegel summed up the responses of people he interviewed as follows:

> Strangely enough, it is not being dead; rather, it is the process of dying. Fears of losing control of your body, suffering increasing pain, losing the ability to do things you love to do, being able to make decisions about your medical care, being separated from

> loved ones: Those are the ways that fears of dying become real. Death is something that pushes the edge of our comprehension. (p. 137)

Death signifies the end of a person's living embodiment. Wanting to die the good death or the ideal death may be everyone's wish at some point in life, but while a person is alive, death often remains a dark secret. Nurses and other healthcare professionals need to envisage dying as a process that everyone must face, and nurses must serve as an advocate for those who are dying. In an article titled "Inventing the Good Death," Brogan (2006) related the story of how the concept of the modern hospice movement was started in 1967 in London by a nurse, Dame Cicely Saunders, who many regard as the Florence Nightingale of the hospice movement. In Saunders's own words about death and dying, she stated:

> I once asked a man who knew he was dying what he needed above all in those who were caring for him. He said, "For someone to look as if they are trying to understand me." I know it is impossible to understand fully another person, but I never forgot that he did not ask for success but only that someone should care enough to try. . . . The suffering of the dying is "total pain" with physical, emotional, spiritual, and social elements. (p. 14)

The suffering man whom Saunders recounted resembles many people's approach to death, meaning that an ideal death does not frequently transpire. Nancy Dubler presented what she called a "cinematic" myth of the "good American death" when she wrote

> [The good death scene] includes the patient: lucid, composed, hungering for blissful release—and the family gathers in grief to mourn the passing of a beloved life. The murmurs of sad good-byes, the cadence of quiet tears shroud the scene in dignity. Unfortunately for many of us, our deaths will not be the spiritual, peaceful "passing" that we might envision or desire. (as cited in Hester, 2010, pp. 3–4)

Lehto and Stein (2009) emphasized the significance of death anxiety and the role of nurses in everyday practice. Nurses need to take into account the possibility that some patients manifest ill effects or behaviors as a result of experiencing death anxiety. For most people, death is a mysterious event to be discovered rather than a comforting scene with the presence of family members and others hovering over them (Hester, 2003). Patients often find themselves, if at all conscious, connected to ventilators and other machines, intravenous lines and meters, and receiving many medications. Technology and medicalization have exacerbated the problem of depersonalization. Family members or significant others experience difficulty communicating with their loved one because of physical, technological, and environmental barriers. During this incomprehensible time, the nursing staff could be a patient's most reliable and consistent contact. When decisions about life and end-of-life need to be made, family members are often faced with uncertainty about the kind of treatment their loved one would want in particular circumstances. Even when patients have adequate decision-making capacity, they may want input from family members or significant others in treatment decisions. Sometimes family members will find it difficult to discuss the uncertainties of treatments with their loved one: they may have restrictions on their visitation because of inflexible hospital policies, or they may feel at a loss to help and do not want their loved one to know how they feel.

Whatever death a person is to experience—a good death; an anticipated death; a sudden, unexpected death; or a painful, lingering death—most of the time, people do not have a choice in how they will die. Individuals, meanwhile, need to shift the focus from thoughts "that we die" toward "how we die" so that people can place substantial thought on future decisions about end-of-life care and what might be best for them (Hester, 2010, p. 3).

The benefit of persons envisioning an ideal death and reflecting on it from time to time is that the image helps them develop a sense of readiness for a peaceful death. The famous American philosopher John Dewey (as cited in Fesmire, 2003) described a similar moral framework that is based on a person's development of intelligent habits through an imaginative dramatic rehearsal. Dewey discussed dramatic rehearsal in terms of creative dialogue between two or more people in a particular scenario. In applying the **imaginative dramatic rehearsal**, a person can imagine one's own death by reconstructing the ideal death scenario; on continued reflection, they may later discover a rich, meaningful experience through this imagination (Fesmire, 2003; Hester, 2003). Persons who imagine an ideal death may have a greater possibility of finding significance at the end of their lives and then, to some extent, may be able to help shape their dying process.

The Concept of Human Suffering of Dying Patients

Philosophers, professionals, researchers, and religious leaders agree that suffering is difficult to condense into one succinct definition. Human suffering can be connected to many episodes, contexts, and events, but a large part of the suffering literature is associated with chronically ill or dying patients and their families.

Hester (2010) emphasized that healthcare professionals should not reduce the concept of suffering to pain, explaining, "When we speak of suffering we mean far more than pain" (p. 18). Kahn and Steeves (1986) stated that an individual could experience suffering following a sense of threat to the being, the self, and existence. Similarly, Eric Cassell (2004) emphasized that suffering involves the whole person and body, but that pain and suffering are separate phenomena. After several years of studying suffering, Eriksson (1997) defined **suffering** as a perceived undesirable inner experience that could threaten the whole existence of being, yet is a necessary element of life, as are joy and happiness. If others show compassion toward a suffering person, one could develop a more meaningful suffering existence.

Stan van Hooft (2000, 2006) has been at the forefront of studying the Aristotelian framework of the human soul as a way to explain human suffering. Aristotle contended that a soul consists of a being with physical and spiritual interconnections. Aristotle (as cited in van Hooft, 2000) described the being as having four inseparable parts:

1. Vegetative: Nonrational biological functions
2. Appetitive: Nonrational desires and the striving for attaining desires
3. Deliberative: Mostly rational and reasoned strategic thinking about how to fulfill self goals
4. Contemplative: A fully rational soul, the spiritual part, and thinking about the things that are unchangeable about the meaning of one's existence and the spiritual soul

Each of these four parts has its own telos (goal), but as interconnected and inseparable parts of a whole being, they have one purpose, which Aristotle labeled as achieving *eudaimonia* (happiness, human fulfillment, and flourishing). If one part cannot reach this would-be goal, the whole being suffers because the mind and body are inseparable insofar as these four parts are concerned. As such, van Hooft (2000) concluded that suffering is the opposite of flourishing.

To differentiate pain from suffering, van Hooft (2000) stated that because pain is a hurtful and unpleasant sensation with a variation of intensities and degrees, it can interfere with individuals' achievement of a flourishing life and therefore will lead to suffering. Pain is a result of malady or an illness of the vegetative or bodily state; pain can steal joy, contentment, and happiness, and cause individuals to suffer and lose a passion for life. Suffering saturates the whole body in all of its four parts.

Catherine Garrett's (2005) life work on the differentiation of pain from suffering contributes to the meaning of suffering, describing the **suffering person** as a tormented being. Suffering is an inevitable but unwelcome component of experiencing life. Suffering is not only subjective, but it is also objective in the sense that a suffering person's symptoms can become recognizable signs to others. Examples include a person who is experiencing death and dying, a chronic illness, or chronic violence.

Responsibility of Nurses toward Suffering Patients

How an individual chooses to understand human suffering is personal. Nurses need to interpret the suffering of their patients in an attempt to alleviate or minimize pain or distress. Examples of official nursing documents that include statements on the need for nurses to reduce and alleviate suffering in patients are highlighted in Box 9.1.

Cassell (2004) made a connection between human suffering on the individual level and a person's need for compassion. Nurses' mindfulness of this connection can enrich their comprehension of patient suffering. Everything that nurses can know about a patient is retrieved from nursing assessments, interviews, and interpersonal interactions. One way for nurses to begin the journey of comprehending others' suf-

BOX 9.1 ETHICAL FORMATIONS: NURSES' MORAL OBLIGATION TOWARD HUMAN SUFFERING

Nursing obligations and responsibilities are published in several official nursing documents. The following comments represent only three of these documents.

- *The ANA Code of Ethics for Nurses with Interpretive Statements* (2001): "Nurses actively participate in assessing and assuring the responsible and appropriate use of interventions in order to minimize unwarranted treatment and patient suffering" (Provision 1.3, p. 8; see Appendix A).
- *The National Council of State Boards of Nursing NCLEX-RN Test Plan 2010* (2009): The goal of nursing is "preventing illness; alleviating suffering; protecting, promoting, and restoring health; and promoting dignity in dying" (p. 2).
- *The International Council of Nurses ICN Code of Ethics for Nurses* (2006): "Nurses have four fundamental responsibilities: to promote health, to prevent illness, to restore health and to alleviate suffering" (p. 1; see Appendix B).

fering is through the context of having compassion. Nurses generally use strategies such as empathy, compassion, and attentive listening to console suffering patients.

Euthanasia

The thought of extended agony and suffering prior to death provokes a sense of dread in most people, but keeping emotional, financial, and social burdens to a minimum and avoiding suffering are not always possible (Munson, 2004). O'Rourke (2002) noted that most people go to extremes to avoid suffering when he stated, "Suffering in all its forms is an evil, and every reasonable effort should be made to relieve it" (p. 221). However, an untold number of people die every day with tremendous suffering and pain. For many years, people have debated whether to legalize euthanasia, a process often referred to as "mercy killing."

Until his conviction on a second-degree murder charge (for which he served eight years in prison, from 1999 to 2007), Dr. Jack Kevorkian assisted with more than 100 suicides or mercy killings (Public Broadcasting System & WGBH Frontline, 1998). From 1990 to 1998, at the request of suffering patients from various parts of the United States, he helped them end their lives; he has been nicknamed "Doctor Death" because of his euthanasia practices. Kevorkian was charged, but later acquitted, on several occasions prior to his conviction for euthanizing Thomas Youk. On November 22, 1998, 15 million viewers of the CBS program *60 Minutes* watched Dr. Kevorkian give a lethal injection to Thomas Youk, age 52, who was dying with Lou Gehrig's disease. Once this program aired, strong debates surfaced in the media and in healthcare, political, and legal systems worldwide. Dr. Kevorkian died in June 2011 with his long-held belief that people have a right to die and a to request death unchanged (Schneider, 2011).

Euthanasia, which has come to mean a good or painless death, has developed a strong appeal in recent years, partly because of the political muddle on the right-to-die issues and the association of these issues with the misery and suffering of dying patients. There are two major types of euthanasia (Munson, 2004). **Active euthanasia** is the intentional and purposeful act of causing the immediate death of another person, such as a person with a terminal illness, a painful disease, or who cannot be cured. **Passive euthanasia**, or letting go, is the intentional withholding or withdrawing of medical or life-sustaining treatments. A debate continues in the United States whether there is a real moral difference between active euthanasia and passive euthanasia, and although withdrawing or withholding medical or life-sustaining treatment has become widely accepted today, active euthanasia has not (Brannigan & Boss, 2001; Jonsen, Veatch, & Walters, 1998).

Other ways that euthanasia has been described are voluntary, nonvoluntary, and involuntary. **Voluntary euthanasia** occurs when patients with decision-making capacity authorize physicians to take their lives. Voluntary euthanasia has become associated most with the term **physician-assisted suicide**, which is defined as the taking of one's own life with a lethal dose of physician-ordered medication. Currently, Oregon, Washington, and Montana have laws approving the practice of physician-assisted suicide. **Nonvoluntary euthanasia** occurs when persons are not able to give express consent to end their lives and are unaware that they are going to be euthanized. For example, a physician could euthanize a patient when a family member who serves as a decision maker gives consent. **Involuntary euthanasia** means that a person's consent may be possible but is not sought, and a physician could euthanize someone without express consent. An example of involuntary euthanasia is the euthanizing of a death-row inmate.

Salvageability and Unsalvageability Principle

In her book, *The Least Worst Death*, Battin (1994) argued that euthanasia is a morally right and humane act on the grounds of mercy, autonomy, and justice. The principle of mercy ("mercy killing") includes two obligations: the duty not to cause further pain and suffering and the duty to act to end existing pain or suffering. The principle of autonomy involves the idea that health professionals ought to respect a person's right to choose a suitable course of medical treatment. The principle of justice is based on how unsalvageable the providers of care believe a permanently unconscious person to be.

Based on this salvageability/unsalvageability principle, however, a healthcare provider could justify performing euthanasia on still competent but dying patients if they were regarded as unsalvageable (Battin, 1994). It is in knowing where to draw the legal and moral line with this principle that providers and families may face difficult decisions. Any decisions must be carefully examined, especially when the acts may go beyond the meaning of the principle of unsalvageability. There are many opponents against this slippery slope euthanasia argument. Battin, who is a supporter of euthanasia for the unsalvageable suffering person, opposes the slippery slope euthanasia argument. She stated:

> But to require the person who chooses to die to stay alive in order to protect those who might unwillingly be killed sometime in the future is to impose an extreme harm—intolerable suffering—on that person, which he or she must bear for the sake of others. [I ask] which is the worse of two evils, death or pain? (p. 119)

Historical Influences on the Definition of Death

In Europe in the 18th and 19th centuries, there was widespread fear of being buried alive because of inadequate methods for detecting when a person was dead; sometimes, when a body was exhumed, claw marks were found on the inside of the coffin lid. There are documented accounts of people being buried alive, but some stories became embellished over time. As a result, many people came to believe exaggerated accounts of premature burial.

Whether stories were embellished or not, great fear persisted during that era, possibly for good reason. Out of fear of being buried alive, the great composer Frédéric Chopin left a request in his will to be dissected after his death and before being buried in order to make certain that he was dead (Bondeson, 2001). Even the dying words of George Washington were "Have me decently buried; and do not let my body be put into the Vault in less than three days after I am dead" (Lear, 1906).

When laws preventing premature burials were enacted, the owners of funeral homes went to the extreme of having their staff monitor dead bodies during the "wait" time. Before the law had taken effect, special signaling devices were installed from inside the coffin to the outside world to help those buried alive to communicate with others above the ground.

For hundreds of years, when a person became unconscious, physicians or others would palpate for a pulse, listen for breath sounds with their ears, look for condensation on an object when it was held close to the body's nose, and check for fixed and dilated pupils (Mappes & DeGrazia, 2001). The invention of the stethoscope in 1819 led to reduced fear, because physicians could listen with greater certainty for a heartbeat through a magnified listening device placed on the chest of the body.

A breakthrough in technology occurred at the beginning of the 20th century when Willem Einthoven, a Dutch physician, discovered the existence of electrical properties of the heart with his invention of the first electrocardiograph (EKG) in 1903 (Benjamin, 2003). The EKG provided sensitive information about whether or not the heart was functioning. From the middle of the 19th century to the middle of the 20th century, there seemed to be a consensus about determination of death, meaning that when the heart stopped beating and the person stopped breathing, the person had ceased to exist.

Society began to change its perceptions of death as technology became integrated into medicine. The 1950s and 1960s brought more uncertainty involving death as physicians kept patients alive in the absence of a natural heartbeat. Once transplants were being performed in the 1960s and 1970s, it became apparent that a diagnosis of death would not necessarily depend on the absence of a heartbeat and respirations. Rather, in the future, the definition of death would need to include brain death criteria.

In 1968, an ad hoc committee at Harvard Medical School attempted to redefine death not only in terms of heart–lung cessation, but added reliable brain death criteria for ventilator-dependent patients with no brain function (described by committee members as patients in an irreversible coma) (Benjamin, 2003). Back then, this definition led to confusion about the term "brain death" and to a widespread misconception about whether the human organism—the person—was actually dead. Somehow, brain death, which technically means death of the brain, came to mean death of a human organism or person. Because of the way some individuals perceived the meaning of the term "brain death," they translated the 1968 definition to mean that two kinds of death existed for human organisms: the traditional heart–lung death and now a new kind of death called brain death. Benjamin emphasized that ethicists and physicians had not given sufficient attention to clarifying this term before the article was published in 1968.

The Definition of Death

Ethicists, physicians, and others continued intense debates about death. It was not until 1981 that members of a President's Commission for the Study of Ethical Problems in Medicine and Biomedical and Behavioral Research wrote in the document *Defining Death* that the body was an organism as a whole:

> Three organs—the heart, lungs, and brain—assume special significance—because their interrelationship is very close and the irreversible cessation of any one very quickly stops the other two and consequently halts the integrated functioning of the organism as a whole. Because they were easily measured, circulation and respiration were traditionally the basic "vital signs." But breathing and heartbeat are not life itself. They are simply used as signs—as one window for viewing a deeper and more complex reality: a triangle of interrelated systems with the brain at its apex. (President's Commission, 1981, p. 33)

The commission members sanctioned a definition of death in 1981 and recommended its adoption (President's Commission, 1981, see Box 9.2 for the definition of death). Debates continue concerning which criteria belong in the definition of death and, more specifically, death of the brain. Since this 1981 definition was adopted, criteria for death of the brain have been adopted by every state.

BOX 9.2 ETHICAL FORMATIONS: DEATH DEFINED IN 1981

The members of the President's Commission defined death in accordance with accepted medical standards. This definition was enacted as the Uniform Determination of Death Act of 1981. A person who is dead is one who has sustained either:

- Irreversible cessation of circulatory and respiratory functions, or
- Irreversible cessation of all functions of the entire brain, including the brain stem.

Source: President's Commission for the Study of Ethical Problems in Medicine and Biomedical and Behavioral Research. (1981). *Defining death: Medical, legal, & ethical issues in the determination of death.* Washington, DC: Government Printing Office, p. 73. Retrieved from http://bioethics.georgetown.edu/pcbe/reports/past_commissions/defining_death.pdf; Youngner, S. J., & Arnold, R. M. (2001). Philosophical debates about the defintion of death: Who cares? *Journal of Medicine and Philosophy, 26*(5), 527–537.

Veatch (2003) has extended the debate on the definition of death by posing an intriguing question regarding the loss of full moral standing for human beings. This statement triggers the question as to when humans should be treated as full members of the human community. Almost every person has reconciled the thought that some persons have full moral standing and others do not, but there is continued controversy about when full moral standing ceases to exist and what characteristics qualify for the cessation of full moral standing. Losing full moral standing is equivalent to ceasing to exist.

Some physicians and bioethicists have recognized three standards for death (DeGrazia, 2007/2011; see Box 9.3). With whole-brain death, the patient may survive physically for an indeterminate duration with a mechanical ventilator. Some patients may seemingly have complete loss of brain function only to have the electrical activity of the brain reappear later, even if it is minimal, which makes the Uniform Declaration of Death Act (UDDA) whole-brain death criteria difficult to use for pronouncing a person dead (Munson, 2004). Veatch (2003) notes the peculiarity of such an event: "A brain-dead patient on a ventilator does, of course, make for an unusual corpse.

BOX 9.3 ETHICAL FORMATIONS: THREE STANDARDS FOR DEATH

- **Cardiopulmonary death:** A person is dead by cardiopulmonary criteria when the cessation of breathing and heartbeat is irreversible.
- **Whole-brain death or permanent brain failure**: Death is regarded as the irreversible cessation of all brain functions, with no electrical activity in the brain, including the brain stem.
- **Higher-brain death:** Human death is considered the irreversible cessation of the capacity for consciousness, which implies that the person is dead even though the continual function of brain stem regulates breathing and heartbeat (such as in a persistent vegetative state).

Source: Degrazia, D. (2007/2011). The definition of death (updated Fall 2011). *Stanford encyclopedia of philosophy.* Retrieved from http://plato.stanford.edu/archives/fall2011/entries/death-definition

On the ventilator, he is respiring and his heart is beating. But if his whole brain is dead, the law in most jurisdictions says that the patient is deceased" (p. 38).

At the point when the person has met brain death UDDA criteria and is pronounced dead, mechanical ventilation and medical treatment can be discontinued (Benjamin, 2003). Because of the variation in the clinical evaluation for brain death from institution to institution, the American Academy of Neurology offered uniform clinical evaluation guidelines for determining brain death (Wijdicks, Varelas, Gronseth, & Greer, 2010, pp. 1911, 1915–1916). See Box 9.4 for these guidelines.

An electroencephalogram (EEG) is a meter device used to measure the electrical activity of the brain (Munson, 2004). If a person is on life-sustaining support when in the process of being pronounced dead, such as in whole-brain death, an EEG is needed in addition to the criteria listed in Box 9.4. Usually, one EEG is sufficient for a physician to pronounce someone brain dead in the United States (Wijdicks et al., 2010), but some jurisdictions require that two EEGs, performed 24 hours apart, show no brain activity before physicians can disconnect them from life-sustaining support. Physicians and nurses must also make certain that loss of brain function is not due to mind-altering medications, hypoglycemia, hyponatremia, or any other cause.

BOX 9.4 ETHICAL FORMATIONS: CLINICAL EVALUATION GUIDELINES FOR DETERMINING BRAIN DEATH BY NEUROLOGIC ASSESSMENT

Coma—patients must lack all evidence of responsiveness.

Eye opening or eye movement to noxious stimuli is absent. Noxious stimuli should not produce a motor response.

Absence of brain stem reflexes.

Absence of pupillary response to a bright light is documented in both eyes.

The pupils are fixed in a midsize or dilated position.

Constricted pupils indicate drug intoxication.

Absence of ocular movements using oculocephalic testing and oculovestibular reflex testing.

There is no movement of the eyes in relation to head movement.

Absence of corneal reflex.

No eyelid movement is observed.

Absence of facial muscle movement to a noxious stimulus.

There is no grimacing or facial movement in response to a noxious stimulus test.

Absence of the pharyngeal and tracheal reflexes.

Apnea—absence of a breathing drive.

Source: Wijdicks, E. F. M., Varelas, P. N., Gronseth, G. S., & Greer, D. M. (2010). Evidence-based guideline update: Determining brain death in adults: Report of the Quality Standards Subcommittee of the American Academy of Neurology. *Neurology, 74*(23), 1911–1918.

With higher-brain death, or loss of higher-brain function, the patient lives in a persistent vegetative state (PVS) indefinitely but without the need for mechanical ventilation. A person with higher-brain death may have some functions permanently lost but not others, which has been the cause of enormous dispute. Even very minimal brain functioning, such as limited reflexes in the brain stem, is cause for a patient to be diagnosed with higher-brain death (Veatch, 2003). It is because of these situations that questions exist regarding whether a person should be treated as one who has full moral standing in the human community.

Society, physicians, and nurses have difficulty defining death by the UDDA definition, especially when they try to incorporate the standards of cardiopulmonary death, whole-brain death, or higher-brain death. No definite criteria for higher-brain have been established for defining death. Meanwhile, Benjamin (2003) posed this question for people to consider: "Exactly what is it that ceases to exist when we say someone like you or me is dead?" (p. 197). Benjamin and Veatch affirmed that there will be no answers to questions like this one until ethicists and others can come to some sort of consensus about what life is, when life begins, when life ends, and who does and does not have full moral standing.

Advance Directives

An **advance directive** is "a written expression of a person's wishes about medical care, especially care during a terminal or critical illness" (Veatch, 2003, p. 119). When individuals lose control over their lives, they may also lose their decision-making capacity, and advance directives become instructions about their future health care for others to follow. Advance directives can be self-written instructions or prepared by someone else as instructed by the patient. Under the federal Patient Self-Determination Act of 1990, states, under mandated authority, have developed state laws to protect the rights of individuals making decisions about end-of-life and medical care. (See Appendix D for an example of a complete legal packet for a healthcare advance directive.) Critical issues that need to be addressed in any advance directive include specific treatments to be refused or that are desired; the time the directive needs to take effect; specific hospitals and physicians to be used; what lawyer, if any, should be consulted; and specific other consultations, such as an ethics team, a chaplain, or a neighbor. There are three types of advance directives: living will, medical care directive, and durable power of attorney.

A **living will** is a formal legal document that provides written directions concerning what medical care is to be provided in specific circumstances (Devettere, 2000). The living will gained recognition in the 1960s, but the Karen Ann Quinlan case in the 1970s brought public attention to the living will and subsequently prompted legalization of the document. Although living wills were a good beginning, today they are not completely adequate. Problems can arise when living wills consist of vague language, contain only instructions for unwanted treatments, lack a description of legal penalties for those people who choose to ignore the directives of living wills, and are legally questionable as to their authenticity.

A **medical care directive** is not a formal legal document, but it provides specific written instructions to the physician concerning the type of care and treatments that individuals want to receive if they become incapacitated. The biggest advantage to medical care directives is that physicians use them as a guide to know what incapacitated patients want in terms of specific healthcare treatments. Convinced that medical care directives are only extended informed consents, attorneys believe that medical care directives are only a minimal improvement over living wills. Other weaknesses of medical care directives are that people cannot possibly anticipate every medical problem that may occur in their future; also, people change over time and may change their mind about future wishes even after they have delineated the instructions for their medical care directive.

The **durable power of attorney** is a legal written directive in which a designated person can make either general or specific healthcare and medical decisions for a patient. This durable power of attorney has the most strength for facilitating healthcare decisions; however, even with a power of attorney, families and healthcare professionals may experience fear about making the wrong decisions regarding an incapacitated patient (Beauchamp & Childress, 2001).

In addition to the weaknesses previously discussed about advance directives, other weaknesses that may arise include the fact that very few people ever complete an advance directive, a surrogate decision maker may be unavailable for decision making, and healthcare professionals cannot overturn advance directives in the event that a decision needs to be made in the best interest of a patient. The existence of advance directives can be a source of comfort for patients and families as long as they realize their limitations and scope. Ensuring the validity of the advance directive, realizing the importance of preserving patients from unwanted intrusive interventions, and respecting the possibility that patients may change their minds about their expressed written wishes are several ways that nurses must demonstrate benevolence toward patients and their families.

Surrogate Decision Makers

When patients can no longer make competent decisions, families may experience difficulty in trying to determine a progressive right course of action. The ideal situation is for patients to be autonomous decision makers, but when autonomy is no longer possible, decision making falls to a surrogate (Beauchamp & Childress, 2009). The **surrogate decision maker**, often known as a proxy, is an individual who acts on behalf of a patient and either is chosen by the patient, such as a family member; is court appointed; or has other authority to make decisions. Family members serving as proxies are generally referred to as surrogates.

Advances in healthcare technology and life-sustaining treatments precipitated the development of the surrogate decision maker role, as it is known today.

Decisions about treatment options and the motives behind these decisions may be complex and destructive. Before the surrogate makes a decision, there needs to be appropriate dialogue among the physicians, the nurses, and the surrogate (Emanuel, Danis, Pearlman, & Singer, 1995). On behalf of the patient, surrogates endure an uncomfortable multistage decision-making process that involves gathering information and engaging the patient (when possible), extended family members, physicians, nurses, and other healthcare professionals. During this process, the surrogate decision makers consider their own subjective views, the perceptions from others on the status of the patient, the medical evidence, and patient preferences (Buckley & Abell, 2009).

Surrogate decision makers sometimes have difficulty distinguishing between their own emotions and the feelings of others or they may have monetary motives for making certain decisions. It is the responsibility of nurses and physicians to be observant for these kinds of motives or concerns and then to look for therapeutic ways to deliberate with the the surrogate. Box 9.5 contains seven principles, called pillars, that form the foundation for surrogate decision makers when deciding to forgo life-sustaining treatment on behalf of incompetent patients. These seven principles are derived from the issues surrounding the 1970s case of Karen Ann

BOX 9.5 ETHICAL FORMATIONS: SEVEN PRINCIPLES FOR SURROGATE DECISIONS WITH INCOMPETENT PATIENTS

1. Competent patients have an autonomy-based right, recognized under the constitution and common law, to refuse treatment, including life-sustaining treatment. Life-sustaining treatment includes artificially provided nutrition and hydration.
2. Incompetent patients have the same panoply [full array] of rights as competent patients, although the manner in which those rights are exercised is different.
3. No right is absolute, but instances in which a patient's right to refuse life support is outweighed by societal interests are rare.
4. Withholding and withdrawing treatment from a terminally ill or permanently unconscious patient allows a natural dying process to take its course. It does not constitute killing or assisted suicide.
5. In making decisions for incompetent patients, surrogate decision makers should seek first and foremost to follow a subjective standard of implementing the patient's wishes. When this test proves inadequate, a best interests standard may be applied.
6. In ascertaining an incompetent patient's wishes, the surrogate, family, and physician should rely on a patient's advance directive if one has been issued.
7. A local process of review in the clinical setting should be employed to facilitate resolution of disagreements. Recourse to the courts should be rare.

Source: Olick, R. S. (2001). *Taking advance directives seriously: Prospective autonomy and decisions near the end of life.* Washington, DC: Georgetown University Press, p. 30.

Quinlan and her family (discussed later in this chapter). As Olick (2001) stated, "In many respects, [these principles] may be said to be a part of the legacy of Karen Ann Quinlan and her family" (p. 30). Of interest too is the influence that these principles had on the Terri Schiavo case and her family. (The Schiavo case is discussed later in this chapter.)

There are three types of surrogate decision-making standards (Beauchamp & Childress, 2009; Veatch, 2003). The **substituted judgment standard** is used to guide medical decisions that involve formerly competent patients who no longer have any decision-making capacity. This standard is based on the assumption that incompetent patients have the exact same rights as competent patients to make judgments about their health care (Buchanan & Brock, 1990). Surrogates make medical treatment decisions based on what the surrogates believe the patients would have decided were the patients still competent and able to express their wishes. In making decisions, the surrogates use their understanding of the patients' previous overt or implied expressions of their beliefs and values (Veatch, 2003). Before losing competency, the patient could have either explicitly informed the surrogate of treatment wishes by oral or written instruction or implicitly made treatment wishes clear through informal conversations.

When more than one sibling is involved in the decisions regarding the care of a dying parent, many times misunderstandings occur and angry feelings over practical, legal, and financial matters become apparent. The siblings will be affected uniquely by their parent's death, depending on several factors: the type of relationship that exists between each sibling and the parent, if and how each sibling has experienced death in the past, each sibling's present life situation and stressors, their past grudges toward siblings, and current sibling relationships. One sibling usually takes charge or the siblings give one sibling the label of speaker for the group. Even when one is empowered, however, the others usually desire an equal voice in the decision-making process. This may be a frustrating process for everyone if the siblings cannot come to a decision. Dialogue is important so that all involved can come to an understanding and avoid further misunderstandings and pain.

The **pure autonomy standard** is based on a decision that was made by an autonomous patient while competent but later drifts to incompetency. In this particular case, the decision is upheld most of the time based on the principle of autonomy extended (Veatch, 2003). The **best interests standard** is an evaluation of what is good for an incompetent patient in particular healthcare situations when the patient has probably never been competent, such as in the case of an infant or mentally retarded adult. The surrogate attempts to decide what is best for the incompetent patient based on the patient's dignity and worth as a human being without taking into consideration the patient's concept of what is good or bad. The surrogate will have no evidence or basis for determining the incompetent patient's desires or what is "best" for that patient, but the surrogate evaluates benefits and burdens for available treatment options. Because the best interests standard is patient-centered, the surrogate must make decisions based on current and future interests (Buchanan & Brock, 1990). These decisions inevitably involve muddy, subjective quality-of-life judgments such as appraising the incompetent patient's simple life pleasures and contentment, sense of social worth, degree of pain and suffering experienced, and the treatment benefits and costs.

According to the American Nurses Association *Code of Ethics with Interpretive Statements* (2001), Provision 1.4, nurses have a moral obligation to respect human dignity and certain patient rights, especially that of patient self-determination. What are some strategies that the nurse can implement to ensure the respect of human dignity and self-determination for an incompetent patient?

Medical Futility

Humpty Dumpty sat on a wall,
Humpty Dumpty had a great fall;
All the King's horses,
And all the King's men,
Could not put Humpty Dumpty together again.

—*Lewis Carroll, 1872,*
Adventures of Alice in Wonderland *and* Through the Looking Glass

The writer of this chapter has posed an analogy between the meaning of medical futility and that of the life of Humpty Dumpty and his broken body after the fall—"All the King's horses and all the King's men could not put Humpty Dumpty together again" (see Figure 9.1). The term *futile* represents pointless or meaningless events or objects (O'Rourke, 2002). **Medical futility** is defined as "the unacceptably low chance of achieving a therapeutic benefit for the patient" (Schneiderman, 1994, para 10). Questions to ask regarding futility as related to the bioethics are:

- What is at stake?
- What weight does the term *futility* carry?
- Is the meaning and weight of the term *futility* appreciated from the broader dominion of bioethics?
- What are healthcare professionals' ethical obligations insofar as thinking that a medical intervention is clearly futile?
- Who makes the final decision—who has the power?
- How can hospitals and other healthcare agencies incorporate a reasonable, fair, objective, and clear policy on futility?

Schneiderman (1994) linked his definition of medical futility to the whole person, the wholeness similar to the way that Aristotle spoke of a human being with four inseparable parts. In other words, a suffering person will seek a cure, healing,

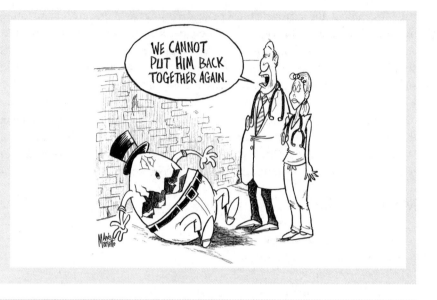

Figure 9.1 Humpty Dumpty Cartoon
Source: Andy Marlette Cartoons.

or care from a provider to become as whole as possible again. In weighing the concept of futility, the nurse must understand that the suffering-healing-provider relationship is integral to the health process and the goals of medicine and nursing. The provider of care is responsible for administering medical treatments and interventions that will benefit the patient as a whole and not just have a small effect on some part of the body or an organ. Integrated throughout this process is the necessity of the patient comprehending and appreciating the benefits of medical treatment. To comprehend these benefits, the person must be conscious at least partially; patients who are in a persistent vegetative state cannot possibly appreciate the beneficiary effects of the treatment. The mere effect is of no benefit if that effect does not help a patient to achieve some degree of life goals or human fulfillment, or the type of *telos* that Aristotle emphasized.

Medical futility goes back in history as long as can be remembered, and in ancient Greece there was an acceptance of physicians refusing to treat people who were overwrought with disease. The futility movement became more important in the 1970s, when medical technology brought about extraordinary life support and life-extending measures. As physicians began asking the questions, "What is a good death?" and "When do we let go?", medical futility emerged as an important concept. Throughout the 1970s and 1980s, philosophers and physicians strongly debated the concept of futility in an effort to define the term and create guidelines for putting it into practice. In the 1990s, definitions began to shift from the theme of blaming providers of care for failures to a focus on more quantitative and qualitative values of treatments that have indicated low probabilities of benefits in the past.

BOX 9.6 ETHICAL FORMATIONS: LANDMARK LEGAL CASES INVOLVING MEDICAL FUTILITY DECISIONS

1988: The Case of Helga Wanglie

An elderly woman, age 85 at that time, fractured her hip when she slipped on a rug and then developed severe ventilator-dependent pneumonia. She was later diagnosed with persistent vegetative state (PVS, or higher-brain death) secondary to hypoxic-ischemic neuropathy and was ventilator dependent secondary to chronic lung disease. (Patients with PVS generally do not require mechanical ventilation because the brain stem is intact. Her dependency on the ventilator related strictly to her chronic lung disease.) Physicians at two facilities agreed that treatment would be futile, but the family members wanted her to be treated and kept alive as long as possible. They believed the physicians were "playing God" but did agree to a DNR physician order with much trepidation. After an intense legal battle, the court on July 1, 1991, authorized Mr. Wanglie, her husband, to be the surrogate decision maker for Ms. Wanglie. However, on July 4, 1991, only 3 days after the final court decision, Ms. Wanglie died.

1993: In the Matter of Baby K

In 1992, Baby K was born with anencephaly, meaning with a brain stem but with no capacity for a conscious life, and statistically was predicted not to be able to survive more than a few days to months. Physicians and ethics committee members argued that it would be futile to keep Baby K alive on ventilator support but the mother insisted that Baby K be kept alive because she believed that all human life is precious and is to be preserved. The federal court supported the mother's claim only if someone would assume the amount of the mother's bills for care of Baby K. The mother found that monetary support, and Baby K lived for 2 years in a nursing home on ventilator support.

1995: *Gilgunn v. Massachusetts General Hospital*

In a rare early case of a court's supporting a physician's claim of medical futility, the jury, after the fact, found that cardiopulmonary resuscitation need not be provided to a patient dying with multiple organ-system failure, as in the case of Ms. Gilgunn, age 71, who was comatose. The family had sought treatment but the physician objected. The jury's decision was the result of a retrospective evaluation of the medical decision. The jury's decision for stopping futile treatment was unique at that time.

There are landmark cases of legal medical futility, including (1) the case of Helga Wanglie, (2) In the Matter of Baby K, and (3) *Gilgunn v. Massachusetts General Hospital*. Box 9.6 contains a brief highlight of these three cases.

Healthcare professionals and most other people have accepted and ethically justified withholding and withdrawing treatments deemed as futile or extraordinary. However, this does not mean that withholding or withdrawing treatment is universally accepted. In the case of Terri Schiavo (*Schindler and Schiavo v. Michael Schiavo*), Terri's case was not primarily about medical futility; rather, it was about Michael's legal, not ethical, responsibility for carrying out Terri's express and previous verbal wishes of not wanting to stay alive in such circumstances. Terri

Schiavo, with all evidential information set forth by the physician who performed the autopsy, met the legal definition of a persistent vegetative state and therefore was a medically futile case regarding treatment.

When a healthcare provider cannot have reasonable hope that a treatment will benefit a terminally ill person, the medical treatment is considered futile care. Treatments often considered medically futile include cardiopulmonary resuscitation (CPR), medications, mechanical ventilation, artificial feeding and fluids, hemodialysis, chemotherapy, and other life-sustaining technologies. When surrogates are the spokespersons for patients, one of the nurse's responsibilities is to make sure that communication remains open between the healthcare team and the decision maker for the family. Everyone needs to have a chance to express feelings and concerns about treatment options viewed as medically futile (Ladd, Pasquerella, & Smith, 2002).

Complete black and white boundaries do not exist regarding medical futility because there are always questionable gray areas, and even Humpty Dumpty's case was questionable. Remember that it was all the King's horses and all the King's men who could not put Humpty Dumpty together again. However, no men or horses from another King's court tried to put Humpty Dumpty together again, contrary to what occurs in real medical futility cases, since a second opinion is an essential component in declaring medical futility.

Grayness will always exist because healthcare providers and other professionals attempt to embrace the patient's hope and consider the patient's values and feelings, even though the patient may not cognitively have feelings. However, healthcare providers acknowledge that all human beings have limits. By the sheer fact that the human component exists on both sides of the futility–value issue, gray areas that blur the boundaries will always exist. Patients, families, judges, patient advocacy groups, the media, sociopoliticos, and the public will challenge these gray boundaries time after time. See Box 9.7 on developing your beliefs and opinions about medical futility.

Palliative Care

Palliative care consists of comfort care measures that patients may request instead of aggressive medical treatments when their condition is terminal. Nurses are probably the most active of all the healthcare professionals in meeting the palliative needs of dying patients. Palliative care has become an organized movement through official associations and organizations since the 1990s. The World Health Organization (WHO, 2011) has defined **palliative care** as an approach that "improves the quality of life of patients and their families facing the problem associated with life-threatening illness, through the prevention and relief of suffering by means of early identification and impeccable assessment and treatment of pain and other problems, physical, psychosocial, and spiritual" (para. 1).

BOX 9.7 ETHICAL FORMATIONS: DEVELOPING YOUR BELIEFS AND OPINIONS ABOUT MEDICAL FUTILITY

Questions to ponder as you develop your beliefs and opinions on the medical futility of a patient, such as one in the last stages of metastasized cancer:

- What ethical theory, approach, or principle provides the rationale for your beliefs on autonomy and medical futility? Explain.
- How far does one go with patient autonomy?
- Do you believe that patient autonomy should have limits?
- Should patient autonomy (and surrogate autonomy) be unlimited, no matter what the physician believes should and should not be done?
- Would the healthcare system's financial burden be a factor for setting limits on patient autonomy (and surrogate autonomy) in your personal opinion or as a societal stance?
- Do patients or families have a moral right to insist on medical treatment that two or more physicians and hospitals have deemed futile? Give your rationale based on your ethical theory, approach, or principle.
- Do providers of care have a moral duty to provide medically futile treatment at the family's request, just because the family wants it?

Understanding what quality of life means to the dying patient is an important part of end-of-life care for nurses, and no matter what stage of dying the patient is experiencing, the main goals of palliative care are to prevent and relieve suffering and to allow for the best care possible for patients and families.

When nurses provide palliative care, they do not hasten or prolong death for these patients; rather, they try to provide patients with relief from pain and suffering and help them maintain dignity in the dying experience. Palliative treatment may include a patient's and family's choice to forgo, withhold, or withdraw treatment. Some patients will have a **do not resuscitate (DNR) order**, which is a written physician's order placed in a patient's chart that indicates that hospital personnel are not to carry out any type of CPR or other resuscitation measures. Each hospital and agency has specific policies and procedures for how a DNR order is to be written and followed. A critical ethical violation to informed consent may occur if a physician writes a DNR order on a patient's record without discussing the order and decision with the patient, family members, or surrogate (O'Rourke, 2002). A DNR physician order needs to be justified by one of three reasons: no medical benefit can come from CPR, a person has a very poor quality of life before CPR, and a person's quality of life after CPR is anticipated to be very poor (Mappes & DeGrazia, 2001).

Unofficial—and unauthorized—"slow codes" have been practiced in the past and can be described as "going through the motions" or as giving half-hearted CPR to a patient whose condition has been deemed futile. At one time, nurses initiated slow codes when a physician had not yet written the DNR order of a terminally ill patient. However, a slow code is an unethical and illegal practice, and physicians and nurses should never initiate them. Slow codes are not recognized as a legal procedure.

The Right to Die and the Right to Refuse Treatment

The right to die is a patient's choice, based on the principle of autonomy. Well-informed patients with decision-making capacity have a right to refuse or forgo recommended treatments in an attempt to avoid a long period of suffering during the dying process. **Right to die** means that a person has an autonomous right to refuse life-sustaining or life-extending treatment measures. Most of the time there are no ethical or legal ramifications if a person decides to forgo treatments; the courts generally uphold the right of competent patients to refuse treatment (Jonsen, Siegler, & Winslade, 2006; Mappes & DeGrazia, 2001). Nevertheless, healthcare professionals need to make certain that the patient's decision is truly autonomous and not coerced. However, healthcare professionals may find it difficult to accept a competent patient's decision to forgo treatment.

Sometimes in a patient's mind, the burdens of medical treatments outweigh the benefits (O'Rourke, 2002). Perceived burden is a concern for nurses, physicians, and patients because physical pain and emotional suffering from treatments or the prolongation and dread of carrying out treatments may be too much to bear. Other views of burden consist of the economic, social, and spiritual burdens on a patient and family. Whether at the end of life or not, adult autonomous patients with competent decision-making capacity may refuse medical treatments at any time in life and may base their refusal on religious or cultural beliefs.

Withholding and Withdrawing Life-Sustaining Treatment

Withholding and withdrawing treatment is the forgoing of life-sustaining treatment that the patient does not desire, either because of a perceived disproportionate burden on the patient or family members or for other reasons. Notable legal decisions led to many questions regarding the right to die and the right to withhold and withdraw life-sustaining treatments. Three landmark legal cases about withholding and withdrawing treatments are presented in this section (Brannigan & Boss, 2001; Jonsen et al., 1998; U.S. District Court for the Middle District of Florida Tampa Division, 2005).

The case of Karen Ann Quinlan in 1975 led to her parents receiving the right to have Karen Ann's mechanical ventilator discontinued (Supreme Court of New Jersey, 1976/1999; Jonsen et al., 1998). Karen Ann, who was age 21, attended a party and ingested diazepam, dextropropoxyphene, and alcohol and then lapsed into a coma. She was placed on a ventilator, and consequently her parents were involved in legal battles for several years to have Karen Ann removed from the ventilator. Physicians would not remove her from the ventilator because they could not establish brain death. Finally, the U.S. Supreme Court district of New Jersey ordered the

BOX 9.8 ETHICAL FORMATIONS: CRITERIA FOR CLINICAL DIAGNOSIS OF A VEGETATIVE STATE

- No awareness of self or environment and an inability to interact with others
- No sustained, reproducible, purposeful, or voluntary responses to visual, auditory, tactile, or noxious stimuli
- No language comprehension or expression
- Intermittent wakefulness exhibited by the presence of sleep–wake cycles
- Preserved autonomic functions to permit survival with medical and nursing care
- Incontinence—bladder and bowel
- Variable degrees of spinal reflexes and cranial-nerve reflexes, such as pupillary, oculocephalic, corneal, vestibulo-ocular, and gag

Source: Multi-Society Task Force on Persistent Vegetative State. (1994). Medical aspects of the persistent vegetative state (p. 1500). *New England Journal of Medicine, 330,* 1499–1508.

physicians to unplug the ventilator. Once unplugged, Karen Ann breathed without the help of the ventilator and continued living for 10 years; her death was a result of pneumonia and its complications. The legacy of Quinlan's case included (1) contributing to the definition of the term **persistent vegetative state (PVS)**; (2) setting precedence for parents (or legal guardians) to have a right to choose; (3) the formation of ethics committees in most healthcare settings, and (4) the creation and implementation of the advance directive. See Box 9.8 for criteria for a clinical diagnosis of a vegetative state.

Nancy Cruzan, age 25, was in a motor vehicle accident in 1983, where she sustained severe injuries that led to a complete loss of consciousness and, later, a persistent vegetative state with continuous artificial nutrition and hydration. Nancy's parents and coguardians filed several cases to have her feeding tube removed on the basis that there was no chance for a return of cognitive capacity. The courts denied each case. After almost 8 years, the Supreme Court of Missouri granted the wishes for the discontinuance of her feeding tube. Nancy died on December 26, 1990, only 3 days after the court's final decision. The judge based the decision on a previous comment by Nancy, who had stated to the housekeeper that she would not want to live in that condition.

Of particular interest is Nancy Cruzan's grave marker. The family members, adapting their idea from a political cartoon about the case, had three dates etched on the grave marker; one date reflects her birth, one reflects her "death" at the time of the accident, and one reflects her actual physical death (Fine, 2005). The etching on the grave marker shows

Born July 20, 1957
Departed January 11, 1983
At Peace December 26, 1990

The grave marker is slightly confusing based on the meanings of the terms "persistent vegetative state" and "brain death." Nancy's persistent vegetative state never equated to the definition of brain death, as the grave marker implies.

At the ruling of Nancy Cruzan, the judges of the Supreme Court of Missouri established three conditions for withdrawing treatments, including artificial nutrition and hydration: (1) the patient has a right to refuse medical treatment; (2) artificial feeding constitutes medical treatment; and (3) when the patient is mentally incompetent, each state must document clear and convincing evidence that the patient's desires had been for discontinuance of medical treatment (Jonsen et al., 1998; Supreme Court of Missouri, 1990).

A more recent case was that of Terri Schiavo, who died on March 21, 2005 (refer to Box 9.9 for a synopsis of the case). There were a total of 21 legal suits, but the last few cases involved her husband Michael's request to have her feeding tube discontinued, which would stop the artificial nutrition and hydration. Terri's parents fought this request. By Florida law, Michael Schiavo as a spouse and guardian had a legal right to serve as a surrogate decision maker for Terri.

Substituted judgment became the ethical and legal standard, with guardianship as the focal point, and a critical factor in decision making regarding Terri Schiavo's care and outcome in light of no advance directive. Surrogates must make unbiased substituted judgments based on an understanding of what patients would decide for themselves, and not the values of the surrogate. As the reader will see in the Ethical Formations Box 9.9, the court obtained documented evidence from Michael Schiavo and other people that Terri had stated she did not want to live in a condition in which she would be a burden to anyone else. This evidence served as the basis for many of the court denials to the Schindlers.

Nurses need to give compassionate and excellent care to patients. No matter what the decision will be, family members and patients need to feel a sense of confidence that nurses will maintain moral sensitivity with a course of right action. In

BOX 9.9 ETHICAL FORMATIONS: FACTS IN THE THERESA "TERRI" MARIE SCHIAVO CASE

In *Theresa Marie Schindler Schiavo and Robert ex relatione [on behalf of] Mary Schindler (plaintiffs) v. Michael Schiavo, Judge George W. Greer, and The Hospice of the Florida SunCoast, Inc.* (defendants) [Civ. Act. No. 8:05-CV-530-T-27TBM]

Major Final Court Rulings

March 21, 2005—A federal court order denied the injunction relief sought by the Schindlers, and the court refused to compel Theresa Schiavo to undergo surgery for reinsertion of the feeding tube.

March 24, 2005—The second federal court denied a motion by the Schindlers for a temporary restraining order against Michael Schiavo and the hospice regarding an alleged violation of Terri's

BOX 9.9 ETHICAL FORMATIONS: FACTS IN THE THERESA "TERRI" MARIE SCHIAVO CASE (continued)

right to artificial nutrition and hydration based on the Americans with Disabilities Act (ADA). The courts ruled that Terri's rights based on the ADA were not violated.

March 24, 2005—The U.S. Supreme Court denied the application by the Schindlers for a stay of enforcement of the Florida judgment.

March 25, 2005—The U.S. Court of Appeals 11th Court District denied an appeal by the Schindlers for a rehearing.

History and Facts of the Case

In 1990, Terri Schiavo's husband, Michael, found Terri unresponsive in the couple's home. Florida physicians affirmed that Terri, at age 26, had experienced prolonged cerebral hypoxia after an acute cardiac arrest. Physicians determined that a severely low potassium level, which was secondary to an eating disorder, brought on her cardiac arrest. Her condition was determined to be consistent with the diagnosis of persistent vegetative state because of the brain insult. In a 1992 medical malpractice suit against her fertility obstetrician, Terri Schiavo was awarded $750,000, which was placed in a trust fund for her future medical care. Michael Schiavo was awarded $300,000 (Cerminara & Goodman, 2005). In 1992, the Schindlers (Terri's parents) and Michael became alienated over the management of Terri's therapy and the money awarded to the Schiavos. In February 1993, the Schindlers unsuccessfully demanded a share of Michael's money from the malpractice settlement.

The first lawsuit filed toward a family member was initiated in 1993 by the Schindlers in an attempt to have Michael removed as Terri's guardian, but the judge dismissed the case. Rehabilitation efforts continued for several years without success. Michael first petitioned the court in 1998 to have Terri's feeding tube removed and artificial nutrition and hydration discontinued, which was vehemently opposed by the Schindlers. Michael testified that before her 1990 event, Terri told him, "If I ever have to be a burden to anybody, I don't want to live like that" (Lynne, 2005). There is court-documented testimony that Terri made similar statements about her wishes to other people. Judge Greer at the 6th Judicial Circuit Court in Clearwater, Florida, avowed that there was clear and convincing evidence of Terri's wishes.

From 1993 to 2005, there were 21 lawsuits and appeals. The majority of the lawsuits were filed after 1998, and most of them upheld Michael's initial contention that he was attempting to carry out Terri's wishes. During the appeals, Terri's feeding tube was removed on three occasions; on the first two occasions, the feeding tube was reinserted and artificial nutrition and hydration was resumed.

Thirteen days after the third and final removal of her feeding tube, Terri died on March 31, 2005, at the age of 41. The ethics and legality of removing the feeding tube were scrutinized until her death through lawsuits, political and media statements, actions of the U.S. Congress, and pleas from high-ranking public figures, such as Pope John Paul II.

Source: Cerminara, K., & Goodman, K. (2005). *Key events in the case of Theresa Marie Schiavo. University of Miami Ethics.* Retrieved from http://www6.miami.edu/ethics2/schiavo/schiavo_timeline.html; Lynne, D. (2005). Life and death tug of war—The whole Terri Schiavo story: 15-year saga of brain-injured woman no clear-cut, right-to-die case. *WorldNetDaily.* Retrieved from http://www.worldnetdaily.com/news/article.asp?ARTICLE_ID=43463

the *Code of Ethics for Nurses with Interpretive Statements*, Provision 1.3, the ANA (2001) emphasized that nurses ethically support the provision of compassionate and dignified end-of-life care as long as nurses do not have the sole intention of ending a person's life. A special statement concerning the Terri Schiavo case was released to the press by the ANA on March 23, 2005, which upheld the decision for the right of the patient or surrogate to choose forgoing artificial nutrition and hydration (see Box 9.10).

In March 2011, the ANA published an updated version of its 1992 position statement on forgoing nutrition and hydration. In the 1992 version, the ANA included the statement that the patient or surrogates, along with guidance from the healthcare team, should make the decision regarding withholding artificial nutrition and hydration, and if discontinued the nurse will continue to provide competent care. This ANA (2011) position statement includes a clear distinction between regular food and water and artificial nutrition and hydration:

> The American Nurses Association (ANA) believes that adults with capacity, or in the event of incapacity, their surrogates are in the best position to weigh the harms and benefits of nutrition and hydration as evaluated and discussed with them by the

BOX 9.10 ETHICAL FORMATIONS: PARTIAL STATEMENTS FROM THE PRESS RELEASE FROM THE AMERICAN NURSES ASSOCIATION: TERRI SCHIAVO CASE

ANA's Press Release on March 23, 2005, on the Terri Schiavo Case

[The] ANA has consistently upheld the right of patients, or if the patient is incapacitated, the right of the designated surrogate, to decide whether to submit to or continue medical treatment.

As nurses, we are ethically bound to assist our patients in maintaining control over their lives and to help them preserve their dignity. The ANA believes that it is the responsibility of nurses to facilitate informed decision making for patients and families who are making choices about end-of-life care. The *Code of Ethics for Nurses* specifically outlines the nurse's obligation to protect the patient's right to self-determination and the role of a designated surrogate in situations where the patient lacks capacity. In this case, Terri Schiavo's physicians, over many years, have declared her to be in a "persistent vegetative state." Furthermore, there is evidence that Terri Schiavo expressed her wishes not to have her life artificially maintained under such circumstances. ANA believes the Congress and the president have acted inappropriately in this case. It is unfortunate that Terri Schiavo has now become the symbol of so many political agendas.

The positive outcome from this case is that it raises the public's awareness of the importance of discussing end-of-life issues with family members and underscores how an advance directive, a living will, and/or durable power of attorney for health care, clarifies and provides evidence of the wishes of an individual regarding end-of-life decisions.

Source: Chosen statements from this press release were quoted from ANA, (2005, March 23). *ANA statement on the Terri Schiavo case.* Statement attributed to B. Blakeney, ANA President. Retrieved from http://www.nursingworld.org/FunctionalMenuCategories/MediaResources/PressReleases/2005/pr03238523.aspx

> healthcare team. The acceptance or refusal of food and fluids, whether delivered by normal or artificial means must be respected. This belief is consistent with the ANA's expressed values and goals relative to respect for autonomy, relief of suffering and expert care at the end of life. . . . Artificial nutrition and hydration are incorporated into the patient's plan of care only when medically appropriate and consistent with the patient's beliefs, circumstances, and goals. Outcomes such as weight gain, increased caloric intake, or changes in laboratory test results do not themselves serve as adequate justification for this intervention . . . [and] are not persuasive reasons to begin or continue to provide nutrition or hydration. (pp. 1, 3)

Alleviation of Pain and Suffering in the Dying Patient

The degree of quality of life contributes to the choices that patients make during the end-of-life process. Attempting to relieve pain and suffering is a primary responsibility for nurses and providers of care, which makes the whole arena of palliative care an ethical concern. Patients fear the consequences of disease—pain, suffering, and the process of dying. Most of the time, it is the nurse who administers the pain medication and evaluates a patient's condition between and during pain injections. In an updated position statement in 2010, the American Nurses Association emphasized that nurses need to provide "aggressive pain control" for suffering patients at the end of life, but should never have the intention of ending a patient's life (p. 2).

Rule of Double Effect

According to Cavanaugh (2006), the **rule of double effect** (RDE) is based on an individual's reasoning that an act causing good and evil is permitted when the act meets the following conditions:

1. The act, considered independently of its evil effect, is not in itself wrong.
2. The agent intends the good and does not intend the evil either as an end or as a means.
3. The agent has proportionately grave reasons for acting, addressing his relevant obligations, comparing the consequences, and, considering the necessity of the evil, exercising due care to eliminate or mitigate it. (p. 36)

Some historians of ethics have attributed the double-effect reasoning to St. Thomas Aquinas's writing about a person's self-defense in a homicide, and other historians have not. Today's double-effect reasoning is inclusive of actions that could cause harm, which is a foreseen but inevitable outcome. The use of the double-effect reasoning is an area of substantial concern when the healthcare professional sees some good in the action but also foresees with certainty that there will be bad in the action. Refer to Box 9.11 for an examination of an instance of each designated condition of the RDE.

When the rule of double effect is applied, nurses need to be aware that the hastening of death must be a possible foreseen, inevitable, but unintended effect. In

BOX 9.11 ETHICAL FORMATIONS: EXAMPLES OF DOUBLE-EFFECT REASONING CONDITIONS

Condition 1:

An example of the first condition of the rule of RDE is applied when a nurse administers a medication that is, "apart from circumstances and intent, neither good [n]or bad" (Jonsen et al., 2006, p. 129).

Condition 2:

The second condition involves the intention of a nurse or physician. An example could be a nurse's intent to relieve pain by administering a medication but not for the patient to be compromised in any way.

Condition 3:

The third condition, said another way, is that the bad effect cannot be the means to the intended good effect; for instance, a nurse cannot administer an opiate-containing or other type of medication to produce the harmful bad effect, such as respiration cessation, in order to achieve the intended good effect, which in this case is pain relief.

Provision 1.3 of the *Code of Ethics for Nurses with Interpretive Statements*, the ANA (2001) supports nurses in their attempts to relieve patients' pain, "even when those interventions entail risks of hastening death" (p. 8).

Nurses may have conflicting moral values concerning the use of high doses of opiate-containing drugs, such as morphine sulfate or even opiate-synthetic medications. In times when nurses feel uncomfortable, they need to explore their attitudes and opinions with their supervisor and, when appropriate, in clinical team meetings. Individually evaluating each patient and circumstance is essential.

Terminal Sedation

Terminal sedation (TS) is an accepted practice in the United States and many other countries. Quill (2001) defined **terminal sedation** as a last resort "when a suffering patient is sedated to unconsciousness, usually through the ongoing administration of barbiturates or benzodiazepines. The patient then dies of dehydration, starvation, or some other intervening complication, as all other life-sustaining interventions are withheld" (p. 181). Terminal sedation is different from usual palliative sedation in that, in TS, the discontinued interventions include other medications and feeding tubes. Some people think that TS hastens death, but Ira Byock stated that TS is used only in the last stages of life, at which point other medications and nutrition and hydration do not prolong life (as cited in Kingsbury, 2008).

When the word "terminal" is used, there is an understanding among the healthcare team and family members that the outcome, and possibly a desired outcome, is death (Sugarman, 2000). The American Nurses Association (2001, 2010) did not directly address TS in the *Code of Ethics for Nurses with Interpretive Statements*, but did address nurses' obligations to give compassionate care at the end of life and not have as their sole intent the ending of a person's life. Understanding the moral and ethical implications will guide nurses in their individualized direction.

Physician-Assisted Suicide

Society has reacted with everything from moral outrage to social acceptance with regard to physician-assisted suicide (PAS). Three states in the United States have made phyisican-assisted suicide legal—Oregon in 1997 and Washington and Montana in 2009 (Lachman, 2010). With certain restrictions, patients who are near death may obtain prescriptions to end their lives in a dignified way. Sugarman (2000) defined physician-assisted suicide as "the act of providing a lethal dose of medication for the patient to self-administer" (p. 213). According to Kopala and Kennedy (1998), PAS must meet three conditions in accordance with the ANA:

1. You (the nurse) must know the person intends to end his or her life.
2. You (the nurse) must make the means to commit suicide available to the person.
3. The person must then end his or her own life. (p. 19)

During a 20-year dispute over euthanasia practices, under certain guidelines, physicians could practice euthanasia in the Netherlands. In February 2002, the Dutch passed a law that permitted voluntary euthanasia and physician-assisted suicide. In the discussions of euthanasia in the United States, the scope has been limited to only physician-assisted suicide, whereas in the Netherlands, the discussion has a much wider perspective.

Special guidelines relating to the Death with Dignity Act in Oregon were written by the Oregon Nurses Association for nurses who care for patients who choose physician-assisted suicide (as cited in Ladd et al., 2002; Kopala & Kennedy, 1998). The guidelines include maintaining support, comfort, and confidentiality; discussing end-of-life options with the patient and family; and being present for the patient's self-administration of medications and during the death. Nurses may not inject the medications themselves, breach confidentiality, subject others to any type of judgmental comments or statements about the patient, or refuse to provide care to the patient.

Rational Suicide

The idea of saving people versus allowing people to die or commit suicide is at the very essence of one of the most debated and controversial dilemmas today. As long as there is difficulty in determining rationality in suicide, this controversy will remain. Moral progress in nursing necessitates that nurses ponder

> *these ethical uncertainties . . . with patients who are contemplating rational suicide. Meanwhile, nurses should never be caught off-guard in relation to the ethical and political changes in health care for fear of losing their power and voice.*
>
> —*RICH & BUTTS, 2004, P. 277*

Rational suicide is a self-slaying based on reasoned choice and is categorized as voluntary active euthanasia. Siegel (1986) stated that the person who is contemplating rational suicide has a realistic assessment of life circumstances, is free from severe emotional distress, and has a motivation that would seem understandable to most uninvolved people in the person's community.

To morally accept a person's act of committing rational suicide seems outrageous to most people, and the very thought of it weighs heavily on their hearts, even today. Should people criticize others for making a choice of rational suicide? More and more people view rational suicide as an acceptable alternative to life, especially when faced with unbearable pain, suffering, or loneliness (O'Rourke, 2002). However, the terms "rational" and "suicide" seem to contradict each other (Engelhardt, 1986; Finnerty, 1987). David Peretz (as cited in O'Rourke, 2002), a noted psychiatrist and suicidologist, gave his interpretation of why rational suicides seem to be occurring and more accepted in society when he stated:

> Under the unprecedented stress of recent decades, denial mechanisms are breaking down and we have become increasingly vulnerable to the threats of intensely painful feelings of anxiety, fear, panic, rage, guilt, shame, grief, longing and helplessness. In order to avoid being overwhelmed, we seek new ways to adapt. . . . I believe that the growing concern with a good death, death with dignity and the right-to-die reflect this search—If our deepest known fear is of being destroyed, and we cannot deal with that fear, we take refuge in planning death and rational suicide. We find comfort in the illusion, "It will not be done to me—I will do it myself." (pp. 206–207)

Peretz believes that this motivation is unethical, dangerous, and harmful because it leads a person to a false sense of omnipotence. Two other elements may contribute to rational suicide but are also unrealistic and unethical, according to Peretz. One element is that people who are advocates of rational suicide believe strongly that personal autonomy is the goal of human life, and therefore, if a person cannot have complete personal autonomy, life is not worth living. The other element is an act of self-destruction, which has a potential to mythologize rational suicide. Peretz stated that by mythologizing an object, it is given false power. Advocates of rational suicide promote self-destruction as a way to realize a false sense of freedom from serious human problems, such as physical suffering, loneliness, or frailty.

For nurses to endorse any suicide seems contradictory to good practice, because traditionally nurses and mental health professionals have intervened to prevent suicide. Many times, cultural, religious, and personal beliefs guide nurses in how they respond to patients who are thinking about suicide. Does a nurse have a right to try to stop a person from committing rational suicide—in other words, to act in the best interest of a patient? Or is a nurse supposed to support a person's autonomous decision to commit rational suicide, even when that decision is morally and religiously incompatible with the nurse's perspective? If the nurse knows of the plan for rational suicide, would care toward that patient be obligatory? Would nurses be obligated to render care despite their own value conflicts? What actions could the nurse take at this point?

According to Rich and Butts (2004), no clear answers exist to this ethical dilemma, but interventions become unique to each situation. Interventions may include everything from providing information regarding Compassion and Choices (a right-to-die organization) to answering questions about lethal injections. Nurses need to consider autonomy and beneficence when deciding on interventions for persons who are planning rational suicide. Nurses are closely involved with more end-of-life ethics as the issue of voluntary active euthanasia is becoming increasingly prevalent.

Nursing Care for Dying Patients

Nurses first must sort out their own feelings about euthanasia and dying before they provide appropriate moral guidance and direction to patients and families. The sights, sounds, and smells of death can be an emotionally draining experience for nurses, but nurses must meet the needs of patients and families. Every day nurses face disturbing moral conflicts and distress, such as whether they should keep giving a continuous morphine sulfate infusion to a dying patient for comfort in light of the risk of depressed respirations or whether they should assist in withdrawing or withholding artificial nutrition and fluids or other life-sustaining interventions. When nurses experience personal value and professional moral distress in decision making, they may find themselves on uncertain moral ground. The substance of decision making in regards to ethical issues and the experience of moral distress needs documenting so as not to lose the richness of the narratives and the degree to which these diagnoses are used.

Barbara Couden (2002), a registered nurse, wrote a beautiful and poignant description of her emotional experiences with loss and death in intensive care, stating that, at times, she just wanted to run away (see Box 9.12). She portrayed her experiences of physical and emotional exhaustion; periods of fatigue, guilt, and sometimes relief when death finally came; the smell of death on her clothes and wetness on her face from crying families pressing against her face; tearfulness and sadness; and her own intense feelings of grief and loss. Couden experienced immeasurable unexpressed grief and unresolved personal losses, along with the losses of

BOX 9.12 ETHICAL FORMATIONS: SOMETIMES I WANT TO RUN

From the words of Barbara A. Couden . . .

Sometimes I want to run. It's work not to recoil from the rawness of life in those rooms. It is probably easier to behave as a starchy, mechanical nurse who staves off discomfort with a cheerful cliché. However, people deserve to experience hospitalization, grief, or even dying at its very best. To provide less isn't care at all. So I give my open heart and plunge into their circumstances, even though really I'm no one special to them—just there by default. In return, they honor me with the privilege of sharing their pain, struggle, and the richness of life, death, and love. In some way, we each live on in the other's memory: endeared by shared suffering, strivings to nurture hope, and our individual attempts to love. So there are nights that I reflect on my heartfelt efforts, smell death on my clothes, and feel dampness where the tears of grieving loved ones have pressed against my face. Sometimes it seems that my role as a nurse is to absorb the feelings of others: pain, sadness, and loss. I'm sitting up in bed tonight, waiting for mine to dissipate.

Source: Quoted from Couden, B. A. (2002). "Sometimes I want to run": A nurse reflects on loss in the intensive care unit. *Journal of Loss and Trauma, 7*(1), p. 41–42.

her patients, until she had no emotions left to express toward her patients and no energy left to spend on them.

After she sought ways to deal with her crisis, she discovered three important aspects of her emotional work. First, she has had to face her own grief and loss, which includes continuous expressions of loss through tears and discussions. Second, she had to find ways to deal with her own intense feelings of grief and loss before she "could dare to give them [her feelings] utterance" (p. 42). She cries and expresses her own grief with patients and, as she does, the environment becomes a unique place for her and her patients as they exchange their emotions. She finds ways to pamper herself. Her third aspect of emotional work involves her mannerisms toward patients and feeling good about the way she responds to her patients. Couden confirmed her feelings about the way she responds to her patients when she saw her therapist emotionally moved by her own stories.

Relationships with patients are at the heart of nursing ethics. Wright (2006) emphasized that nursing at its best is good for the souls of the patient and nurse, and stated, "For the heart is the seat of the soul, and when we nurse another, we nurse a soul too. Soulful work requires soulful individuals and communities" (p. 23). Without this soulful work, patients will feel disconnected. Maeve (1998) stated that relationships can become quite complex because of the accompanied interrelational experiences and emotions.

Most nurses share in patients' emotional experiences of pain, suffering, and joy and do not just give superficial care and then forget about it. The care that nurses provide to their dying patients becomes an essential component of their own lives, and the stories that they remember about their patients become interwoven into their own life stories. Maeve (1998) studied nine nurses who worked with suffering and dying patients. As Maeve listened to the nurses' stories, she realized that moral issues about practice and relationships were dominant where suffering and dying patients were concerned.

Three major themes were identified from the study (Maeve, 1998). One was "tempering involvement," which meant that nurses had a dilemma or conflict about becoming involved: how much involvement, setting limits, setting boundaries to distinguish their lives from their patients' lives, and becoming embodied, such as when nurses may actually live in the experience with their patients (p. 1138). The second theme was "doing the right thing/the good thing," which involved education, experience, courage, moral dilemmas, and past regrets for a few of their performances or decisions with patients (p. 1139). "Cleaning up" was the third theme that emerged, and this theme marked the end of the involvement with the patient (p. 1140). During this time, the nurse needs to reflect on experiences and clean up grief.

In one Japanese study of 160 nurses, Konishi, Davis, and Aiba (2002) studied withdrawal of artificial food and fluid from terminally ill patients. The majority of the nurses supported this act only under two conditions: if the patient requested withdrawal of artificial food and fluids and if the act relieved the patient's suffering. Nurses agreed that comfort for the patient was of great concern. One nurse in the study stated: "[Artificial food and fluid] only prolongs the patient's suffering. When withdrawn, the patient showed peace on the face. I have seen such patients so many times" (p. 14). In the same study, another nurse who was experiencing moral conflict with a decision to withdraw artificial food and fluid stated: "Withdrawal is killing and cruel. I feel guilty" (p. 14).

Other end-of-life issues may be reasons for moral conflicts, as well. Georges and Grypdonck (2002) conducted a literature review on the topic of ethical issues in terms of how nurses perceive their care of dying patients. There has been a deficiency of systematic research on this topic specific to nurses' moral conflicts and distress. However, Georges and Grypdonck outlined some of the moral dilemmas that nurses perceive as particularly critical to end-of-life care. Some of the moral problems of nurses found in the literature were:

- Communicating truthfully with patients about death because they were fearful of destroying all hope in the patient and family
- Managing pain symptoms because of fear of hastening death
- Feeling forced to collaborate with other health team members about medical treatments that, in the nurses' opinion, are futile or too burdensome
- Feeling insecure and not adequately informed about reasons for treatment

- Trying to maintain their own moral integrity throughout relationships with patients, families, and coworkers because of the feeling that they are forced to betray their own moral values

Although a nurse has an obligation to provide compassionate and palliative care, the nurse has a right to withdraw from treating and caring for a dying patient as long as another nurse has assumed that care. When care is such that the nurse perceives it as violating personal and professional morality and values, the professional nurse must pursue alternative approaches to care.

Nursing care for dying patients needs to be enriched over time, as new nurses and nurses not routinely caring for dying patients are not automatically skilled in this type of care. Nurses must acquire expertise and skills in end-of-life care as in any other area of practice. As we will see, compassionate care is an essential component of nursing care of dying patients.

The Compassionate Nurse with a Dying Patient

Nurses find themselves on uncertain moral ground when attempting to sustain dying patients, but they must be honest with patients and give sufficient information concerning advance directives and medical treatment options. However, the most important aspect is to offer support to dying patients by relating to their fear of death and by alleviating pain and suffering. Family members need to support their loved one and they can often learn support strategies from talking with nurses and observing how nurses interact with the patient. When dying patients experience the compassionate acts of nurses and family members, death can be a positive experience for them. Nurses must remember that the little things are what make a big difference in the care of dying patients. Medical treatments aimed at relieving pain and suffering can coexist with palliative care, and nurses' compassionate acts are essential to this cohesive coexistence (Ciccarello, 2003). One particular compassionate act is for nurses to teach individuals and patients in community and hospital settings about treatment decisions at the end of life, such as life-sustaining treatments and palliative care with symptom management. Nurses can teach patients about advance directives and surrogate decision making. The case of Terri Schiavo could possibly have a positive influence on the need for understanding and having advance directives.

Physical and Emotional Pain Management

Understanding and actually upholding aggressive pain management precepts may be the most challenging moral dilemma that nurses face when caring for dying patients. The lack of understanding regarding the issues and fears of patient addiction or death causes nurses and physicians to undertreat pain and suffering in many cases. Miller, Miller, and Jolley (2001) emphasized the importance for nurses to apply three basic precepts when controlling pain: (1) nurses and physicians need to follow the WHO's "pain ladder" protocol for palliative pain management (see *Types of Pain*); (2) nurses and physicians need to treat pain early because once out of control, pain is more difficult to treat; and (3) nurses and physicians need to explain to terminally ill patients that addiction should not be feared and dying patients rarely develop an addiction to properly administered pain medications.

Types of Pain

Miller et al. (2001) described two major types of pain: nociceptive and neuropathic. Nociceptive pain involving tissue damage occurs with two types of pain: somatic (musculoskeletal pain) and visceral (organ pain—the most common type of pain). Once nurses have performed a thorough pain assessment, the WHO's pain ladder (2011) is an excellent approach for providers of care. The WHO's pain ladder is a step-by-step approach to managing pain with palliative care of patients. At the first sign of a patient's pain, nurses should administer oral nonopioid medications or adjuvant therapy, as ordered by the primary care provider. The next progressive step involves use of opioids, such as codeine, for mild to moderate pain, in addition to interventions in the first step. Finally, the last step involves use of strong opioids, such as morphine sulfate, for moderate to severe pain, in addition to interventions in the previous steps of the ladder.

Nurses need to be aware of the moral conflicts that patients and family members experience when it comes to the relief of pain and suffering during end times. Sharing in each patient's experience of pain and emotional suffering will provide a better experience for nurses and their patients during the death process.

Core Principles for End-of-Life Care

Benner, Kerchner, Corless, and Davies (2003) delineated core principles for end-of-life nursing care that are based on a central thought of "death as a human passage" (p. 558). The core ethical principles reflect a summary of the work of Benner et al. on the Expert Panel on End-of-Life Care at the American Academy of Nursing. The group's core principles are ethical approaches that nurses can apply when caring for dying patients. The core principles are as follows:

- Because death is an essential human passage, nurses must acknowledge and respect the passage. Nurses, significant others, and patients themselves have an impact on how that passage occurs.
- Always consider if patients actually desire an optimal level of pain management and sedation to relieve pain and suffering and respect their wishes. Patients may wish for a balance between alertness and level of comfort so that they can chat and feel the presence of others.
- Palliative care should be comprehensive and flexible for pain and symptom management. Nurses should provide treatments to enhance quality of life.

- Avoid offering treatment options or any other options that are unrealistic. Dying patients are very limited as to their choices and options and do not need to be offered treatment options that do not have any beneficial effects.
- Be respectful of the time that patients and family members need for coming to terms with the realization of death. Each person and family member is unique.
- Be respectful of time that is needed for family members or significant others to grieve, to come to terms with their loved one's death, and for their own spiritual practices.
- Give attentive end-of-life care to dying patients so that the ones who are grieving can witness the nurse's impact on the facilitation of human passage. The sight of well-cared-for dying loved ones promotes emotional and physical well-being among the grieving family members and significant others.
- Avoid universal prescriptions and expectations for dying patients. Every death and death narrative is unique.

Spiegel (1993) captured the importance of following these core principles in end-of-life care. The following passage describes how people feel about unfinished business and caring for one another during the dying process.

> There is such an absoluteness to death. Harsh words cannot be taken back. Promises unfulfilled can never be completed. One cannot even say goodbye. Facing the absoluteness of death can be a tremendous stimulus to life. If it is important, do it now. . . . Say what you mean to say. Settle old grievances. Accomplish what needs doing, sooner rather than later. . . . Death is so overwhelming that it is rather humbling. There seems to be so little one can do about it. Strangely enough, we always resort to the same comfort: our sense of caring about one another. In some sense, we huddle together. Our bond of caring forms a kind of talisman against the power of death. Although, ultimately, each of us has to face death alone, it is a tremendous relief to do some of the work with someone else. A good hug or some shared tears may not save a life, but it will make you feel more alive. (pp. 144–145)

Spiritual Considerations

Spirituality is one of the most important aspects of end-of-life nursing care, but often nurses feel helpless when it comes to providing the right type of spiritual care for their patients. Meaningful experiences, especially at the end of life, are important for nurses in their care of patients because nurses feel that they touch patients' lives in some way through generous or compassionate acts. One such way may be the facilitation of spirituality. Spirituality has become more essential to nursing care since it has been included in the definition of palliative care. Most Americans believe that end-of-life spiritual care is an important part of the dying process, and at the same time, they believe that nurses and others do not effectively provide spiritual care.

In her book, *Spiritual Care: Nursing Theory, Research, and Practice*, Taylor (2002) defined **spirituality** as a deeply personal and integral part of a person's life. Several definitions of spirituality exist in nursing (see, for example, Dossey & Guzzetta, 2000; Taylor, 2002; Narayanasamy, 1999). Spirituality, as defined by Dossey and Guzzetta, is "a unifying force of a person; the essence of being that permeates all of life and is manifested in one's being, knowing, and doing; the interconnectedness with self, others, nature, and God/Life Force/Absolute/Transcendent" (p. 7).

Taylor (2003) studied the expectations of patients and family members regarding spiritual needs and care from nurses. In-depth, tape-recorded interviews were conducted with 28 adult patients with cancer and their family caregivers. Six categories, and consequently specific nursing interventions, are listed in the priority of responses; they are: "kindness and respect," "talking and listening," "prayer," "connecting," "quality temporal nursing care," and "mobilizing religious or spiritual resources" (Taylor, 2003, p. 588).

The category with the most responses was kindness and respect, and a few responses regarding this theme included "just be nice," "giving loving care," and "a smile does a lot" (Taylor, 2003, pp. 587–588). For the next category, talking and listening, the responses varied widely because some patients enjoyed the superficial chatter, whereas others were pleased about nurses sharing their own deep religious experiences as comforting measures. Another category, prayer and the nurse's offering to pray with patients, varied widely in responses according to individualized beliefs. The category of connecting relates to certain characteristics, such as nurses being authentic and genuine, having physical presence, and having symmetry with patients. (Symmetry with patients means that patients want to have a sense of working with nurses in a notion of friendship.) Giving quality temporal nursing care, another category, relates to the mechanisms that support the spirit of the person, such as keeping the room clean and not allowing the patient to suffer. The last category is mobilizing religious or spiritual resources. Nurses can facilitate mobilization by consulting chaplains, having Bibles in the room, and having other religious materials available as needed.

There are no completely "right" ways to help a person die because dying processes are individual experiences (Benner et al., 2003). Nursing care depends on each situation. Stories told by family members and dying patients are particularly significant to the understanding of death and are central to paying proper tribute to human passage. As Benner et al. pointed out, "death forever changes the world of those who experience the loss of the person dying" (p. 558). The involvement of nurses in decisions about death becomes more complex every day as more technology emerges in the dying process. Family members and patients must be involved with all ethical decisions.

KEY POINTS

- Whatever death a person is to experience—a good death; an anticipated death; a sudden, unexpected death; or a painful, lingering death—most of the time, people do not have a choice of how they will die.
- Suffering is defined as something that all human beings and every living thing experiences, and because of the multidimensional aspects of humans, suffering affects every part of people's lives—physical, mental, emotional, social, and spiritual.
- Types of euthanasia include active, passive, voluntary, nonvoluntary, and involuntary. Physician-assisted suicide is a type of voluntary euthanasia.
- Death was legally defined in 1981 in the Uniform Determination of Death Act.
- Three standards for death—cardiopulmonary, whole-brain, and higher-brain—emerged as a result of the landmark legal decisions associated with these terms.
- Nurses need to develop awareness and knowledge of the types of advance directives in order to provide education to patients.
- The surrogate decision maker, often known as a proxy, is an individual who acts on behalf of a patient and either is chosen by the patient, such as a family member; is court appointed; or has other authority to make decisions.
- The standards used in deciding for others include the substituted judgment standard, pure autonomy standard, principle of autonomy extended standard, and best interest standard.
- Before physicians estimate that treatments are medically futile to a patient, they must ponder questions such as, "How far does one go with patient autonomy?" and "What is the potential outcome of treatments for the patient?"
- Palliative care and terminal sedation are accepted practices in most countries, including the United States.
- The landmark legal cases of Karen Ann Quinlan, Nancy Cruzan, and Terri Schiavo brought recognition to the concepts of patient (or surrogate) self-determination as related to the right to die or refuse treatment, withholding and withdrawing life-sustaining treatment such as artificial nutrition and hydration and mechanical ventilation, and persistent vegetative state and brain death.
- The states of Oregon, Montana, and Washington have legally approved physician-assisted suicide.
- Death and dying can result in a more positive experience if nurses give compassionate care during the process.
- The American Nurses Association emphasized that nurses need to provide aggressive pain control for suffering patients at the end of life, but should never have the intention of ending a patient's life.
- The American Nurses Association supports nurses in their attempts to relieve patients' pain even when the interventions leads to risks of hastening death.

CASE STUDY: END OF LIFE WITH MARY LOU WARNING

www

Tom Warning, the oldest son, took his mother, Mary Lou Warning, a 73-year-old widow, to the emergency department (ED) after he found her disoriented and confused. He was going to her house to drop off her refilled prescriptions on his way home from work. The ED physician and her primary provider agreed that they could not rule out a stroke and therefore wanted to admit her for "observation only." Tom thought, "This seems minor enough!" Tom went home to rest for the night once he signed the papers for his mother's admission. She went to a regular room. During the night, alone in her room, her stroke extended, and, when the registered nurse made one of her visits, she found Ms. Warning breathing but unresponsive to commands and pain. She immediately called the ED physician to check her and asked another nurse to call her primary physician and her son. Ms. Warning had five sons and one daughter, all of whom lived out of town except for Tom.

An occlusive stroke was the diagnosis after CT and MRI scans. Treatment was probably not going to be helpful because of the degree of damage. The ED and primary physicians planned to send her to the intensive care unit (ICU) and prepared themselves for how they were going to approach Tom. The primary physician informed Tom that she might not live, but, if she did, he and his siblings had to make some decisions about whether or not they wanted her to be on a mechanical ventilator, if it came to that decision. He also told Tom that currently she was in an unconscious state, which could mean an indefinite existence, and they needed to think about what types of treatment, if any, they wanted for her. The physician thoroughly explained the treatment options and the siblings' options to withdraw or withhold treatment for their mother. He explained to Tom that her prognosis was poor and that, if she lived, she probably would never regain consciousness.

Meanwhile, Tom frantically called all of his siblings to tell them to "come fast" and that decisions needed to be made "now" regarding their mother's end-of-life care. Tom was pacing back and forth with distress and fear because no one in his family had ever discussed these issues among themselves or with his mother. When all of the siblings arrived the next day, they made a decision for the physician to withdraw all medications and intravenous fluids and requested no treatments of any kind. The physician wrote a DNR order on Ms. Warning's chart.

Case Study Questions

Apply a nursing theory, approach, or principle to justify your answers and decisions in this case study.

1. You are the nurse who is caring for Ms. Warning in the ICU. Before bedtime, you keep a daily journal of all of your experiences. The day you had to discontinue all of her treatments, you went home to reflect and write down the day's event and your feelings in an effort to express pent-up emotions concerning the day. Imagine becoming part of this experience, then dramatically rehearse this whole event as if you were that nurse, experiencing the event, seeing the sights and sounds, and feeling the intense emotions. Please complete this journaling process as an exercise.
2. What is the role that medical futility plays in this situation and in the family's decision?
3. The primary physician mentioned to Tom that Ms. Warning could need a mechanical ventilator at some point. Clarify this statement by explaining the difference in

(*continues*)

CASE STUDY: END OF LIFE WITH MARY LOU WARNING (continued)

the levels of care (nonmechanical ventilation care and mechanical ventilation-dependent care) and the significance of brain death. Discuss nursing ethical implications involved with each level.

4. What ethical role could you as a nurse take to help support Tom and his siblings?
5. How could an advance directive have helped Tom's distressed state of mind when the physician presented him with "options"? Which one of the advance directives would have been the most suitable in Ms. Warning's case? Please explain.
6. What type of nursing care does Ms. Warning need to receive? In answering this question, explore the ethical issues that you as a nurse must face. Please explain your answer.
7. In Ms. Warning's case, the siblings came to a unified decision. However, if the siblings had not come to a consensus about a course of action for their mother, there could have been disagreement and arguing between them. Consider the nature of "equal voice" for each of the siblings when discussing how they might view the equality of their input compared with the other siblings. If they could agree on one spokesperson for them, what approach might they take to channel their equal voice to one sibling spokesperson? Do you think the siblings would consider appointing the eldest son, Tom, to be the spokesperson to represent them? Please discuss this issue.
8. Which principle serves as the basis for surrogate decision making in Ms. Warning's case? Please define this principle and discuss why this particular principle is best for this particular patient.

References

Albom, M. (1997). *Tuesdays with Morrie: An old man, a young man, and life's greatest lesson.* New York, NY: Random House—Broadway Books.

American Nurses Association. (2001). *Code of ethics for nurses with interpretive statements.* Silver Spring, MD: Author.

American Nurses Association. (2005). *ANA statement on the Terri Schiavo case.* Statement attributed to Barbara A. Blakeney, MSN, RN, President. Silver Spring, MD: Author. Retrieved from http://www.nursingworld.org/FunctionalMenuCategories/MediaResources/PressReleases/2005/pr03238523.aspx

American Nurses Association. (2010, June 14). *Registered nurses' roles and responsibilities in providing expert care and counseling at the end of life.* Silver Spring, MD: Author. Retrieved from http://www.nursingworld.org/MainMenuCategories/EthicsStandards/Ethics-Position-Statements/etpain14426.aspx

American Nurses Association. (2011, March 11). *Revised position statement: Forgoing nutrition and hydration, April 2, 1992.* Silver Spring, MD: Author. Retrieved from http://nursingworld.org/MainMenuCategories/HealthcareandPolicyIssues/ANAPositionStatements/EthicsandHumanRights/prtetnutr14451.aspx

Battin, M. P. (1994). *The least worst death: Essays in bioethics on the end of life.* New York, NY: Oxford University Press.

Beauchamp, T. L., & Childress, J. F. (2001). *Principles of biomedical ethics* (5th ed.). New York, NY: Oxford University Press.

Beauchamp, T. L., & Childress, J. F. (2009). *Principles of biomedical ethics* (6th ed.). New York, NY: Oxford University Press.

Benjamin, M. (2003). Pragmatism and the determination of death. In G. McGee (Ed.), *Pragmatic bioethics* (2nd ed., pp. 193–206). London, UK: Bradford Book, MIT.

Benner, P., Kerchner, S., Corless, I. B., & Davies, B. (2003). Attending death as a human passage: Core nursing principles for end-of-life care. *American Journal of Critical Care, 12*(6), 558–561.

Bondeson, J. (2001). *Buried alive: The terrifying history of our most primal fear.* New York, NY: W. W. Norton.

Brannigan, M. C., & Boss, J. A. (2001). *Healthcare ethics in a diverse society.* Mountain View, CA: Mayfield.

Brogan, G. (2006). Inventing the good death. *Registered Nurse: Journal of Patient Advocacy, 102*(7), 10–14.

Buchanan, A. E., & Brock, D. W. (1990). *Deciding for others: The ethics of surrogate decision making.* New York, NY: Cambridge University Press.

Buckley, J. W., & Abell, N. (2009). Factors affecting life-sustaining treatment decisions by health care surrogates and proxies: Assessing benefits and barriers. *Social Work in Health Care, 48*, 386–401.

Cassell, E. J. (2004). *The nature of suffering and the goals of medicine* (2nd ed.). New York, NY: Oxford University Press.

Cavanaugh, T. A. (2006). *Double-effect reasoning: Doing good and avoiding evil.* Oxford, UK: Clarendon Press.

Cerminara, K., & Goodman, K. (2005). *Key events in the case of Theresa Marie Schiavo. University of Miami Ethics.* Retrieved from http://www6.miami.edu/ethics2/schiavo/schiavo_timeline.html

Ciccarello, G. P. (2003). Strategies to improve end-of-life care in the intensive care unit. *Dimensions of Critical Care Nursing, 22*(5), 216–222.

Connelly, R. (2003). Living with death: The meaning of acceptance. *Journal of Humanistic Psychology, 43*(1), 45–63.

Couden, B. A. (2002). "Sometimes I want to run": A nurse reflects on loss in the intensive care unit. *Journal of Loss and Trauma, 7*(1), 35–45.

Degrazia, D. (2007/2011). The definition of Death (updated Fall 2011). *Stanford encyclopedia of philosophy.* Retrieved from http://plato.stanford.edu/archives/fall2011/entries/death-definition

Devettere, R. J. (2000). *Practical decision making in health care ethics: Cases and concepts* (2nd ed.). Washington, DC: Georgetown University Press.

Dossey, B. M., & Guzzetta, C. E. (2000). Holistic nursing practice. In B. M. Dossey, L. Keegan, & C. E. Guzzetta (Eds.), *Holistic nursing: A handbook for practice* (3rd ed., pp. 5–26). Rockville, MD: Aspen.

Emanuel, L. A., Danis, M., Pearlman, R. A., & Singer, P. A. (1995). Advance care planning as a process: Structuring the discussions in practice. *American Geriatrics Society, 43*, 440–446.

Engelhardt, H. T. (1986). Suicide in the cancer patient. *Cancer, 36*(2), 105–109.

Eriksson, K. (1997). Understanding the world of the patient, the suffering human being: The new clinical paradigm from nursing to caring. *Advanced Practice Nursing Quarterly, 3*(1), 8–13.

Fesmire, S. (2003). *John Dewey and moral imagination.* Bloomington, IN: Indiana University Press.

Fine, R. L. (2005). From Cruzan to Schiavo: Medical, ethical, and legal issues in severe brain injury. *Baylor University Medical Center Proceedings, 18*(4), 303–310.

Finnerty, J. L. (1987). Ethics in rational suicide. *Critical Care Nursing Quarterly, 10*(2), 86–90.

Frank, R., & Anselmi, K. K. (2011). Washington v. Glucksberg: Patient autonomy v. cultural mores in physician-assisted suicide. *Journal of Nursing Law, 14*(1), 11–16.

Garrett, C. (2005). *Gut feelings: Chronic illness and the search for healing* (At the Interface/Probing the Boundaries series, Vol. 16). Amsterdam, Netherlands: Rodopi.

Georges, J. J., & Grypdonck, M. (2002). Moral problems experienced by nurses when caring for terminally ill people: A literature review. *Nursing Ethics, 9*(2), 155–178.

Hester, D. M. (2003). Significance at the end of life. In G. McGee (Ed.), *Pragmatic bioethics* (2nd ed., pp. 121–136). London, UK: Bradford Books, MIT.

Hester, D. M. (2010). *End of life care and pragmatic decision making: A bioethical perspective.* New York, NY: Cambridge University Press.

International Council of Nurses. (2006). *The ICN code of ethics for nurses.* Geneva, Switzerland: Author. Retrieved from http://www.icn.ch/about-icn/code-of-ethics-for-nurses/

Jonsen, A. R., Siegler, M., & Winslade, W. J. (2006). *Clinical ethics* (6th ed.). New York, NY: McGraw-Hill.

Jonsen, A. R., Veatch, R. M., & Walters, L. (1998). *Source book in bioethics.* Washington, DC: Georgetown University Press.

Kahn, D. L., & Steeves, R. H. (1986). The experience of suffering: Conceptual clarification and theoretical definition. *Journal of Advanced Nursing, 11*, 623–631.

Kingsbury, K. (2008, March 21). Time health: When is sedation really euthanasia? *Time Magazine.* Retrieved from http://www.time.com/time/health/article/0,8599,1724911,00.html

Konishi, E., Davis, A. J., & Aiba, T. (2002). The ethics of withdrawing artificial food and fluid from terminally ill patients: An end-of-life dilemma for Japanese nurses and families. *Nursing Ethics, 9*(1), 7–19.

Kopala, B., & Kennedy, S. L. (1998). Requests for assisted suicide: A nursing issue. *Nursing Ethics, 5*(1), 16–26.

Lachman, V. (2010). Ethics, law, and policy: Physician-assisted suicide: Compassionate liberation or murder? *MedSurg Nursing, 19*(2), 121–125. Retrieved from http://www.nursingworld.org/DocumentVault/Ethics_1/Physician-Assisted-Suicide.aspx

Ladd, R. E., Pasquerella, L., & Smith, S. (2002). *Ethical issues in home health care.* Springfield, IL: Charles C. Thomas.

Lear, T. (1906). Tobias Lear's journal account of George Washington's last illness and death, 14–25 December 1799. *Letters and recollections of George Washington: Being letters to Tobias Lear and others between 1790 and 1799, showing the first American in the management of his estate and domestic affairs, with a diary of Washington's last days, kept by Mr. Lear* (pp. 129–141). New York, NY: The Papers of George Washington Exhibits. Retrieved from http://gwpapers.virginia.edu/project/exhibit/mourning/lear.html

Lehto, R. H., & Stein, K. F. (2009). Death anxiety: An analysis of an evolving concept. *Research and Theory for Nursing Practice: An International Journal, 23*(1), 23–41.

Lustig, A. (2003). End-of-life decisions: Does faith make a difference? *Commonweal, 130*(10), 7.

Lynne, D. (2005). Life and death tug of war—The whole Terri Schiavo story: 15-year saga of brain-injured woman no clear-cut, right-to-die case. *WorldNetDaily.* Retrieved from http://www.worldnetdaily.com/news/article.asp?ARTICLE_ID=43463

Maeve, M. K. (1998). Weaving a fabric or moral meaning: How nurses live with suffering and death. *Journal of Advanced Nursing, 27*, 1136–1142.

Mappes, T. A., & DeGrazia, D. (2001). *Biomedical ethics* (5th ed.). Boston, MA: McGraw-Hill.

Miller, K. E., Miller, M. M., & Jolley, M. R. (2001). Challenges in pain management at the end of life. *American Family Physician, 64*(7), 1227–1234.

Munson, R. (2004). *Intervention and reflection: Basic issues in medical ethics* (7th ed.). Victoria, Australia: Wadsworth-Thomson.

Multi-Society Task Force on Persistent Vegetative State. (1994). Medical aspects of the persistent vegetative state. *New England Journal of Medicine, 330*(21), 1499–1508.

Narayanasamy, A. (1999). ASSET: A model for actioning spirituality and spiritual care education and training in nursing. *Nurse Education Today, 19*, 274–285.

National Council of State Boards of Nursing. (2009). *NCLEX-RN examination 2010: Test plan for the National Council Licensure Examination for Registered Nurses*. Chicago, IL: Author. Retrieved from https://www.ncsbn.org/2010_NCLEX_RN_TestPlan.pdf

Olick, R. S. (2001). *Taking advance directives seriously: Prospective autonomy and decisions near the end of life*. Washington, DC: Georgetown University Press.

O'Rourke, K. (2002). *A primer for health care ethics: Essays for a pluralistic society* (2nd ed.). Washington, DC: Georgetown University Press.

President's Commission for the Study of Ethical Problems in Medicine and Biomedical and Behavioral Research. (1981, July). *Defining death: Medical, legal, and ethical issues in the determination of death*. Washington, DC: Government Printing Office. Retrieved from http://bioethics.georgetown.edu/pcbe/reports/past_commissions/defining_death.pdf

Public Broadcasting System & WGBH/Frontline. (1998). The Kevorkian verdict: The chronology of Dr. Jack Kevorkian's life and assisted suicide campaign. Retrieved from http://www.pbs.org/wgbh/pages/frontline/kevorkian/chronology.html

Quill, T. E. (2001). *Caring for patients at the end of life: Facing an uncertain future together*. New York, NY: Oxford University.

Rich, K. L., & Butts, J. B. (2004). Rational suicide: Uncertain moral ground. *Journal of Advanced Nursing, 46*(3), 270–283.

Schneider, K. (2011, June 3). Jack Kevorkian dies at 83: A doctor who helped end lives. *The New York Times* (p. A1). Retrieved from http://www.nytimes.com/2011/06/04/us/04kevorkian.html?pagewanted=all

Schneiderman, L. J. (1994). Medical futility and aging: Ethical implications. *Generations, 18*(4), 61–64.

Siegel, K. (1986). Psychosocial aspects of rational suicide. *American Journal of Psychotherapy, 40*(3), 405–418.

Spiegel, D. (1993). *Detoxifying dying. Living beyond limits: New hope and help for facing life-threatening illness*. New York, NY: Random House, Times Books.

Sugarman, J. (2000). *20 common problems: Ethics in primary care*. New York, NY: McGraw-Hill.

Supreme Court of Missouri. (1990). *Cruzan by Cruzan v. Missouri Department of Health* [497 U.S. 261]. Reprinted and summarized (n.d.) by Cornell University Law School. Retrieved from http://www.law.cornell.edu/supct/html/historics/USSC_CR_0497_0261_ZS.html

Supreme Court of New Jersey. (1976/reprinted in 1999). *In re Quinlan—In the matter of Karen Ann Quinlan, an alleged incompetent* [70 N.J. 10; 355 A.2d 647; 1976 N.J. LEXIS 181; 79 A.L.R.3d205]. Lexus-Nexus, a division of Elsevier Reed. Retrieved from http://euthanasia.procon.org/sourcefiles/In_Re_Quinlan.pdf

Taylor, E. J. (2002). *Spiritual care: Nursing theory, research, and practice*. Upper Saddle River, NJ: Prentice Hall.

Taylor, E. J. (2003). Nurses caring for the spirit: Patients with cancer and family caregiver expectations. *Oncology Nursing Forum, 30*(4), 585–590.

U.S. District Court for the Middle District of Florida Tampa Division. (2005, March 21). *Theresa Marie Schindler Schiavo and ex relatione Robert Schlinder and Mary Schindler (plaintiffs) v. Michael Schiavo, Judge George W. Greer, and The Hospice of the Florida Suncoast, Inc. (defendants).* (Civ. Act. No. 8:05-CV-530-T-27TBM). Retrieved from http://fl1.findlaw.com/news.findlaw.com/hdocs/docs/schiavo/hus32105opp.pdf

van Hooft, S. (2000). The suffering body. *Health, 4*(2), 179–195.

van Hooft, S. (2006). *Caring about health* (Ashgate Studies in Applied Ethics series). Burlington, VT: Ashgate.

Veatch, R. M. (2003). *The basics of bioethics* (2nd ed.). Upper Saddle River, NJ: Prentice Hall.

Wijdicks, E. F. M., Varelas, P. N., Gronseth, G. S., & Greer, D. M. (2010). Evidence-based guideline update: Determining brain death in adults: Report of the Quality Standards Subcommittee of the American Academy of Neurology. *Neurology, 74*(23), 1911–1918.

World Health Organization. (2011). WHO definition of palliative care. Retrieved from http://www.who.int/cancer/palliative/definition/en/

World Health Organization. (2011). WHO's pain ladder. Retrieved from http://www.who.int/cancer/palliative/painladder/en/

Wright, S. (2006). The heart of nursing. *Nursing Standard, 20*(47), 20–23.

Yalom, I. D. (1980). *Existential psychotherapy.* New York, NY: Basic.

Youngner, S. J., & Arnold, R. M. (2001). Philosophical debates about the definition of death: Who cares? *Journal of Medicine and Philosophy, 26*(5), 527–537.

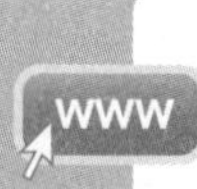

For a full suite of assignments and additional learning activities, use the access code located in the front of your book to visit this exclusive website: http://go.jblearning.com/butts. If you do not have an access code, you can obtain one at the site.

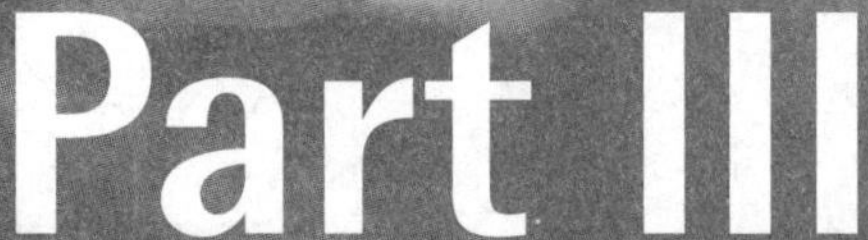

Part III

Special Issues

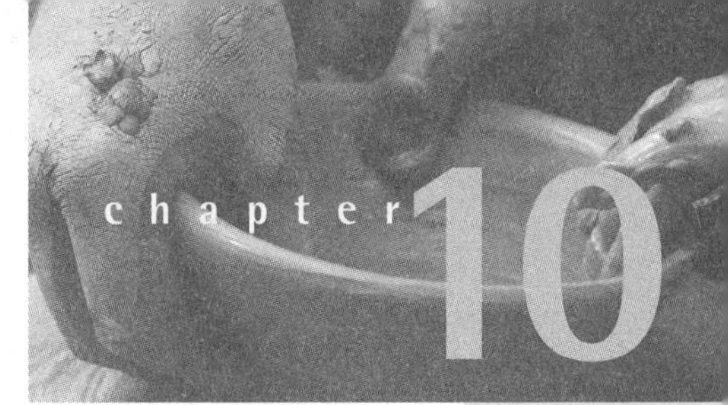

Psychiatric/Mental Health Nursing Ethics

Karen L. Rich

Nasruddin became prime minister to the king. Once, while he wandered through the palace, he saw a royal falcon. Now Nasruddin had never seen this kind of a pigeon before. So he got out a pair of scissors and trimmed the claws, the wings, and the beak of the falcon. "Now you look like a decent bird," he said. "Your keeper had evidently been neglecting you. You're different so there's something wrong with you!"

—*Anthony de Mello,* The Song of the Bird, *1982, p. 7*

OBJECTIVES

After reading this chapter, the reader should be able to:

1. Identify how personal and professional values affect psychiatric/mental health nursing.
2. Discuss the ethical implications of diagnostic labeling.
3. Examine ways that psychiatric patients are stigmatized by both healthcare professionals and the general public.
4. Adhere to appropriate boundaries in nurse–patient relationships.
5. Discuss the differences among privacy, confidentiality, and privileged communication as they apply to psychiatric/mental health nursing.
6. Describe psychiatric patients' rights in directing their care.
7. Use humanistic theories in psychiatric/mental health nursing practice.
8. Discuss the American Nurses Association's (ANA's) *Code of Ethics for Nurses* in relation to psychiatric/mental health nursing.

Characteristics of Psychiatric Nursing

Although psychiatric/mental health nursing does not have what some nurses perceive to be the excitement of other nursing specialties, such as intensive care and emergency department nursing, mental health care is extremely important. Most nurses are inspired when they realize that psychiatric/mental health nursing care is focused on the very nucleus of personal identity. However, this realization brings with it an awesome moral responsibility.

According to Radden (2002a), there are three areas that distinguish psychiatry from other medical specialties: the characteristics of the therapeutic relationship, the characteristics of psychiatric patients, and what Radden called the "therapeutic project." Keltner, Schwecke, and Bostrom (2003) proposed that psychiatric nursing can be divided into three components: "the psychotherapeutic nurse–patient relationship (words), psychopharmacology (drugs), and milieu management (environment), all of which must be supported by a sound understanding of psychopathology" (p. 14). Ethical implications involved with these different aspects of psychiatric care and special issues in mental health are addressed in this chapter.

In general, professional healthcare practices are made credible because of formal expert knowledge used in professional-patient relationships, but the nature of professional–patient relationships, the first distinguishing area of psychiatry, may be even more important in mental health care than in other healthcare specialties (Radden, 2002a; Sokolowski, 1991). One reason is that facilitative relationships are often the key to therapeutic effectiveness with psychiatric patients. The nurse–patient relationship in psychiatry has been characterized from the perspective of the nurse's "therapeutic use of self," which has been defined as "the ability to use one's personality consciously and in full awareness in an attempt to establish relatedness and to structure nursing intervention" (Travelbee, 1971, p. 19). Radden compared the therapeutic relationship to a "treatment tool analogous to the surgeon's scalpel" (2002a, p. 53). When nurses are using their personalities to effect changes in patients, it becomes very important that the nurses' behaviors reflect moral character.

The second distinguishing feature of psychiatry involves the characteristics of psychiatric patients. Psychiatric patients may be more vulnerable than other patients to exploitation, dependence, and inequality in relationships (Radden, 2002a). A presumed decrease in psychiatric patients' ability to exercise judgment and the stigma associated with mental illness lead to this special vulnerability. A central issue in psychiatric ethics is vulnerability with regard to "treatment refusal, involuntary hospitalization for care and protection, responsibility in the criminal setting, and the set of issues surrounding the criterion of competence (competence to stand trial, competence to refuse and consent to treatment, competence to undertake legal contracts, for example)" (Radden, 2002b, p. 400).

The third distinguishing feature of psychiatric care proposed by Radden (2002a), the therapeutic project, is an important part of the overall relationship between ethics and mental health. The therapeutic project is a major undertaking that involves "reforming the patient's whole self or character, when these terms are understood in holistic terms as the set of a person's long-term dispositions, capabilities and social and relational attributes" (p. 54). As with the nurses' use of self, nurses have an important moral responsibility in working with psychiatric patients in regard to the therapeutic project. Radden stated that there are only a few other societal projects that compare with the impact of the therapeutic project; one is the raising of children, which also places great responsibility on the person who is in a position of power with vulnerable others.

A Value-Laden Specialty

We do not know our own souls, let alone the souls of others.
—Virginia Woolf, "On Being Ill," 1926

The Greek philosopher Socrates said the unexamined life is not worth living. This thought underlies the aim of much of the care that patients receive from psychiatric/mental health nurses. However, one might add two supplementary statements to the famous statement made by Socrates:

1. Many people are unable to adequately examine their lives, but these lives are still worth living.
2. Even for people who try to examine the content and context of their lives, understanding often is elusive.

Although personal values pervade all discussions of nursing ethics, an emphasis on values is even more relevant to psychiatric/mental health nursing because it is largely involved with subjective experiences rather than objective diseases. According to Dickenson and Fulford (2000), psychiatry is sometimes referred to as a moral discipline rather than a medical discipline. Human values are generally shared values with regard to the experiences and behaviors addressed by physical medicine. However, in psychiatry, values relating to experiences and behaviors are usually diverse. These diverse values among mental health professionals and patients focus on motivation, desire, and belief as opposed to an overall agreement about objective findings, such as an agreement that cancer and heart disease are bad conditions. Problems arise in psychiatric/mental health care when nurses do not know how to use practical wisdom in navigating through value disparities and disagreements with patients and other healthcare providers.

Seedhouse (2000) proposed that there often is a fundamental values difference between what nurses are traditionally taught about the goals of nursing care and the priorities of the medical model in psychiatry (see Box 10.1). According to Seedhouse, the psychiatric system often relegates nursing priorities to the rank of secondary importance. In mental health organizations, professionals other than nurses may view it as an irritation when nurses try to reinforce the personal worth of patients by trying to find meaning in the patients' behaviors and experiences rather than just providing medicalized treatment. However, the acknowledgement of this problem is not intended to mean that nurses should make negative generalizations about the psychiatric healthcare system as a whole; instead, nurses' knowledge of the views of other healthcare professionals should encourage them to be aware of the values that influence the systems in which they function.

It is important for psychiatric/mental health nurses to remember that truly knowing oneself is hard and that understanding what underlies the emotions, words, and behaviors of other people often is even more difficult. Ethical practice in psychiatry generally is consistent with a foundationally nonjudgmental attitude. This does not mean, however, that nurses should not have thoughts, values, and considered judgments or opinions. It is unrealistic to believe that nurses' values do not affect their work—that is, that the work of nurses can be completely value neutral. The key to moral care is to have moral values. Nurses are responsible for using practical wisdom in their judgments, for being truthful with themselves about their own values, and for being compassionately truthful in their work with patients (see ANA [2001] *Code of Ethics for Nurses with Interpretive Statements*, provisions 5.3 and 5.4; see Appendix A). Nurses need to take care that their attitude does not degenerate into one of condescension or pity. Keeping a "there but for the grace of God go I" attitude when working in a psychiatric/mental health setting often contributes to compassionate care.

The Practice Area of Mental Health: Unique Characteristics

Some people believe that psychiatry is the one healthcare specialty in which 19th-century philosophies continue to exert a strong influence on today's approach to

BOX 10.1 ETHICAL FORMATIONS: POSSIBLE PRIORITY DISPARITIES

Nursing Priorities

[Nurses are] supposed to be respectful of all other people's beliefs, treat people as equals, care personally to the extent that [they enter] patients' subjective worlds, uphold their dignity, ensure their privacy, be ethical at all times, nurture all patients and—of course—work for their health (in this case work for their mental health).

Psychiatric [System] Priorities

The psychiatrist is trained to diagnose and treat mental illnesses supposedly as real and independent of the psychiatrist as [if treating] cold sores and bronchitis.

Source: Seedhouse, D. (2000). *Practical nursing philosophy: The universal ethical code.* Chichester, UK: John Wiley & Sons, p. 138.

practice (Beresford, 2002). Even in the 21st century, "bad" is often equated with "mad," and many people closely associate dangerous and murderous activities with mental illness. Until the discovery of new drug therapies revolutionized the field of psychiatry, mentally ill patients were frequently warehoused in asylums, often for very long periods of time or even for life (Hobson & Leonard, 2001). Research in the 1950s and 1960s produced new psychotropic medications that ushered in a metamorphosis in psychiatry. The new medications provided a way to manage psychiatric symptoms that had been difficult or impossible to manage before, but these drugs still caused many serious side effects related to their use.

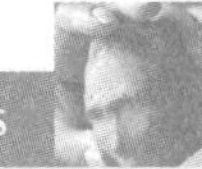

WWW Ethical Reflections

- How has mental health care been shaped by the values of Western societies?
- In what ways do you believe that nurses' values have critical ethical implications in psychiatric nursing?
- How can nurses reconcile disparities in care priorities among psychiatric healthcare professionals?

Because of the discovery of new drugs, there was a wide-scale release of patients from mental institutions in the 1960s and 1970s, and many of these people eventually became homeless or were jailed (Hobson & Leonard, 2001; Keltner et al., 2003). When patients were released from hospitals, the doors were almost literally locked and barred behind them. The patients were assured that they would receive adequate treatment for their mental illnesses in the community, but society and the medical community did not keep their promises to these patients. Satisfactory community treatment never materialized, and access to care is still a problem in mental health today. Although healthcare professionals often use the term mental health when speaking about the specialty of psychiatry, the system of psychiatric care continues to be based on mental illness (Beresford, 2002).

After the 1970s, patients still were not well managed with the new psychotropic drugs, and psychoanalysis had started to lose favor. When in the 1980s and 1990s health maintenance organizations further constrained the care and treatment of psychiatric patients, holistic care almost fell apart (Hobson & Leonard, 2001). The payment that psychiatrists received to conduct therapy sessions with their patients was no longer an incentive to provide these services; psychiatrists have been pushed in the direction of focusing on biomedical treatment, while nonphysician therapists provide counseling but no prescriptions for medications. This trend in treatment began a severe fragmentation in the environment of psychiatric care. Physicians and therapists traditionally have not communicated well among themselves and sometimes fight turf battles that further impede the quality of patient care.

Although there have continued to be many more improvements in the psychiatric medications that are available, medications still provide, at best, a symptom-only treatment, not a cure. Generally, there continues to be a fragmentary divide between professionals who treat mental illnesses biomedically and professionals who provide psychological therapy and counseling (Hobson & Leonard, 2001). This fragmentation, or treatment gap, has ethical implications for the quality of care that patients receive. It is in filling this treatment gap that nurses can move forward from a moral perspective.

Nurses are in a crucial bridge, or in-between, position to advance the holistic care of psychiatric patients by assessing their behavior and responses to medications and by providing education and valuable psychological and spiritual care, counseling, and support. Advanced-practice psychiatric/mental health nurse practitioners can prescribe medications as well as provide therapeutic and supportive counseling. However, one of the primary ways that all mental health nurses can affect the ethical environment of psychiatric/mental health care is to act as patient advocates within the imperfect system.

Advocacy

There often is a fragmentation in mental healthcare when patient treatment is separated into the biomedical sphere of psychiatrists and the psychological sphere of therapists such as psychologists and social workers. Nurses are in a unique position to act as patient advocates in bridging this fragmentary divide. Advocacy in nursing has been defined as "the active support of an important cause" (Fry & Johnstone, 2002, p. 37). According to Seedhouse (2000), "more than any other branch of nursing, mental health nursing exposes the rift between nursing's nurturing instincts and medicine's/society's insistence that aberrant behaviors are contained" (p. 153).

Nurses must try to bring to the forefront the idea that there need not be a sharp distinction between physical or biomedical health promotion and prevention and mental health promotion and prevention. This integration can be accomplished by nurse-led dialogue among the whole team of healthcare providers caring for psychiatric patients. Nurses must be open to listening and sensing the feelings, emotions, and goals of all members of the team, while practicing existential advocacy as described by Sally Gadow. According to Gadow (as cited in Bishop & Scudder, 2001), "the nurse as existential advocate does not merely help patients choose what they want—for example, the drug user who wants to be as 'high' as possible while in the hospital. The existential advocate is there to help patients recognize and realize their best selves, given their situation" (pp. 76–77).

Ethical Implications of Diagnosis

Although it is not always a case of such serious proportions, through the use of mental illness diagnostic categories "people may be locked up, subjected to compulsory (and health damaging) 'treatment' and have their rights restricted" (Beresford, 2002, p. 582). This issue is closely tied to considerations of the stigma that psychiatric patients face. Pipher (2003), a psychologist, acknowledged that ethical guidelines in clinical mental health practice do not address some of the important moral issues. Disagreement about the application of psychiatric diagnoses is one of these issues. In a qualitative study conducted by Watts and Priebe (2002), the psychiatric patient participants expressed that they perceived the psychiatric system and the labeling involved with psychiatric diagnoses as "an attack on their identity" (p. 446).

Corey (2005) cautioned counselors that cultural differences must be considered when patients are diagnosed with mental disorders:

> Certain behaviors and personality styles may be labeled neurotic or deviant simply because they are not characteristic of the dominant culture. Thus, counselors who work with African Americans, Asian Americans, Latinos, and Native Americans may erroneously conclude that a client is repressed, inhibited, passive, and unmotivated, all of which are seen as undesirable by Western standards. (p. 45)

Because psychiatric diagnoses often represent the boundaries of what is categorized as normal versus abnormal in society, psychiatric diagnoses, along with cultural, gender, and class biases, can perpetuate oppressive power relationships (Crowe, 2000). Consequently, the psychiatric diagnosing of patients is a morally charged issue. Psychiatric/mental health advanced-practice nurses are in a position to assign a psychiatric diagnosis to patients, but the assigning of diagnoses is an ethical issue about which generalist nurses also must be aware. Crowe proposed that even when nurses are not responsible for assigning a diagnosis to a patient, they are collaborators in the diagnostic process when they:

- Provide data and descriptions of observations to enable a diagnosis
- Integrate the nomenclature of diagnosis into the language of mental health nursing practice
- Administer medications that have been determined by psychiatric diagnosis
- Engage in service user and family education based on psychiatric diagnosis and treatment (Crowe, 2000, p. 585)

In psychiatry, there often are no definitive tests that can be used to diagnose illness, which has led to arguments over the years about the subjectivity of diagnosing mental illness (Kahn, 2001). However, the third edition of the Diagnostic and Statistical Manual of Mental Disorders (DSM-III), published in 1980, radically changed how psychiatric diagnoses were categorized, which began to satisfy some of the critics. The DSM-III was the first in a series of the DSM manuals to use research as a basis for categorizing diagnoses. The developers of the DSM-IV went even further in using biological data for diagnostic categories. Diagnosing with the DSM-IV-TR (4th edition, text revision) was intended to be based on observed data rather than on what is subjective or merely based on theory. Although some practitioners disagree with this assumption, many professionals believe that the DSM system is a good one. Practitioners generally identify the same diagnoses when using the system (that is, the system is reliable), but some people contend that the DSM diagnoses are not always valid (correct). Seedhouse (2000) suggested that people who take an antipsychiatric view (see Box 10.2) believe that the DSM-IV is a "house of cards" (p. 126) based on

BOX 10.2 ETHICAL FORMATIONS: ANTIPSYCHIATRY

Practitioners who have an antipsychiatry view want:

> To focus more on the beliefs and values of their patients and to include the spiritual, political, and socio-cultural dimensions of experience in their practice. This approach indicates that the concept of illness is far too restrictive to assist us in understanding insanity and reminds us that in order to understand mental illness some deconstruction of what constitutes mental illness is necessary.

Source: O'Brien, O., Woods, M., & Palmer, C. (2001). The emancipation of nursing practice: Applying anti-psychiatry to the therapeutic community. *Australian and New Zealand Journal of Mental Health Nursing, 10,* 4.

speculative assumptions. Kahn (2001) proposed that practitioners are best served if they remain openminded when using the DSM system for diagnosing patients; in other words, the system is useful, but not infallible.

When mental health professionals are forced by insurance companies to assign a diagnosis to patients, ethical dilemmas may arise (Corey, 2005). In suggesting that there are ethical implications and problems with subjectivity in identifying the psychiatric diagnoses of patients, Pipher (2003) presented a story about a young boy with an apparent obsessive-compulsive disorder. The boy's hands were chafed from frequent handwashing, and he insisted that all of his possessions be rigidly organized. The young man might even have qualified for special services at school based on his having a specific diagnosis, but there was a question about whether the diagnosis would ultimately help or hurt the boy. How would a label affect the child's self-perception and the perception of other people who might learn about the diagnosis? In the end, Pipher decided that a diagnosis was not necessary in this boy's case. Distraction was used as a treatment, and the child's family physician was available to prescribe appropriate medications as needed.

The point of Pipher's story is that clinicians must be very careful in labeling patients because healthcare professionals often are unable to determine what additional problems might be triggered by a psychiatric label. According to Pipher (2003), clinicians would do well to ask the following questions before diagnosing psychiatric patients: "Why are we doing this? Will a diagnosis allow clients to get the help they need? Can the diagnosis hurt the client?" (p. 143).

Diagnoses often are generated or changed based on information gathered and reported by nurses. Staff nurses must remember that loosely applied diagnoses that the nurse might offhandedly repeat to other people, whether these people are coworkers, the patient, families, or healthcare insurers, can be harmful to the best interests of patients—in other words, a psychiatric diagnosis is not something to be applied without skillful and reflective consideration by professionals who are specially educated to do so. Even then, nurses must be aware that often the determination of psychiatric diagnoses is a subjective and inexact science and sometimes can be detrimental to a patient's well-being.

Stigma

> *The days of telling your patients to "pull themselves together" should be over. It is not our patients who should be pulling themselves together: we should look at ourselves.*
>
> —*J. Bolton, "Reducing the Stigma of Mental Illness," 2003, pp. 104–105*

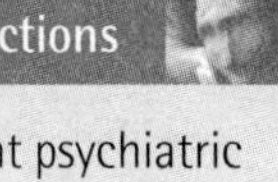

Ethical Reflections

- Do you believe that psychiatric nursing is more of an art or a science? Explain.
- What factors make an objective diagnosis difficult in the field of psychiatry? What are some of the moral implications related to this difficulty? How might this issue affect nursing care?

It is common knowledge that people with psychiatric illnesses and conditions are stigmatized by a broad spectrum of society (Bolton, 2003; Green, Hayes, Dickinson, Whittaker, & Gilheany, 2003; Knight, Wykes, & Hayward, 2003; Rosen, Walter, Casey, & Hocking, 2000; Wahl, 2003). In fact, some people believe that this stigma even extends to the professionals, such as nurses and physicians, who care for psychiatric patients (Bolton, 2003; Halter, 2002). Rosen et al. (2000) defined psychiatric **stigma** as "the false and unjustified association of individuals who have a mental illness, their families, friends and service providers with something shameful" (p. 19). This negative perception is perpetuated by the media and frequently results in hostility in communities and discrimination by service providers and employers. Fears are exacerbated and illnesses are left untreated.

When referring to people with mental illnesses, the U.S. Surgeon General stated: "Stigma tragically deprives people of their dignity and interferes with their full participation in society" (U.S. Department of Health and Human Services [DHHS], 1999, p. viii). The National Alliance on Mental Illness (NAMI, 2006) cited a study that revealed people's reluctance to use psychiatric drugs when they are needed because people are afraid of the stigma that they will endure (see Box 10.3). Healthcare professionals and patients from some cultures, especially Asian cultures, may be reluctant to give or accept a psychiatric diagnosis. Galanti (2008), a cultural anthropologist, presented related examples from her work with nurses and physicians (see Box 10.4).

Unfortunately, even healthcare professionals perpetuate the stigma of mental illness (see Box 10.5). Bolton (2003), a hospital liaison psychiatrist, voiced his distress with regard to healthcare professionals' negative perceptions of patients with mental illnesses. He stated that professionals who refer patients to him often say things such as "we've got another nutter for you" (pp. 104–105). Bolton followed up this concern by saying that he no longer accepts this sort of language and stigmatization without tactfully educating the user of such language about its inappropriateness.

BOX 10.3 ETHICAL FORMATIONS: A HISTORY OF STIGMA

The Greeks . . . originated the term *stigma* to refer to bodily signs designed to expose something unusual and bad about the moral status of the signifier. The signs were cut or burnt into the body and advertised that the bearer was a . . . blemished person, ritually polluted, to be avoided, especially in public places.

Source: Goffman, E. (1963). *Stigma: Notes on the management of spoiled identity.* New York, NY: Simon & Schuster, p. 1.

BOX 10.4 ETHICAL FORMATIONS: THE STIGMA OF MENTAL ILLNESS IN ASIA

As a Korean student explained to me, mental illness is thought to be inherited. If it were known that someone in the family was mentally ill, no one would want to marry into that family . . . students from other Asian countries have nodded in agreement. This is consistent with the fact that in Asian cultures the group is the primary unit. It is not just individuals who marry, but families.

When I was teaching a class of nurses from mainland China in the 1980s, they were quite astounded to learn that many Americans sought psychotherapy for minor problems. They believed that you were either sane or hopelessly mentally ill. There was no middle ground, no category of "neurotic," only that of "psychotic." I once met a Chinese psychiatrist in Los Angeles. When I mentioned that it was surprising to me to hear the combination of "Chinese" and "psychiatrist," he nodded understandingly and said that his parents were ashamed that he was a psychiatrist due to his association with the mentally ill. To hide their shame, they told their friends only that he was a "doctor."

Source: Galanti, G. A. (2008). *Caring for patients from different cultures* (4th ed.). Philadelphia, PA: University of Pennsylvania Press, p. 188.

BOX 10.5 ETHICAL FORMATIONS: STIGMATIZING BELIEFS

Stigmatizing Beliefs about Mental Illness

- People with mental illnesses are dangerous to others.
- Mental illness is feigned or imaginary.
- Mental illness reflects a weakness of character.
- Disorders are self-inflicted.
- Outcome is poor.
- Disorders are incurable.
- It is difficult to communicate with people with mental illness.

Source: Bolton, J. (2003). Reducing the stigma of mental illness. *Student British Medical Journal, 11*, 104–105.

Goffman (1963), a sociologist, did landmark work regarding stigma, contrasting the normals of society with stigmatized people, or people who may be called the discreditables. He proposed that people with a particular stigma, such as mental illness, have common experiences in terms of how they learn to view their stigma and their very conception of self. Goffman described this phenomenon as a common moral career. These common experiences, or moral careers, involve four phases that range from having an inborn stigma to developing a stigma later in life. However, regardless of the progression of the moral careers of stigmatized persons, it is a significant point in time when these persons realize that they possess the stigma and are exposed to new relationships with others who also have the same stigma. Goffman proposed that on first meeting other people who the stigmatized person must accept as "his own," there often is a feeling of ambivalence, but eventually a sense of identity develops.

It is important for nurses who practice in mental health settings to understand the meaning of relationships among psychiatric patients. If nurses become sensitive to the lived experiences of psychiatric patients and the therapeutic value of these patients' relationships with other people who are mentally ill, it ultimately may help to create a more supportive environment for these patients. Psychiatric patients who are marked with a stigma by society, their own families, and even healthcare professionals, may feel a sense of camaraderie with other people who have experienced similar moral careers.

Frequently, nurses find patient-to-patient camaraderie disconcerting and sometimes attempt to minimize the support that psychiatric patients develop among themselves. However, psychiatric patients often find encouragement in these relationships, as illustrated by the comments of a former psychiatric patient, Irit Shimrat (see Box 10.6). Although sound judgment on the part of nurses is essential when assessing safety factors and the therapeutic value of relationships among psychiatric patients, compassionate nursing care involves being sensitive to the stigma experienced by psychiatric patients and how this stigma affects patients' perceptions of other people who have lived through similar experiences.

Reducing Stigma

With regard to stigma, Goffman (1963) proposed that people who are stigmatized often have a turning point in their lives. Sometimes this turning point is recognized when it occurs, but sometimes it is recognized only in retrospect. Goffman stated that the turning point is an

> isolating, incapacitating experience, often a period of hospitalization, which comes later to be seen as the time when the individual was able to think through his problem, learn about himself, sort out his situation, and arrive at a new understanding of what is important and worth seeking in life. (p. 40)

BOX 10.6 ETHICAL FORMATIONS: A COMMON MORAL CAREER

Former psychiatric patient Irit Shimrat stated:

> What saved me was the help I got from other patients, and the fact that I was able to help them. By showing each other compassion, by listening to each other, against all odds, we were able to remember that we were still alive. . . . When I'm feeling terrified of the world, I can talk to someone else who's been terrified of the world, but who isn't right now, and they can free me from that terror. The stories we tell ourselves about the world and our place in it have a huge influence on how we feel and what we're capable of. When people who have been labeled mentally ill can talk to each other about these stories, without fear of being judged, the feedback we get, and give, can be enormously liberating.

Source: Shimrat, I. (2003, July/August). Freedom. *Off Our Backs, 55*, 18.

Because nurses are unaware of when patients are ready to undergo such a significant or potentially life-changing event, nurses must constantly cultivate a humanistic environment or milieu that facilitates the personal growth of patients. Smart (2003) stated that he has realized that it is best to think of sanity as occurring along a continuum rather than as a "them versus me" event. Bolton (2003) suggested other ways that stigma can be reduced (see Box 10.7).

Borderline Personality Disorder

> *And it seems to me you lived your life like a candle in the wind*
> *never knowing who to cling to when the rain set in.*
> —Elton John and Bernie Taupin, "Candle in the Wind"

Borderline personality disorder (BPD) is probably the most stereotyped and stigmatized psychiatric disorder in North America (Nehls, 1998); therefore, it warrants special consideration in terms of mental health stigma. It has been proposed that the very term, BPD, creates a prejudice and stigma that necessitate a need for changing the name of the diagnostic label (as was done in the past with the term hysteria). However, as Nehls proposed, merely changing the name of the disorder will not prevent the same stigma from being attached to a subsequent label.

The behaviors exhibited by persons with BPD—poor judgment, overdramatizing situations, relational inconsistency, not keeping appointments and then demanding immediate attention, and so on—tend to "engender feelings of anger, irritation, confusion, helplessness, and hopelessness in providers" (McCann & Ball, 2001, p. 194). These feelings may prompt healthcare professionals to exhibit nontherapeutic behaviors such as:

- Blaming the patient for lack of improvement

BOX 10.7 ETHICAL FORMATIONS: WAYS TO REDUCE STIGMA

- Examine our own attitudes.
- Update our knowledge of mental illness.
- Listen to what our patients say about mental illness and its consequences.
- Watch out for stigmatizing language.
- Be an advocate for those with mental illness.
- Add political activism to our daily work.
- Challenge stigma in the media.

Source: Bolton, J. (2003). Reducing the stigma of mental illness. *Student British Medical Journal, 11*, 104–105.

- Believing that the patient would be better off dead
- Failing to return phone calls
- Failing to carefully assess the ongoing risk of prescribing medications
- Labeling the patient's motivation as the cause of treatment failure
- Overzealous use of potentially addictive medications
- Arguing with patients
- Arguing with other professional staff regarding the patient (McCann & Ball, 2001, p. 194)

Nurses need to be self-aware of the personal emotions that are engendered by all psychiatric patients, while being particularly cognizant of these emotions when they arise in response to interactions with persons diagnosed with BPD. Lynn Williams (1998), a woman who professed to have experienced "world-class" symptoms of BPD, but whose condition improved, wrote a poignant article intended to help healthcare professionals understand some of the experiences of the disorder (see Box 10.8). Remembering that patients with BPD are worthy of nurses' concern and worthy of the best nursing care is important with regard to moral psychiatric practice.

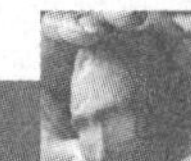

www Ethical Reflections

After returning from the Iraq War, soldiers stated that they were not comfortable seeking psychiatric treatment for posttraumatic stress disorder. One soldier interviewed on National Public Radio stated that his officers pressured him to cancel his mental health counseling appointments in order to participate in scheduled military maneuvers.

- What might be the source of the discrimination and stigma associated with soldiers' postwar psychiatric treatment?
- What role do nurses have in regard to this issue? Does the ANA's *Code of Ethics for Nurses* provide guidance for nurses? Explain.

Boundaries

A discussion of boundaries is particularly relevant to psychiatric/mental health nursing because of the particular vulnerability of mentally ill patients and the importance of trust in supporting therapeutic nurse–patient relationships. Boundary violations occur when a nurse or patient exceeds the therapeutic limits of the nurse–patient relationship. Professional boundaries are specifically covered in provision 2.4 of the *Code of Ethics for Nurses with Interpretive Statements* (ANA,

BOX 10.8 ETHICAL FORMATIONS: BORDERLINE PERSONALITY DISORDER

Someone answering to my name was once a terrified, angry person who was showing up in emergency rooms nearly every night and throwing up into a basin, or was being looked for regularly by the police when threatening suicide. . . . But that wasn't the real me. That's not who I want to be. Nor are the other people who are seen through the pathology of borderline personality disorder showing their real selves. As frustrating as these acutely ill people may be, please don't write them off. Maybe, just maybe, you'll be able to help one of them. I'm living proof that—over time—we can be helped.

Source: Williams, L. (1998). A "classic" case of borderline personality disorder. *Psychiatric Services, 49*(2), 174.

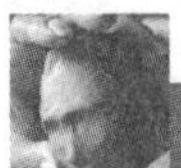

Ethical Reflections 

- What words or phrases have you heard being used that are stigmatizing to people with mental illnesses? What are the ethical implications when healthcare professionals use stigmatizing talk?
- In what ways do you believe that the media has contributed to the stigma of mental illness? In what ways might this media influence also affect the way the public views mental health nurses?
- How can nurses help to change negative perceptions of mental illness?

2001; see Appendix A). By keeping in mind that the primary concern of nurses' care is "preventing illness, alleviating suffering, and protecting, promoting, and restoring the health of patients" (ANA, 2001, p. 11), nurses can find guidance in maintaining professional boundaries. Nurses must ask themselves if the actions that they take, the words that they say, and the behaviors that they model are in the best interest of patients; in other words, nurses must be very conscious of how their behavior might affect patients and be interpreted by them. It cannot be assumed that psychiatric patients will react the same way that other patients might react to the behaviors of the nurse.

Concepts that underlie nurse–patient boundaries include power, choice, and trust (Maes, 2003). The asymmetry of power in favor of the nurse can place nurses in a position of influencing the decisions of patients. Patients need complete information to make choices, and nurses must help patients receive the information that they need. Though psychiatric patients may try to test nurses' good judgment by pushing nurse–patient boundaries to inappropriate limits, overall, patients trust nurses to have the knowledge, prudence, and skill necessary to provide them with ethical and competent care. Nurses must be faithful to that trust.

Potential violations of nurse–patient boundaries can involve gifts, intimacy, inappropriate limits, neglect, abuse, and restraints (Maes, 2003). Gifts often are nontherapeutic in psychiatric/mental health nurse–patient relationships, and gifts given to nurses by patients need to be considered in terms of why the gift was given, its value, and whether the gift might provide therapeutic value for the patient. Gifts should not influence the type of care provided by the nurse or the quality of the nurse–patient relationship. General guidelines for the inappropriate acceptance of gifts from patients include situations in which the gift is expensive; the patient is seeking approval by giving the gift; the gift is given early in the relationship, which may set the stage for lax boundaries; the nurse does not feel comfortable accepting the gift but does so because of not wanting to hurt the patient's feelings; or the nurse is having difficulty setting boundaries (Corey, Corey, & Callanan, 2003). Nurses should never accept money as tips or gifts.

The cultural implications of gift giving also need to be considered. For example, patients from Asian cultures may view giving an inexpensive gift as a sign of gratitude and respect, whereas nurses responding from a Western perspective may view the taking of a gift from a patient as a boundary violation. If a nurse refused an inexpensive gift from an Asian patient, the patient may be insulted (Corey et al., 2003). It is important for nurses to keep ethical boundaries in mind, but sometimes inflexibility is damaging to therapeutic relationships. Each situation must be evaluated individually and in accordance with the policies of the employing healthcare facility.

In addition to an obvious violation of intimacy through inappropriate sexual relationships, a violation of intimacy might occur if a nurse inappropriately shares information with other people in ways that violate a patient's privacy. The nature of nurses' work with both patients and colleagues has a very personal element, but nurse–patient relationships are not to be confused with the common definition of friendship (*Code of Ethics for Nurses* provision 2.4 in Appendix A). Nurses are not discouraged from having a caring relationship with patients, patients' families, or colleagues; however, caring and jeopardizing professional boundaries are two very distinct issues. Although carefully chosen self-disclosure is sometimes therapeutic, revealing personal information to psychiatric patients often is detrimental to patient care. Nurses are cautioned to observe limits that prevent either the nurse or the patient from becoming uncomfortable in their relationship (ANA, 2001). Psychiatric patients are best helped when they remain the focus of nursing care rather than when attention is diverted to the personal experiences of nurses.

Physically, chemically, and environmentally restraining patients, which is discussed in most psychiatric/mental health nursing textbooks, can provide a major pitfall for nurses in terms of boundary violations (ANA, 2001). Nurses are responsible for providing safe, reasonable, and compassionate care to all patients according to appropriate ethical codes, professional standards, state nurse practice acts, and organizational policies. Nurses must do everything possible to prevent or stop patient abuse in whatever form it occurs, whether the abuse is perpetrated by a patient's family or a member of the healthcare team. The safe and appropriate use of physical, chemical, and environmental restraints is a particularly important issue about which nurses continuously must be aware during patient care. It is essential that nurses know the policies of their employer as well as the standards set by professional organizations and accrediting agencies to safeguard patients (see Box 10.9).

BOX 10.9 ETHICAL FORMATIONS: AMERICAN PSYCHIATRIC NURSES ASSOCIATION [APNA] POSITION STATEMENT ON THE USE OF SECLUSION AND RESTRAINT

- Individuals have the right to be treated with respect and dignity and in a safe, humane, culturally sensitive and developmentally appropriate manner that respects individual choice and maximizes self-determination.
- Seclusion or restraint must never be used for staff convenience or to punish or coerce individuals.
- Seclusion or restraint must be used for the minimal amount of time necessary and only to ensure the physical safety of the individual, other patients or staff members and when less restrictive measures have proven ineffective.
- Individuals who are restrained must be afforded maximum freedom of movement while assuring the physical safety of the individual and others. The least number of restraint points must be utilized and the individual must be continuously observed.
- Seclusion and restraint reduction and elimination requires preventative [sic] interventions at both the individual and milieu management levels using evidence-based practice.
- Seclusion and restraint use is influenced by the organizational culture that develops norms for how persons are treated. Seclusion and restraint reduction and elimination efforts must include a focus on necessary culture change.
- Effective administrative and clinical structures and processes must be in place to prevent behavioral emergencies and to support the implementation of alternatives.
- Hospital and behavioral healthcare organizations and their nursing leadership groups must make commitments of adequate professional staffing levels, staff time and resources to assure that staff are adequately trained and currently competent to perform treatment processes, milieu management, de-escalation techniques and seclusion or restraint.
- Oversight of seclusion and restraint must be an integral part of an organization's performance improvement effort and these data must be open for inspection by internal and external regulatory agencies. Reporting requirements must be based on a common definition of seclusion and restraint. Specific data requirements must be consistent across regulatory agencies.
- Movement toward future elimination of seclusion and restraint requires instituting and supporting less intrusive, preventative[sic], and evidence-based interventions in behavioral emergencies that aid in minimizing aggression while promoting safety.

Source: APNA. (2007). *2007 Position Statement on the Use of Seclusion and Restraint.* Retrieved from http://www.apna.org/files/public/APNA_SR_Position_Statement_Final.pdf

Whose Needs Are Being Served?

An issue closely tied to relationship boundaries and the restraint of patients is the ethical obligation of determining whose needs are being served in professional–patient relationships. When discussing counselor–client relationships, Corey (2005) proposed that counselors need to be aware of when they may be placing their own needs before those of their client. This type of assessment and awareness of needs is equally applicable in nurse–patient relationships. It is easy for nurses to unintentionally become absorbed in their own self-interests during day-to-day patient care. Personal needs of the nurse that may be placed before the patient's needs include:

- The need for control and power
- The need to be nurturing and helpful
- The need to change others in the direction of our own values
- The need to persuade
- The need for feeling adequate, particularly when it becomes overly important that the client confirm our competence
- The need to be respected and appreciated (Corey, 2005, p. 38)

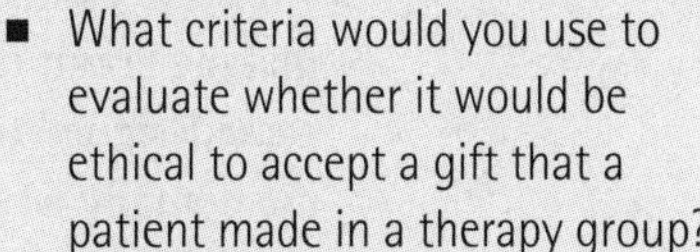

Ethical Reflections

- What criteria would you use to evaluate whether it would be ethical to accept a gift that a patient made in a therapy group?
- What would you say to a patient who offered you his dead mother's pearl necklace?
- What would you do if a coworker told you that she accepted jewelry from a patient?

Nurses may have to take special care to keep in mind that patients' needs are to be placed first. As is stated in the second provision of the ANA (2001) *Code of Ethics for Nurses with Interpretive Statements*, "the nurse's primary commitment is to the patient, whether an individual, family, group or community" (p. 9). Because of the psychological nature of their conditions, psychiatric/mental health patients may be particularly vulnerable to nurses placing them in dependent positions.

Psychotropic drugs sometimes make patients more manageable for nurses, which raises the question of whose needs are being served: the nurse's or the patient's? Similar to the point made with regard to nurses' complicity in the diagnostic labeling of patients, nurses have a very important role in determining the type and amount of medications that are ordered for and administered to psychiatric patients, particularly in hospital settings. Nurses are the professionals who spend the most time with hospitalized psychiatric patients, and physicians often base treatment decisions on nurses' formal or informal comments, reports, and documentation. Nurses must be very aware of whose needs are being served and must use careful reflection in determining how they choose to represent patients' behaviors and conditions to other people.

Ethical Reflections

- What questions might nurses ask to evaluate their motives before giving p.r.n. medications to psychiatric patients?
- What could a nurse do to positively influence a coworker who tends to oversedate patients because she likes patients to be "easy to handle"?

Privacy, Confidentiality, and Privileged Communication

Although privacy, confidentiality, and privileged communication are similar concepts, there are important differences to be considered. Confidentiality and privileged communication are both issues of a patient's right to privacy; confidentiality usually is more associated with ethics, whereas privileged communication pertains more to the legal nature of provider–patient relationships (Corey et al., 2003).

Privacy

The concept of privacy began receiving attention in the 1920s, when the U.S. Supreme Court addressed the liberty interest of families with regard to decision making about their children (Beauchamp & Childress, 2009). The court's rulings were designed to protect part of a person's private life from state intrusion, which incidentally was also the foundation for overturning restrictive abortion laws in 1973. However, the right to **privacy** cannot be reduced to a narrow context of having a right to act autonomously. In addition to autonomy, the rights that fall within the boundaries of privacy include a person's right to be protected from no more than limited physical and informational access by others.

Allen (as cited in Beauchamp & Childress, 2009) described four types of privacy that address limited personal access:

1. Informational privacy: Communication of information
2. Physical privacy: With regard to personal spaces
3. Decisional privacy: With regard to personal choices
4. Proprietary privacy: Property interests, including interests with regard to bodily tissues, one's name, etc.

Beauchamp and Childress added a fifth type of privacy to Allen's list: relational or associational privacy. This type of privacy represents an admission that people make decisions within the context of intimate relationships and depend on significant others to be involved with their private decisions.

The value placed on privacy varies among situations and people. Sometimes, for example, persons may feel comfortable with other people knowing that they have a psychiatric condition, but they are not comfortable with sharing the exact nature of the condition. Nurses need to err on the side of strictly maintaining a patient's privacy unless there is a justifiable reason for privacy to be violated, such as a duty to warn (see the following *Privileged Communication* section).

Confidentiality

In healthcare ethics, confidentiality is one of the oldest moral commitments, dating back to the Hippocratic oath (Gillon, 2001). **Confidentiality**, or nondisclosure of information, involves limits on the communication of "any information a nurse obtains about a patient in the context of the nurse–patient relationship" (Killion, 2006b, p. 36). It includes limits on the communication of information related to any of the five types of privacy previously listed. The Joint Commission on Accreditation of Healthcare Organizations (1998) defined confidentiality as "an individual's right, within the law, to personal and informational privacy, including his or her healthcare records" (p. 139). Confidentiality is one of the most important ethical precepts in psychiatric/mental health nursing because the therapeutic nurse–patient relationship is grounded in trust.

Privileged Communication

Whereas confidentiality involves a professional duty not to disclose certain information, **privilege** provides relief from having to disclose information in court proceedings (Smith-Bell & Winslade, 2003). Patients have a legal right to believe that their communication with nurses will be kept confidential, but there are limits to confidentiality in psychiatric/mental health practice. Limits to both confidentiality and privilege would permit disclosure of information by the nurse when:

- Patients are a threat to themselves (suicide, for example) or to identifiable others
- Statutes require the disclosure of certain happenings, such as abuse, rape, incest, or other crimes
- The patient consents to release of the information
- A court mandates the release
- The information is needed for other caregivers to provide care to the patient—that is, when certain people have a "need to know" information (Corey, 2005; Killion, 2006b)

Nurses cannot disclose patient information to unidentified or unauthorized telephone callers or to relatives, significant others, or friends of the patient without the patient's consent (Killion, 2006b).

Duty to Warn

In some cases, nurses may have a **duty to warn**, which involves "a duty to disclose confidential information to protect an identifiable victim" (Killion, 2006b, p. 37). Documentation by nurses of patient threats is necessary, but this may not be enough in some cases. Nurses also may have a duty to warn appropriate authorities about threats made by patients or even to warn the specific person(s) targeted by the threats. This duty is weighed by viewing it as a dilemma between respecting a patient's privacy and respecting society's need to be informed about acts that are dangerous to citizens (Everstine et al., 2003). The duty to warn is based on the case of *Tarasoff v. Board of Regents of the University of California* (see Box 10.10).

Decisional Capacity

According to Beauchamp and Childress (2009), some people distinguish competence and capacity based on who is making the determination; that is, capacity is assessed by healthcare professionals, and competence is determined within the court system. Singer (2003) defined competence "as a group of capacities" (p. 152). However, some people propose that for all practical purposes, the consequences of the determination of capacity versus competence are basically the same (Grisso & Appelbaum, 1998). In psychiatric care, both capacity and competence are related to questions of whether patients have a right to consent to and refuse treatment, and are closely associated with the issue of autonomy.

BOX 10.10 ETHICAL FORMATIONS: *TARASOFF V. BOARD OF REGENTS OF THE UNIVERSITY OF CALIFORNIA*

In August 1969, a voluntary outpatient, Prosenjit Poddar, was being counseled at the student health center at the University of California, Berkeley campus. The patient threatened to kill a woman (Tatiana Tarasoff) who was unnamed, but who was identifiable to the therapist. The therapist warned the campus police about the threat, but the police spoke with Poddar and deemed him to be "rational" and did not take action to warn Ms. Tarasoff. The therapist continued to pursue the issue, but Ms. Tarasoff was not warned of the threat and was later killed by Poddar. Her family sued the Board of Regents and the university staff for failing to warn the victim. In 1976, the California Supreme Court ruled in favor of the parents. The court proclaimed: "The protective privilege ends where the public peril begins" (*Tarasoff v. Board of Regents of the University of California*, 1976, p. 347).

Source: Corey, G., Corey, M. S., & Callanan, P. (2003). *Issues and ethics in the helping professions.* Pacific Grove, CA: Wadsworth Group-Brooks/Cole.

Statutory Authority to Treat

Involuntary commitment poses ethical as well as legal problems for psychiatric healthcare professionals. Based on a general social policy of deinstitutionalization, involuntary hospitalization decisions can be made only after less restrictive options have failed or have carefully been determined not to be a viable option (Corey et al., 2003). The decision usually is made based on a person being a danger to self, a danger to others, and, in some states, being gravely disabled. Each state jurisdiction has statutes that allow psychiatrists to hold persons involuntarily for psychiatric treatment, and healthcare professionals are responsible for following their state's particular laws and regulations (Corey et al., 2003; Jonsen, Siegler, & Winslade, 2010; Videbeck, 2006). If a patient is determined by a psychiatrist to be incompetent, state statutes can be followed for a temporary involuntary commitment. Court proceedings are then initiated to extend the involuntary treatment or commitment. This legal process is expedited while the person is being (temporarily) held involuntarily.

This process begins with a presumption of competency (Dempski, 2009). However, when it is determined by a psychiatrist that the person exhibits a lack of decision-making capacity, a petition is filed with the court to determine competency. The person receives a court-appointed guardian or legal counsel and undergoes psychological testing procedures. A hearing is scheduled, and evidence is presented with regard to the person's ability to handle personal affairs and to understand the consequences of personal decisions. Negotiations are conducted with the aim of determining the least restrictive alternative for the person's care and treatment. Outcomes of the hearing can result in a dismissal of the petition, the appointment of limited guardianship, or an appointment of complete guardianship.

These outcomes may be appealed, and a restoration hearing can be held later if the person's circumstances change and warrant a removal of guardianship. This process is often inappropriately called a "medical hold" (Jonsen et al., 2010, p. 92). The psychiatric commitment process does not automatically include an authorization to treat a patient involuntarily for medical, in addition to psychiatric, conditions. A legally authorized appointee also must be specially assigned to make medical decisions other than those that are determined to be for a life-saving emergency, in which an implied consent is sufficient.

Competence and Informed Consent

Competence and informed consent are intricately connected. Informed consent, as required by legal authorities, is impossible in situations involving incompetent patients (Singer, 2003). A patient, even when involuntarily committed, has a right to refuse treatment, such as psychotropic medications, until or unless the patient has been deemed incompetent by formal legal proceedings. In the case of *Rivers v. Katz,* the New York State Court of Appeals established that there are limited circumstances in which a patient's right to refuse unwanted treatment can be overridden: only on the determination that a patient is a danger to self or other people. Patients may not be prevented from refusing medications based on healthcare professionals' desire to create a therapeutic environment, for the convenience of hospital staff, or to facilitate the process of deinstitutionalization.

There are no uniform standards that can be used to determine competence, although it is accepted that incompetence is founded on cognitive impairment (Berg, Appelbaum, & Grisso, as cited in Singer, 2003). Brody (1988) outlined general criteria of competency that also are applicable with regard to psychiatric patients. These criteria include:

- The ability to receive information from surroundings
- The capacity to remember the information received
- The ability to make a decision and give a reason for it
- The ability to use the relevant information in making the decision
- The ability to appropriately assess the relevant information (pp. 101–102)

To this list, Singer (2003) added the capacity to participate constructively in discussions with the caregiver regarding treatment, including the "ability to engage in mutual questioning and answering" (p. 153). Singer called this supplementary capacity of communicative interchange "dialogic reciprocity" (see Box 10.11).

Psychiatric Advance Directives

The Patient Self-Determination Act (PSDA) enacted by the federal government in 1990 has drawn focused attention to patients' right to autonomy in making healthcare decisions. The psychiatric advance directive (PAD) developed as an outcome

BOX 10.11 ETHICAL FORMATIONS: DIALOGIC RECIPROCITY

Dialogic "reciprocity... involves mutual respect for the autonomy and authority of all the participants in a discussion, a respect that . . . should be accorded to them as a matter of right. . . . Respecting a person's authority in this sense can be thought of as a type of empowerment: empowerment to have one's contribution to the discussion taken seriously, even if it may be subsequently rejected or overridden. . . . In the exercise of dialogic reciprocity we reflect autonomously and critically on our own judgments as well as those of the others with whom we are in dialogue. Therefore, we are open to change, even though the dialogue may result in strengthening our original position."

Source: Singer, B. J. (2003). Mental illness: Rights, competence, and communication. In G. McGee (Ed.), *Pragmatic Bioethics* (pp. 158–159). Cambridge, MA: Massachusetts Institute of Technology.

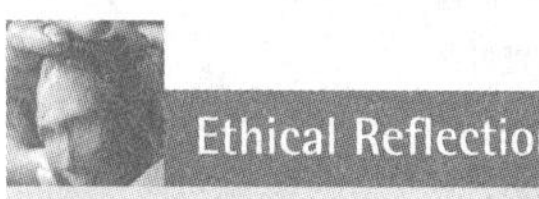

- Partner with a peer and develop a patient case scenario that involves the use of a PAD. Trade cases with other peers and determine the ethical issues involved. Compare answers.

of the PSDA and is legal in 25 states (National Resource Center on Psychiatric Advance Directives, 2011). A **psychiatric advance directive** may be completed by competent psychiatric patients who want to direct their psychiatric care when and if they later lose their capacity to voice their treatment choices.

Treatment issues that can be addressed in the PAD include choices regarding medication administration, hospital admission, and electroconvulsive therapy. There are limits to the PAD, such as directives that might conflict with laws, life-threatening needs, and professional practice standards. In addition to treatment directives, a proxy for directing one's psychiatric care can be designated in the PAD. Psychiatric patients often find having a PAD to be an important means of supporting their sense of autonomy and feelings of self-worth. Box 10.12 contains statements from psychiatric patients about their PADs.

Mental Illness and Children

When nurses are considering ethical issues surrounding the subject of mental illness and children, one of the primary considerations should be nurses' own sensitivity in recognizing signs of problems with a child's mental health. Mental illness, along with an impairment diagnosable disorder, occurs in one in five children and adolescents (Mental Health America, 2011). A report in the *New York Times* (Duff, 2010) revealed the following:

- More than 500,000 children and adolescents in America are now taking antipsychotic drugs, according to a September 2009 report by the Food and Drug Administration. Their use is growing not only among older teenagers, when schizophrenia is believed to emerge, but also among tens of thousands of preschoolers. (para. 7)

BOX 10.12 ETHICAL FORMATIONS: PATIENTS SPEAK ABOUT PADS

Selected and edited statements from research interviews with participants in a study of PADs at Duke University Medical Center:

> We talked about what was in my PAD. The doctor didn't treat me like a "nut case" because some hospitals do. He said, "You've got rights and it's great that you know you have them—and we'll try to respect those completely." He did a lot for my health, too.
>
> This time, with a PAD, I did not receive any treatments that I did not want. They were very respectful. I really felt like the hospital took better care of me because I had my PAD. In fact, I think it's the best care that I've ever received.
>
> My healthcare agent is a real close friend and she knows about my illness. She's been around my illness for so long and basically, she knows what's going on with me. I trust her judgment.

Source: National Resource Center on Psychiatric Advance Directives. (2011). *PAD stories.* Retrieved from http://www.nrc-pad.org/index.php?option=com_content&task=view&id=141&Itemid=55

- A Columbia University study recently found a doubling of the rate of prescribing antipsychotic drugs for privately insured 2- to 5-year-olds from 2000 to 2007. Only 40 percent of them had received a proper mental health assessment, violating practice standards from the American Academy of Child and Adolescent Psychiatry. (para. 8)

Any nurse who works with children is obliged to be educated, at the very least, regarding the basic signs and symptoms of mental illness in childhood, such as the symptoms of depression, which can manifest differently in children than in adults. Children and adolescents often have more difficulty expressing feelings that are indicative of depression and may exhibit more irritability than depressed adults (Keltner et al., 2003). In some instances, a nurse may be the primary link between preventing a child's suicide and helping the child imagine a meaningful future.

Another ethical issue involves nurses being active in helping children with mental disorders deal with stigma and the consequent development of what Goffman (1963) referred to as the stigmatized person's moral career. One childhood mental disorder that is particularly surrounded by stigma, confusion, and misinformation is attention deficit hyperactivity disorder (ADHD).

Attention Deficit Hyperactivity Disorder

The assessment and treatment of ADHD in children is a controversial issue in the United States. Some healthcare professionals and people in the general public have voiced concerns about a possible trend toward the overidentification of behavioral problems being labeled and treated as ADHD. According to the Centers for Disease Control and Prevention (CDC) (2011), 5.3 million children in the United

States between the ages of 3 and 17 years old have at some point been diagnosed with ADHD. A report of data gathered through the 2007 National Survey of Children's Health indicated "that the percentage of children aged 4–17 years with a parent-reported ADHD diagnosis (ever) increased from 7.8% to 9.5% during 2003–2007, representing a 21.8% increase in 4 years" (CDC, 2010, para. 2).

When ADHD is recognized, a debate often ensues about whether the disorder should be treated with medication or behavioral therapy (Powell, Welch, Ezell, Klein, & Smith, 2003).

Dodson (2001) listed the following possible causes for the perception by many people that ADHD may be overdiagnosed and overtreated:

- Increased awareness of the condition by the public
- Acceptance of a broader set of diagnostic criteria
- Greater appreciation of the course of the illness and its ultimate impact on adult life, which justifies lengthier and uninterrupted treatments
- Diminished concern about growth retardation, predisposition to drug use, and long-term effects of stimulant-class medications
- Increased treatment of adults (p. 304)

Nurses and other healthcare professionals need to keep in mind that, as with almost any mental disorder, ADHD can be over- or under-diagnosed and treated. Nurses working with children, such as nurses who work in schools, need to seek a thorough understanding regarding the appropriate assessment of ADHD, referral to other healthcare professionals, and treatment options. Some children who have ADHD are required to take their medication during the school day, although new, long-acting medications make this situation less common. However, having to take medications at school or be monitored for a physical or psychological disorder can be a source of stigma for any child, separating the child from the so-called normals within the social structure of the school (see Box 10.13). The ethical responsibility of nurses and other healthcare professionals with regard to ADHD and all childhood mental illnesses involves an interest in the careful and individualized evaluation, treatment, and follow-up of each child, as well as being alert and active in trying to minimize stigma.

BOX 10.13 ETHICAL FORMATIONS: ABOUT NORMAL

Right now, I don't know what Normal is anymore. That's because Normal has been changing so much, so often, lately. For a long while of lately. I'd like Normal to be okayness. Good health . . . emotional health, medical health, spiritual health. I'd like Normal to be like that. I'd like Normal to stay, like that. For now though, I know that Normal won't be normal for a little while . . . but somehow, sometime, even if things are not Normal, they'll be okay. That's because I believe in the great scheme of things and life.

Source: Stepanek, M. J. T. (2002). *Hope through heartsongs.* New York, NY: Hyperion.

Humanistic Nursing Care in Psychiatric/Mental Health Nursing

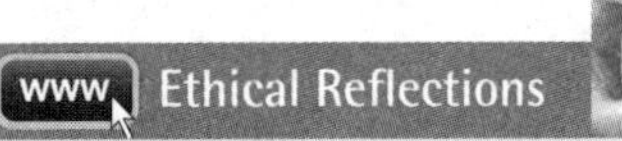

- What specific actions can school nurses take to reduce the stigma of children who are not among the "normals" of the school?
- What interventions can a nurse provide if a mother cries and expresses feelings of guilt with regard to her child's diagnosis of ADHD?
- How and why would the nature of these interventions be ethically related?

As was mentioned at the beginning of this chapter, some people say that psychiatry is a moral discipline rather than a medical discipline (Dickenson & Fulford, 2000). Ethics in nursing has been distinguished as a special area of ethics based on its grounding in relationships (Austin, Bergum, & Dossetor, 2003; Nortvedt, 1998; Scott, 2003). Humanistic care is provided from the perspective that all humans are of equal worth and deserving of respect. Yalom (1995), when discussing humanistic or person-centered therapy as advanced by Carl Rogers, said, "experienced therapists today agree that the crucial aspect of therapy, as Rogers grasped early in his career, is the therapeutic relationship" (p. ix). Psychiatric/mental health nursing is morally enriched by humanistic nurse–patient relationships that lead to human flourishing. Three humanistic approaches that were developed in the 1960s and 1970s, but are still relevant to psychiatric nursing care today, have been included in the discussion of humanistic nursing care.

Person-Centered Approach

The concepts of humanistic psychology and existentialism form the basis of psychologist Carl Rogers's person-centered approach (Corey, 2005). According to Rogers (1980), the development of "person" is the central goal of any person-centered relationship. For a growth-promoting environment to exist in the relationship, three conditions are necessary: (1) genuineness or realness; (2) acceptance, caring, or prizing; and (3) empathic understanding. The nurse who employs the element of genuineness or realness does not maintain a distant professional facade with the patient—the nurse truly experiences the feelings that are occurring in the relationship. The nurse who is exhibiting Rogers's second condition of a therapeutic relationship maintains an attitude of unconditional positive regard for a patient. The patient is prized in a total way and whatever feelings are occurring are accepted. Acceptance of the patient is not conditional. The last of Rogers's facilitative factors, empathic understanding, is a deep sensitivity to the patient's feelings, both those feelings on the level of awareness and those below. The professional nurse is able to sense the personal meanings of the patient's experience and communicates this understanding to the patient.

Humanistic Nursing Practice Theory

Paterson and Zderad first published their humanistic nursing practice theory in 1976, when nurses were in the midst of assertiveness training as a result of the women's movement in the United States (Moccia, 1988). Moccia proposed that the power that is supported by Paterson and Zderad's theory involves authentic dialogue with patients, students, and other healthcare professionals. According to Paterson and Zderad (1988), humanistic nursing emphasizes both the art and science of nursing. "Humanistic nursing embraces more than a benevolent technically competent subject–object one-way relationship guided by a nurse in behalf of another" (p. 3). Nursing, rather, involves a responsible searching for nurse–patient two-way interactions that receive their meaning from and are grounded in the nurse's and patient's existential experiences, or the experiences of living. A brief overview of Paterson and Zderad's perspectives about the domain of nursing—person, nurse (nursing), health, environment—provides some clarification of their theory, which can be used imaginatively by nurses in moral psychiatric/mental health practice.

Persons (including patients and nurses) have the freedom to make choices. Persons have individual, unique views of the world; are adequate, having the capacity to hope and envision alternatives to what is immediately apparent; have the capacity for authentic presence and intersubjective relatedness; and have meaningful personal histories, although their histories do not control them.

Nursing is an art–science, meaning that nursing is derived from subjective, objective, and intersubjective experiences. Nursing is a form of unique knowledge that is developed through dialogical human processes. Finally, nursing is both being and doing, with focus on being present with another and engaging in two-way dialogue.

Health does not always mean the absence of disease. The nurse's aim is to provide comfort to patients, with comfort conceptualized as being all that one can be at a particular point in time. Nurses try to promote well-being and more-being of others, emphasizing that persons are adequate as they are (well-being) but are free to become more than they are (more-being).

Environment, the final part of the domain, focuses on time and space, the here and now, or the connectedness of past, present, and future. It also focuses on the nursing situation, which includes the whole world of people and things, a world that is more than just the patient and the nurse—the "all-at-once" or an awareness of all of the emotions, values, and experiences that work together to increase wisdom, a community of persons striving toward a common center, and a complementary synthesis or living out the tension between the objective scientific world and the subjective and intersubjective domains of nursing (O'Connor, 1993; Paterson & Zderad, 1988).

Human-to-Human Relationship Model

The human-to-human relationship model, developed by Joyce Travelbee, was based on her experiences in psychiatric nursing and grounded in the philosophy of existentialism. Travelbee (1971) proposed that (1) nurses must possess a body of knowledge and know how to use it, and (2) nurses must learn to use themselves therapeutically if helping relationships are to be established. The phases that lead to the establishment of human-to-human relationships, as described by Travelbee, can be used for ethical practice in psychiatric/mental health nursing. These phases are:

1. The phase of the original encounter: First impressions of both the patient and nurse are perceived. The nurse must be aware of value judgments and feelings.
2. The phase of emerging identities: A bond is established between the nurse and the patient. There is again an emphasis on awareness by the nurse of how the patient is being perceived. Nurses must develop an awareness and a valuing of the uniqueness of others.
3. The phase of empathy: This is a conscious process of sharing in another person's experiences.
4. The phase of sympathy: In this phase, the nurse progresses further than empathy and wants to alleviate a patient's distress.
5. The phase of rapport: Rapport is the end goal of all nursing endeavors; it is a process, an experience, or a happening; it is the human-to-human relationship.

(Rangel, Hobble, Lansinger, Magers, & McKee, 1998; Travelbee, 1971)

WWW Ethical Reflections

- Box 10.14 contains examples from the ANA's (2001) *Code of Ethics for Nurses with Interpretive Statements*. How are these examples relevant to psychiatric/mental health nursing?
- What other provisions and statements in the ANA's *Code of Ethics for Nurses* are particularly pertinent to psychiatric/mental health nursing (see Appendix A)? Discuss these provisions and provide examples of how they apply to nursing practice.

BOX 10.14 ETHICAL FORMATIONS: *CODE OF ETHICS FOR NURSES*

- The nurse respects the worth, dignity, and rights of all human beings irrespective of the nature of the health problem (1.3, p. 7).
- Each nurse has an obligation to be knowledgeable about the moral and legal rights of all patients to self-determination (1.4, p. 8).
- The nurse recognizes that there are situations in which the right to individual self-determination may be outweighed or limited by the rights, health, and welfare of others (1.4, p. 9).
- When acting within one's role as a professional, the nurse recognizes and maintains boundaries that establish appropriate limits to relationships (2.4, p. 11).
- The patient's well-being could be jeopardized and the fundamental trust between patient and nurse destroyed by unnecessary access to data or by the inappropriate disclosure of identifiable patient information (3.2, p. 12).
- Duties of confidentiality are not absolute and may need to be modified in order to protect the patient, other innocent parties, and in circumstances of mandatory disclosure for public health reasons (3.2, p. 12).
- As an advocate for the patient, the nurse must be alert to and take appropriate action regarding any instances of incompetent, unethical, illegal, or impaired practice by any member of the healthcare team or the healthcare system or any action on the part of others that places the rights or best interests of the patient in jeopardy (3.5, p. 14).

CASE STUDY: IS THERE A DUTY TO WARN?

www

Kendrick M. is a 25-year-old man hospitalized with a paranoid delusional disorder. When Kendrick was admitted, he was very angry and vehemently verbalized that he believed that his ex-mother-in-law had been spreading lies about him around town, and he accused her of getting him fired from his last job. When Kendrick's sister, Rose, visited him at the hospital, he gave consent for you, his nurse, and his psychiatrist to talk with her about his condition. At that time, Rose stated that Kendrick's ideas about his ex-mother-in-law were delusional thinking and that there was no basis in fact regarding his beliefs. Kendrick's condition has improved with adjustments of his psychotropic drugs (he is no longer actively exhibiting angry and paranoid behavior), and he is being discharged today. When you are talking with Kendrick today in preparation for his discharge, he tells you "I'm still not finished with my ex-mother-in-law." You ask him to explain this statement, and he is evasive but answers with cryptic statements that seem to indicate veiled threats against the woman.

Case Study Questions

1. As Kendrick's nurse, how would you evaluate the duty to warn in this situation?
2. Do you believe that Kendrick still should be discharged today? Please provide a rationale for your answer and discuss the information that would be needed to make this decision.
3. What actions would you take?
4. Discuss ethics-related principles, precedents, and concepts that are relevant to this case.

Recognizing Inherent Human Possibilities

Rogers (1980) believed that there is an underlying movement toward inherent possibilities that all human beings exhibit. He proposed that it is a self-actualizing tendency for complete development and that life is an active process that moves toward maintaining, enhancing, and reproducing, even when conditions are not favorable. Rogers compared this view of human flourishing to a story about sprouting potatoes that he observed in his youth. He noticed that even when potatoes were stored in the basement during winter, they would produce pale (as opposed to healthy green) sprouts that twisted toward what little light they might have. Life was still trying to flourish, although conditions were not favorable. Rogers's words very eloquently compare how these potatoes can be likened to psychiatric patients, or any patients, whose lives nurses touch. Rogers (1980) said:

> In dealing with clients whose lives have been terribly warped, in working with men and women on the back wards of state hospitals, I often think of those potato sprouts. So unfavorable have been the conditions in which these people have developed that their lives often seem abnormal, twisted, scarcely human. Yet, the directional tendency in them can be trusted. The clue to understanding their behavior is that they are striving, in the only ways that they perceive as available to them, to move toward growth, toward becoming. To healthy persons, the results may seem bizarre and futile, but they are life's desperate attempt to become itself. (p. 119)

KEY POINTS

- Psychiatry may be thought of as a moral discipline rather than a medical discipline because it is often involved with subjective experiences and relationships rather than objective tests and diseases.
- Nurses must be sensitive to the moral implications of using diagnostic labels when referring to patients, because diagnostic labels can be a source of harm and distress for patients.
- People in society often stigmatize mentally ill persons, and healthcare professionals sometimes perpetuate this stigma. Even those people who care for mentally ill persons are often stigmatized.
- Confidentiality and privileged communication are issues of a patient's right to privacy. Confidentiality is usually thought of in ethical terms, whereas privileged communication pertains more to legal protection.
- In some situations, there are limits to a patient's right to confidentiality and privileged communication, such as when healthcare professionals have a duty to warn identifiable others of threats made by patients.
- The decision to involuntarily hospitalize a person is usually based on the person being a danger to self, a danger to others, and in some states, being gravely disabled.
- Humanistic nursing care is grounded in the belief that through genuine, intersubjective experiences and relationships, nurses can help patients to be free to become all that they can be.

References

American Nurses Association. (2001). *Code of ethics for nurses with interpretive statements.* Silver Spring, MD: Author.

Austin, W., Bergum, V., & Dossetor, J. (2003). Relational ethics: An action ethic as a foundation for health care. In V. Tschudin (Ed.), *Approaches to ethics: Nursing beyond boundaries* (pp. 45–52). Edinburgh, UK: Butterworth-Heinemann-Elsevier Science.

Beauchamp, T. L., & Childress, J. F. (2009). *Principles of biomedical ethics* (6th ed.). New York, NY: Oxford University Press.

Beresford, P. (2002). Thinking about "mental health": Towards a social model. *Journal of Mental Health, 11*(6), 581–584.

Bishop, A., & Scudder, J. (2001). *Nursing ethics: Holistic caring practice* (2nd ed.). Sudbury, MA: Jones and Bartlett.

Bolton, J. (2003). Reducing the stigma of mental illness. *Student British Medical Journal, 11,* 104–105.

Brody, B. A. (1988). *Life and death decision making.* New York, NY: Oxford University Press.

Centers for Disease Control and Prevention. (2010). Increasing prevalence of parent-reported attention-deficit/hyperactivity disorder among children—United States, 2003 and 2007. *Morbidity and Mortality Weekly Report, 59* (44), 1439–1443.

Centers for Disease Control and Prevention. (2011). *Attention deficit hyperactivity disorder (ADHD).* Retrieved from http://www.cdc.gov/nchs/fastats/adhd.htm

Corey, G. (2005). *Theory and practice of counseling and psychotherapy* (7th ed.). Belmont, CA: Brooks/Cole-Thomson Learning.

Corey, G., Corey, M. S., & Callanan, P. (2003). *Issues and ethics in the helping professions.* Pacific Grove, CA: Wadsworth Group-Brooks/Cole.

Crowe, M. (2000). Psychiatric diagnosis: Some implications for mental health nurse care. *Journal of Advanced Nursing, 31*(3), 583–589.

Dempski, K. (2009). Emergency psychiatric admissions. In S. J. Westrick & K. Dempski (Eds.), *Essentials of nursing law and ethics* (pp. 126–129). Sudbury, MA: Jones and Bartlett.

Dickenson, D., & Fulford, K. W. M. (2000). *In two minds: A casebook of psychiatric ethics.* New York, NY: Oxford University Press.

Dodson, W. W. (2001). Attention-deficit hyperactivity disorder. In J. L. Jacobson & A. M. Jacobson (Eds.), *Psychiatric secrets* (2nd ed., pp. 302–309). Philadelphia, PA: Hanley & Belfus.

Duff, W. (2010, September 1). Child's ordeal shows risks of psychosis drugs for young. *New York Times.* Retrieved from http://www.nytimes.com/2010/09/02/business/02kids.html?pagewanted=1&_r=1&ref=health

Everstine, L., Everstine, D. S., Heymann, G. M., True, R. H., Frey, D. H., Johnson, H. G., . . . Richard, H. (2003). Privacy and confidentiality in psychotherapy. In D. N. Bersoff (Ed.), *Ethical conflicts in psychology* (3rd ed., pp. 162–164). Washington, DC: American Psychological Association.

Fry, S., & Johnstone, M. J. (2002). *Ethics in nursing practice: A guide to ethical decision making* (2nd ed.). Oxford, UK: Blackwell Science.

Galanti, G. A. (2008). *Caring for patients from different cultures* (4th ed.). Philadelphia, PA: University of Pennsylvania Press.

Gillon, R. (2001). Confidentiality. In H. Kuhse & P. Singer (Eds.), *A companion to bioethics* (pp. 425–431). Oxford, UK: Blackwell.

Goffman, E. (1963). *Stigma: Notes on the management of spoiled identity.* New York, NY: Simon & Schuster.

Green, G., Hayes, C., Dickinson, D., Whittaker, A., & Gilheany, B. (2003). A mental health service users' perspective to stigmatization. *Journal of Mental Health, 12*(3), 223–234.

Grisso, T., & Appelbaum, P. S. (1998). *Assessing competence to consent to treatment: A guide for physicians and other health care professionals.* New York, NY: Oxford University Press.

Halter, M. J. (2002). Stigma in psychiatric nursing. *Perspectives in Psychiatric Care, 38*(1), 23–28.

Hobson, J. A., & Leonard, J. A. (2001). *Out of its mind: Psychiatry in crisis—A call to reform.* Cambridge, MA: Perseus.

Joint Commission on Accreditation of Healthcare Organizations. (1998). *Ethical issues and patient rights: Across the continuum of care.* Oakbrook Terrace, IL: Author.

Jonsen, A. R., Siegler, M., & Winslade, W. J. (2010). *Clinical ethics* (7th ed.). New York, NY: McGraw-Hill.

Kahn, M. W. (2001). Introduction to DSM-IV. In J. L. Jacobson & A. M. Jacobson (Eds.), *Psychiatric secrets* (2nd ed., pp. 18–20). Philadelphia, PA: Hanley & Belfus.

Keltner, N. L., Schwecke, L. H., & Bostrom, C. E. (2003). *Psychiatric nursing* (4th ed.). St. Louis, MO: Mosby.

Knight, M. T. D., Wykes, T., & Hayward, P. (2003). "People don't understand": An investigation of stigma in schizophrenia using interpretative phenomenological analysis (IPA). *Journal of Mental Health, 12*(3), 209–222.

Maes, S. (2003). How do you know when professional boundaries have been crossed? *Oncology Nursing Society News, 18*(8), 3–5.

McCann, R. A., & Ball, E. M. (2001). Borderline personality disorder. In J. L. Jacobson & A. M. Jacobson (Eds.), *Psychiatric secrets* (2nd ed., pp. 190–197). Philadelphia, PA: Hanley & Belfus.

Mental Health America. (2011). *Children's mental health statistics.* Retrieved from http://www.nmha.org/go/information/get-info/children-s-mental-health/children-s-mental-health-statistics

Moccia, P. (1988). Preface. In J. G. Paterson & L. T. Zderad, *Humanistic nursing* (pp. iii–v). New York, NY: National League for Nursing.

National Alliance on Mental Illness. (2006). *Study confirms that stigma still a barrier to psychiatric care.* Retrieved from http://www.nami.org/Template.cfm?Section=20065&Template=/ContentManagement/ContentDisplay.cfm&ContentID=31897

National Resource Center on Psychiatric Advance Directives. (2011). *Do all states specifically have PAD statutes?* Retrieved from http://www.nrc-pad.org/content/view/41/25/

Nehls, N. (1998). Borderline personality disorder: Gender stereotypes, stigma, and limited system of care. *Issues in Mental Health Nursing, 19*, 97–112.

Nortvedt, P. (1998). Sensitive judgment: An inquiry into the foundations of nursing ethics. *Nursing Ethics, 5*(5), 385–392.

O'Brien, O., Woods, M., & Palmer, C. (2001). The emancipation of nursing practice: Applying anti-psychiatry to the therapeutic community. *Australian and New Zealand Journal of Mental Health Nursing, 10*, 4.

O'Connor, N. (1993). Paterson and Zderad: *Humanistic nursing theory*. Newbury Park, CA: Sage.

Paterson, J. G., & Zderad, L. T. (1988). *Humanistic nursing*. New York, NY: National League for Nursing.

Pipher, M. (2003). *Letters to a young therapist: Stories of hope and healing.* New York, NY: Basic Books.

Powell, S. E., Welch, E., Ezell, D., Klein, C., & Smith, L. (2003). Should children receive medication for symptoms of attention deficit hyperactivity disorder? *Peabody Journal of Education, 72*(3), 107–115.

Radden, J. (2002a). Notes towards a professional ethics for psychiatry. *Australian and New Zealand Journal of Psychiatry, 36*, 52–59.

Radden, J. (2002b). Psychiatric ethics. *Bioethics, 16*(5), 397–411.

Rangel, S., Hobble, W. H., Lansinger, T., Magers, J. A., & McKee, N. J. (1998). Joyce Travelbee: Human-to-human relationship model. In A. M. Tomey & M. R. Alligood (Eds.), *Nursing theorists and their work* (4th ed., pp. 364–374). St. Louis, MO: Mosby.

Rogers, C. R. (1980). *A way of being*. Boston, MA: Houghton Mifflin.

Rosen, A., Walter, G., Casey, D., & Hocking, B. (2000). Combating psychiatric stigma: An overview of contemporary initiatives. *Australasian Psychiatry, 8*(1), 19–26.

Scott, A. P. (2003). Virtue, nursing and the moral domain of practice. In V. Tschudin (Ed.), *Approaches to ethics: Nursing beyond boundaries* (pp. 25–32). Edinburgh, UK: Butterworth-Heinemann-Elsevier Science.

Seedhouse, D. (2000). *Practical nursing philosophy: The universal ethical code.* Chichester, UK: John Wiley & Sons.

Shimrat, I. (2003, July/August). Freedom. *Off Our Backs, 55*, 18.

Singer, B. J. (2003). Mental illness: Rights, competence, and communication. In G. McGee (Ed.), *Pragmatic bioethics* (2nd ed., pp. 151–162). Cambridge, MA: Massachusetts Institute of Technology.

Smart, D. (2003, April 7). Take action now to banish mental health prejudices. *Pulse-I-Registrar, 63*(14), 60.

Smith-Bell, M., & Winslade, W. J. (2003). Privacy, confidentiality, and privilege in psychotherapeutic relationships. In D. N. Bersoff (Ed.), *Ethical conflicts in psychology* (3rd ed., pp. 157–161). Washington, DC: American Psychological Association.

Sokolowski, R. (1991). The fiduciary relationship and the nature of professions. In E. D. Pellegrino, R. M. Veatch, & J. P. Langan (Eds.), *Ethics, trust, and the professions: Philosophical and cultural aspects* (pp. 23–43). Washington, DC: Georgetown University.

Stepanek, M. J. T. (2002). *Hope through heartsongs.* New York, NY: Hyperion.

Travelbee, J. (1971). *Interpersonal aspects of nursing.* Philadelphia, PA: F. A. Davis.

U.S. Department of Health and Human Services. (1999). *Mental health: A report of the Surgeon General—Executive summary.* Rockville, MD: Author.

Videbeck, S. L. (2006). *Psychiatric mental health nursing* (3rd ed.). Philadelphia, PA: Lippincott, Williams, & Wilkins.

Wahl, O. F. (2003). Depictions of mental illnesses in children's media. *Journal of Mental Health, 12*(3), 249–258.

Watts, J., & Priebe, S. (2002). A phenomenological account of users' experiences of assertive community treatment. *Bioethics, 16*(5), 439–454.

Williams, L. (1998). A "classic" case of borderline personality disorder. *Psychiatric Services, 49*(2), 173–174.

Yalom, I. D. (1995). Introduction. In C. R. Rogers (Ed.), *A way of being* (pp. vii–xiii). Boston, MA: Houghton Mifflin.

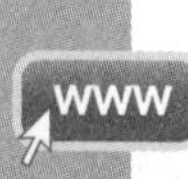

For a full suite of assignments and additional learning activities, use the access code located in the front of your book to visit this exclusive website: http://go.jblearning.com/butts. If you do not have an access code, you can obtain one at the site.

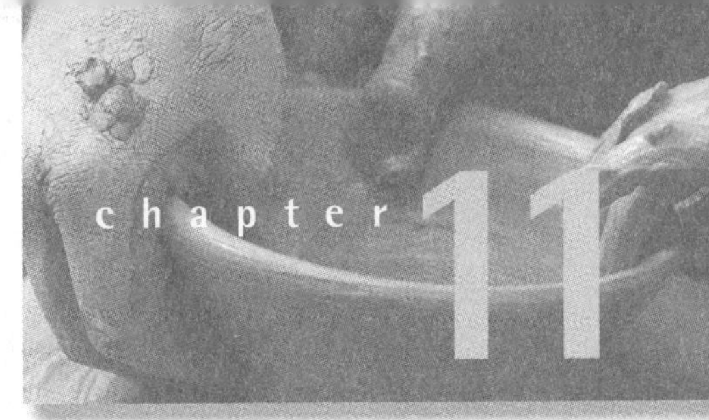

Public Health Nursing Ethics

Karen L. Rich

To be a [person] is, precisely to be responsible. It is to feel shame at the sight of what seems to be unmerited misery. . . . It is to feel, when setting one's stone, that one is contributing to the building of the world.

—ANTOINE DE SAINT-EXUPERY,
A GUIDE FOR GROWN-UPS: ESSENTIAL WISDOM FROM THE COLLECTED WORKS

OBJECTIVES

After reading this chapter, the reader should be able to:

1. Distinguish a moral community from a population.
2. Apply different ethical approaches to public health nursing (PHN) issues.
3. Discuss healthcare disparities and identify populations at risk.
4. Analyze communicable disease-related ethical issues.
5. Analyze ethical issues that may arise during disasters.
6. Identify ethical issues and questions that are outcomes of the human genome project.
7. Explain what it means for a nurse to be a servant leader.
8. Discuss the ANA (2001) *Code of Ethics for Nurses with Interpretive Statements* in relation to public health nursing.

Introduction

In their own way, public health (PH) nurses are contributors to the building of the world. "Public health nurses integrate community involvement and knowledge about the entire population with personal, clinical understandings of the health and illness experiences of individuals and families within the population" (American Public Health Association [APHA], 2011, para. 1). "The practice is population-focused with the goals of promoting health and preventing disease and disability for all people through the creation of conditions in which people can be healthy" (American Nurses Association [ANA], 2007, p. 5). The following eight principles outlined in the ANA's (2007) *Public Health Nursing: Scope and Standards of Practice* distinguish public health nursing (PHN) from other nursing specialties. Because of the nature of these principles, PHN, like all types of nursing, is inherently ethical in nature.

1. The client or unit of care is the population.
2. The primary obligation is to achieve the greatest good for the greatest number of people or the population as a whole.
3. The processes used by public health nurses include working with the client as an equal partner.
4. Primary prevention is the priority in selecting appropriate activities.
5. Public health nursing focuses on strategies that create healthy environmental, social, and economic conditions in which populations may thrive.
6. A public health nurse is obligated to actively identify and reach out to all who might benefit from a specific activity or service.
7. Optimal use of available resources to assure the best overall improvement in the health of the population is a key element of the practice.
8. Collaboration with a variety of other professions, populations, organizations, and other stakeholder groups is the most effective way to promote and protect the health of the people. (pp. 8–9)

The fundamental purpose of PHN is consistent with the overarching goals articulated by the U.S. Department of Health and Human Services (USDHHS, 2011) in *Healthy People 2020*, the nation's public health agenda. The first goal of this national agenda is to help the U.S. population "attain high-quality, longer lives free of preventable disease, disability, injury, and premature death" (para. 5). Public health nurses share this goal and other *Healthy People 2020* goals, with the common hope being to "achieve health equity, eliminate disparities, and improve the health of all groups [and to] create social and physical environments that promote good health for all" (para. 5).

Population is the term used to describe the recipients of the health promotion and disease and disability prevention care that is the primary focus of PHN. In this chapter, a **population** is defined as a group of people who share at least one common descriptive characteristic but who do not necessarily have a collective commitment to a common good. The name used to denote a population often is related to the common characteristic(s) of the people who make up the population, such as male alcoholics or pregnant teenagers. People within populations may or may not interact or share in a collective dialogue.

The word *community* means different things to different people (see Box 11.1). A **community** is a group of people who have a shared interest in a common good, and members of the group have the potential to share in a collective dialogue about their common good. Membership in the community forms some part of each member's identity. The sharing in a commitment to promote the community's well-being, which transcends individual interests and goals, makes personal relationships within the community moral in nature. A **moral community** is formed by members who care about collectively alleviating the suffering and facilitating the well-being of other members of the community and who may take action in doing so. Individual persons may be active or inactive members of a moral community.

A moral community can be as large as the global community, whose members are generally committed to the common good and prosperity of the inhabitants of the Earth, or as small as a community of senior nursing students at a university. The common good of a community of nursing students might be the collective concern about obtaining professional nursing licensure while maintaining individual physical and psychological well-being. The student community accomplishes its goals through the members' shared commitment to providing emotional support to members and to helping one another move toward the successful completion of the National Council Licensure Examination (NCLEX). An even smaller community is a family that is committed to common goals beyond the individual personal goals of family members.

Members of a community may or may not share close geographic boundaries; however, if members of a community share some type of geographic boundaries, the primary moral connection among the members typically is not based solely on that geography. Nurses, patients, and other people in society are usually members of more than one community. A nurse is a member of the community of registered nurses who are collectively committed to the common good of alleviating patients'

BOX 11.1 ETHICAL FORMATIONS: COMMUNITY

Community. A word of many connotations—a word overused until its meanings are so diffuse as to be almost useless. Yet the images it evokes, the deep longings and memories it can stir, represent something that human beings have created and recreated since time immemorial, out of our profound need for connection among ourselves and with Mother Earth.

Source: Forsey, H. (1993). *Circles of strength: Community alternatives to alienation.* Philadelphia, PA: New Society, p. 1.

suffering and promoting patients' well-being. The same nurse also may be a member of a faith community, a member of a geographic neighborhood community that is interested in the common good and safety of the neighbors; and a member of a parent–teacher community that is committed to the common good of a population of children.

Ethical Approaches to Public Health

As it is with all sorts of ethical considerations regarding nurses' personal and professional beliefs and behaviors, it is difficult to limit one's philosophy to only one ethical theory or approach in public health practice. At varying times and in varying situations, one of a number of important ethical approaches and theories may help guide nurses' actions and the development of public health policies.

According to the ANA (2007), public health nurses must adhere to the ethical principles outlined in the *Code of Ethics for Nurses with Interpretive Statements* (ANA, 2001), the *Principles of the Ethical Practice of Public Health* (Public Health Leadership Society, 2002), and the *Environmental Health Principles for Public Health Nursing* (APHA, 2006) (see Boxes 11.2 and 11.3). Public health nurses are charged with honoring "the diverse values, beliefs and cultures present in the population served" (ANA, 2007, p. 9) and providing information necessary for members of populations to discuss healthcare choices and make uncoerced healthcare decisions. Because of the scope of PHN, ethical practice is especially focused on social justice and the rights of various populations.

BOX 11.2 ETHICAL FORMATIONS: PRINCIPLES OF THE ETHICAL PRACTICE OF PUBLIC HEALTH

1. Public health should address principally the fundamental causes of disease and requirements of health, aiming to prevent adverse health outcomes.
2. Public health should achieve community health in a way that respects the rights of individuals in the community.
3. Public health policies, programs, and priorities should be developed and evaluated through processes that ensure an opportunity for input from community members.
4. Public health should advocate and work for the empowerment of disenfranchised community members, aiming to ensure that the basic resources and conditions necessary for health are accessible to all.
5. Public health should seek the information needed to implement effective policies and programs that protect and promote health.

Source: Public Health Leadership Society. (2002). *Principles of the ethical practice of public health*, p. 4. For a complete list of principles, go to http://www.apha.org/codeofethics/ethicsbrochure.pdf

BOX 11.3 **ETHICAL FORMATIONS: ENVIRONMENTAL HEALTH PRINCIPLES FOR PHN**

1. Safe and sustainable environments are essential conditions for the public's health.
2. Environmental health is integral to the role and responsibilities of all public health nurses.
3. All public health nurses should possess environmental health knowledge and skills.
4. Environmental health decisions should be grounded in sound science.
5. The precautionary principle is a fundamental tenet for all environmental health endeavors.
6. Environmental justice is a right of all populations.
7. Public awareness and community involvement are essential in environmental health decision making.
8. Communities have a right to relevant and timely information for decisions on environmental health.
9. Environmental health approaches should respect diverse values, beliefs, cultures, and circumstances.
10. Collaboration is essential to effectively protect the health of all people from environmental harm.
11. Environmental health advocacy must be rooted in scientific integrity, honesty, respect for all persons, and social justice.
12. Environmental health research addressing the effectiveness and public health impact of nursing interventions should be conducted and disseminated.

Source: American Public Health Association: Public Health Nursing Section. (2006). *Environmental health principles for public health nursing.* Retrieved from http://www.apha.org/membergroups/newsletters/sectionnewsletters/public_nur/winter06/2550.htm (para. 5)

Kantian Ethics (Deontology)

Kantian ethics emphasizes that all rational persons are autonomous, ends-in-themselves and worthy of dignity and respect. (See Chapter 1 for a more complete discussion of Kantian ethics.) Kantianism is highly valued in Western medicine because of the focus on individual rights and informed consent. In the U.S. healthcare system and in Western bioethics, the choices of rational individuals are generally respected. However, in public health, practitioners often must balance the rights of individuals with the rights of populations and communities. Sometimes, navigating this delicate balance can be controversial or generate dilemmas, such as considering appropriate actions when a person with a communicable disease may jeopardize the health of other people. This situation results in a need to balance respecting the autonomy and protecting the confidentiality of one person while trying to protect the safety and rights of other persons.

Utilitarianism (Consequentialism)

As discussed in Chapter 1, utilitarianism is an ethical approach based on maximizing the good, happiness, or moral consequences of one's decisions and actions. Although there are variations in utilitarian theories, when utilitarianism is used in health care, the goal or intended consequence generally is to produce the greatest good for the greatest number of people. Because of the emphasis on population-focused care, utilitarianism is one of the most widely used ethical approaches in public health practice. The second distinguishing element of PHN outlined in the ANA's (2007) *Public Health Nursing: Scope and Standards of Nursing* is that "the primary obligation is to achieve the greatest good for the greatest number of people or the population as a whole" (p. 8). This directive for PH nurses is a classic example of utilitarianism.

Communitarian Ethics

> *There is no power for change greater than a community discovering what it cares about.*
>
> —*Margaret Wheatley,* Turning to One Another

The philosophy of communitarian ethics is in opposition to rights theories that promote liberal individualism (Beauchamp & Childress, 2009). **Communitarian ethics** derives from "communal values, the common good, social goals, traditional practices, and cooperative virtues" (p. 356). Communitarian ethics is relevant to moral relationships in any community, and this ethical approach is particularly useful in the practice of PHN because of the focus on populations and communities rather than on the care of individuals.

The notion that communitarian ethics is based on the model of friendships and relationships that existed in the ancient Greek city-states as described by Aristotle was popularized in modern times by the philosopher and ethicist Alasdair MacIntyre (1984) in his book, *After Virtue.* In general societal ethics and in bioethics, the valuing and consideration of community relationships has come to mean different things to different people. Communitarian ethics as an ethical approach is distinguished because the epicenter of communitarian ethics is the community, rather than any one individual (Wildes, 2000). Populations, in general, and moral communities, in particular, also are the starting points for PHN practice.

The value of discussing and articulating an approach to communitarian ethics lies in the benefit that can be gained through illuminating and appreciating the relationships and interconnections between people that often are overlooked in everyday life. Although personal moral goals, such as the pursuit of personal well-being, are significant, the importance of forming strong communities and identifying the moral goals of communities must not be neglected if both individuals and communities are free to flourish.

An important distinction that legitimately can be drawn between communitarian and other popular ethical approaches, such as deontological or rule-based ethics, is based on communitarian ethicists' proposal that it is natural for humans to favor the people with whom they live and have frequent interactions, while

Kantian deontologists base their ethics on an impartial stance toward the persons who experience the effects of their morally related actions. However, using a communitarian ethic and valuing partiality as a way of relating to other people does not have to exclude caring about people who are personally unknown to moral agents. Although it is often easier for people to care about and have compassion for people who are relationally closest to them, it is not unrealistic to believe that people also can develop empathy or compassion toward people who are personally unknown to them. Such behavior and expectations are an integral part of Christian and Buddhist philosophies, for example. Accepting the notion that humans usually are more partial to people with whom they are most closely related, while at the same time believing that it is possible to expand the scope of their empathy and compassion to unknown others, broadens the sphere of morality in communitarian ethics.

Nussbaum (2004) suggested that people often develop an us-versus-them mentality, especially when significant ethnic and cultural differences separate them. People are able to generate sympathy, or fellow-feeling, when they hear about epidemics, disasters, and wars occurring on continents that are far away, but it often is difficult for people to sustain their sympathy for more than a short period of time after media coverage diminishes. People tend to stop and notice the needs of other people and then soon turn back to their own personal lives. According to Nussbaum, humanity will "achieve no lasting moral progress unless and until the daily unremarkable lives of people distant from us become real in the fabric of our own daily lives" (p. 958) and until people include others that they do not know personally within the important sphere of their lives (see Box 11.4). Public health nurses need to expand their scope of concern to consistently include people affected by healthcare disparities, diseases, epidemics, and ethnic violence and wars all over the world every day, not only when issues are highlighted in the media.

"All communities have some organizing vision about the meaning of life and how one ought to conduct a good life" (Wildes, 2000, p. 129). Public health nurses have an important role in bringing populations and communities together to work toward a common humanitarian good. Transforming a community from an

BOX 11.4 ETHICAL FORMATIONS: THE DELUSION OF SEPARATENESS

A human being is a part of the whole called by us "universe," a part limited in time and space. He experiences himself, his thoughts, and feelings as something separated from the rest, a kind of optical delusion of his consciousness. This delusion is a kind of prison for us, restricting us to our personal desires and to affection for a few persons nearest to us. Our task must be to free ourselves from this prison by widening our circle of compassion to enhance all living creatures and the whole of nature in its beauty.

Source: Einstein, A. (1930). *What I believe.* Retrieved from http://home.earthlink.net/~johnrpenner/Articles/Einstein3.html

us-versus-them mentality to one that seeks a common good is possible through education (Nussbaum, 2004): "Children [and people] at all ages must learn to recognize people in other countries as their fellows, and to sympathize with their plights. Not just their dramatic plights, in a cyclone or war, but their daily plights" (p. 959). This need for empathetic understanding also is important in one's own country, state, city, town, or neighborhood. Many people of all ages are suffering in the United States and throughout the world because they lack adequate health care, proper food, a sanitary environment, and good housing.

The education of communities often occurs through role modeling (Wildes, 2000). Members of communities learn about what is and is not accepted as moral through personal and group interactions and dialogue within their communities. Narratives are told by nurses about the lives of exemplars, such as Florence Nightingale and Lillian Wald, to illustrate moral living. By her efforts to improve social justice and health protection through environmental measures and her efforts to elevate the character of nurses, Nightingale exhibited moral concern for her local society, the nursing profession, and people remote from her local associations, such as the population of soldiers affected by the Crimean War. Likewise, Lillian Wald was an excellent role model for members of communities because of her efforts to improve social justice through her work at the Henry Street Settlement. When learning from the example of Nightingale and Wald, communitarian-minded PH nurses are in an excellent position to educate the public and other nurses and healthcare professionals about why they should assume the role of being their brothers' and sisters' keepers.

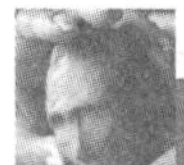

Ethical Reflections 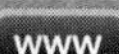

- To what communities do you belong? What can be identified as the common good of each of these communities?
- Have you noticed us-versus-them thinking among members of the nursing community? Among members of the larger community of healthcare professionals? If so, what effect has this thinking had on relationships among members of the particular community?
- Can a community really exist when there is us-versus-them thinking among the members? Why or why not?
- What patient populations might be particularly susceptible to having people approach them in an us-versus-them way? What evidence did you use for your answer? How can nurses change this type of separatist thinking?
- Explore information about the lives of Florence Nightingale and Lillian Wald. What did these two women do to promote the common good of the populations that they served?

Social Justice

As discussed in Chapter 1, **social justice** is related to the fair distribution of benefits and burdens among members of a society. However, in our U.S. society, it has been argued that market justice has been the dominant model (Beauchamp, 1999; Riegelman, 2010) and remains so today. **Market justice** is based on the principle that the benefits and burdens of a society should be distributed among its members according to the members' individual efforts and abilities. In a market justice system, money for health care tends to be invested in technology and curing diseases rather than in health promotion and disease prevention.

Major public health problems usually are concentrated among a small minority of the U.S. population. For social justice to be achieved, members of U.S. society who are not directly experiencing problems, such as a lack of access to health care, poverty, poor quality of housing, and malnutrition, may have to significantly reduce their share of societal benefits and increase their share of societal burdens. Therefore, public health and social justice involve important ethical decisions about how members of societies choose to distribute their resources and provide for the well-being of their fellow citizens.

Health Disparities

> *If we gloss over the difficulties that people face in their communities, we cannot hope to build a better world.*
>
> —*Helen Forsey*, Circles of Strength: Community Alternatives to Alienation, *p. 50*

Health disparities are inequalities or differences in healthcare access and treatment that result in poor health outcomes for persons and populations. Health disparities occur because of some characteristic(s) of the persons or population affected. After the first goal of helping people "attain high-quality, longer lives free of preventable disease, disability, injury, and premature death" (USDHHS, 2011, para. 5), the second goal of *Healthy People 2020* is to "achieve health equity, eliminate disparities, and improve the health of all groups" (para. 5). Eliminating health disparities is a moral issue for PH nurses because social justice and communitarian ethics are based on building flourishing communities that support the common good of all community members.

According to nurse-anthropologist Lundberg (2005), "social and cultural factors give context and meaning to health, illness, and injury. The experience is more than that of the patient. It also reflects the worldview of the individuals helping the person in distress" (p. 152). A major concern of bioethicists is that people's health and access to health care is adversely affected in proportion to their lack of power and privilege in a society (Sherwin, 1992). Consequently, poverty and the placement of people within the margins of society are key factors in the determination of public health. When any community members are suffering or are in need, all people in the community are affected, even if it is in imperceptible ways. One must only think about the hypothetical Net of Indra (see Box 1.4 in Chapter 1) to imagine how this situation might be a reality.

Racial and ethnic minorities suffer serious health disparities in access to care and health outcomes. The USDHHS has selected six target areas of focus to try to minimize disparities among minorities (Centers for Disease Control [CDC], 2009). The six areas of emphasis are infant mortality, cancer screening and management, cardiovascular disease, diabetes, HIV infections/AIDS, and immunizations. Several of the many specific examples of health disparities experienced by minorities include a black-to-white infant mortality ratio of 2.5 to 1, diabetes being 2.6 times more likely to be diagnosed in American Indians and Alaska Natives than in non-Hispanic whites, and the influenza and pneumococcal vaccine being less likely to be received by people age 65 and older who are Hispanic or African American than by non-Hispanic white people.

Public health nurses need to play a role in helping members of communities to collectively accept responsibility for their own health and to develop the capacity to help themselves in resolving problems that lead to health disparities. One coordinated plan to address public health disparities involves four phases or themes: community participation, community mobilization, commitment to social justice, and the leadership challenge (Berkowitz et al., 2001).

Public health nurses can support members of communities by participating in the validation of suspected problems through investigation and research and by building partnerships to collaborate on policy development. Public health nurses facilitate community mobilization by educating members of the community about health promotion and health protection measures that are likely to improve the lives of people in the community. Teaching people in the community about how

BOX 11.5 ETHICAL FORMATIONS: THREE PARTS OF A LEGISLATIVE MEETING

During meetings with legislators, nurses can use the following strategies to effect change:

1. Hook: Briefly explain who you are.
2. Line: Briefly explain your issue and why you care about it. Present a strong argument, a personal story, or both. Try to put a face on your issue.
3. Sinker: Clearly present your specific request and try to get a commitment. It is very important to stay focused on your message and to listen attentively to feedback.

Other suggestions:

- Plan for the meeting to last no more than 15 minutes.
- Arrive 10 to 15 minutes early for your appointment.
- Before the meeting, assign responsibilities among your colleagues, such as deciding who will begin and end the meeting.
- Rehearse your talking points before the meeting.
- Exchange business cards during the meeting.
- At the end of the meeting, thank everyone who met with you or helped schedule the meeting. Send a thank you note shortly after the meeting.

Source: Kush, C. (2004). *The one hour activist: The 15 most powerful actions you can take to fight for the issues and candidates you care about.* San Francisco, CA: Jossey-Bass.

to begin grassroots political efforts to obtain needed resources is an important advocacy role of PH nurses. Being committed to social justice requires PH nurses to speak out about health disparities to other nurses and healthcare professionals, to a wide group of community members, and to politicians (see Box 11.5). In helping communities increase participation, mobilize action, and expand social justice, the leadership challenge for PH nurses is to "act as a resource, consultant, facilitator, educator, advocate, and role model" (Berkowitz et al., 2001, p. 53).

A widely accepted approach to organizing communities to address their health disparity and social justice problems has been based on the idea that healthcare professionals must appeal to the self-interest of the community and its members (Minkler & Pies, 2002). However, Minkler and Pies argue that this traditional approach often only further divides groups of people by emphasizing the notion of individualism and separateness that is already a divisive way of thinking in Western societies. This approach does not support a community's interest in a common good.

Minkler and Pies (2002) adapted a feminist approach to social change as an agenda for trying to eliminate disparities in the equitable distribution of community resources. Historically, feminist philosophers and activists have approached their agenda in terms of the disparities experienced by women, but a feminist approach often can be used with other marginalized populations. This approach can be used to build a bridge that connects local community efforts to eliminate disparities with efforts to address more global social concerns. Nurses and other healthcare professionals working with community members who are involved in organizing to facilitate change can ask:

> (1) Does [the community's organizing effort] materially improve the lives of community members and if so, which members and how many? (2) Does [participating in the organizing process] give community members a sense of power, strength and imagination as a group and help build structures for further changes? and (3) Does the struggle . . . educate community members politically, enhancing their ability to criticize and challenge the system in the future? (Minkler & Pies, 2002, pp. 132–133)

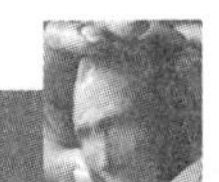

www Ethical Reflections

- What is meant by the term "marginalized populations"? Identify populations in your community that may be marginalized and experience health disparities and discuss why this may be so.
- Reflect on and discuss why appeals to self-interest in addressing health disparities might divide people and communities.
- Review critical theory in Chapter 1. Why is this theory relevant to the issue of health disparities? Provide one example of how a public health nurse could use critical theory in addressing health disparities in a specific population.
- Identify issues and problems that PH nurses might address via a meeting with a state or national legislator.

The Precautionary Principle

The ANA noted that the precautionary principle is a good guide to use in supporting social justice and populations' rights. The **precautionary principle** is based on the German word *vorsorgeprinzip*, which means the principle of forecaring. The word *forecaring* conveys more than being cautious: it means that one uses foresight and preparation, and it is aligned with the principle of "first do no harm" (nonmaleficence) and the adage "better safe than sorry" (Science & Environment Health Network [SEHN], 2011). In 1998, a multinational, multiprofessional group met at the Wingspread conference, sponsored by the SEHN, to discuss using the precautionary principle as the basis of international agreements, especially those related to the environment and health. The participants at the conference developed a statement to guide actions by governmental and nongovernmental agencies. The group stated: "When an activity raises threats of harm to the environment or human health, precautionary measures should be taken even if some cause and effect relationships are not fully established scientifically" (para. 1).

According to SEHN (1998), "the key element of the principle is that it incites us to take anticipatory action in the absence of scientific certainty" (para. 1). Advocates of the precautionary principle contend that people should not wait until they have "certain evidence" from traditional science to show the causal connection between various actions or toxins and their harmful effects. Minimum standards for citing evidence of cause and effect relationships via traditional science are usually very high (SEHN, 2011), and it can take a long time to gather the large amounts of evidence required. The type of science needed to support the precautionary principle has been called appropriate science, as distinguished from traditional science (Kriebel, Tickner, & Crumbley, 2003). Appropriate science is based on the context of the problem at hand rather than requiring that scientific pursuits be forced into a preconceived idea of necessary rigor.

People who oppose the precautionary principle believe that if science has not provided certain evidence that a particular activity or substance is harmful to humans and/or the environment, then the activity or substance is assumed to be safe until shown to be otherwise. However, proponents of using the precautionary principle answer with the argument that by the time harmful causal relationships are established with certainty, much, sometimes irreparable, damage already may have occurred. An example cited by proponents of the precautionary principle is the harmful connection between cigarette smoking and lung cancer: "Smoking was strongly suspected of causing lung cancer long before the link was demonstrated conclusively" (SEHN, 2011, para. 3). Fortunately, many smokers had stopped smoking based on precautionary measures rather than waiting on scientific certainty to confirm the harmful effects.

Today, there is evidence that the incidence of chronic illnesses, birth defects, infertility, cancer, Alzheimer's disease, and autism are increasing, while certain causal links to these conditions are lacking. Advocates of using the precautionary principle strongly propose that society should limit exposure to potentially harmful substances even before those substances are shown to have direct causal links to human health problems.

For PH nurses to practice ethically, it is recommended in the ANA's (2007) *Public Health Nursing: Scope and Standards of Practice* that PH nurses use the precautionary principle. As a follow-up to the Wingspread conference, another community of philosophers, scientists, and environmentalists, called the Blue Mountain group, met to discuss the ethics that underlie the precautionary principle. This group's consensus was that the precautionary principle is an integration of science and ethics (Raffensperger & Myers, 2001). Whereas traditional science tries to separate evidence from values, the precautionary principle supports the integration of the two, and the precautionary principle is "an ethic of survival" (para. 8). The Blue Mountain group contended that emotions and "values such as compassion, sympathy, gratitude, and even humor are based on sound instinct" (para. 8). Societal values become societal actions. The group argued that people must live in a positive reciprocal relationship with nature as well as with one another if society is to survive.

Environmental Justice

Environmental justice relates to distributing environmental benefits and burdens in an equitable manner. The U.S. Environmental Protection Agency (USEPA, 2011a) more specifically defines environmental justice as "the fair treatment and meaningful involvement of all people regardless of race, color, national origin, or income with respect to the development, implementation, and enforcement of environmental laws, regulations, and policies" (para. 1). It is the goal of the EPA for all people in the United States to have a voice in environmental policymaking and to be protected from environmental hazards that affect their health and well-being. Three fundamental principles of environmental justice developed by the U.S. Department of Transportation are listed in Box 11.6.

Environmental racism is a particular type of environmental injustice that affects populations of color. It has been demonstrated that people of color generally experience a disproportionate amount of environmental burdens; for example, children of color are more likely than white children to experience the effects of environmental hazards, such as exposure to lead. These environmental disparities are likely to result from power and privilege differentials within a society or community (Friis, 2007). However, it primarily was people of color themselves who advanced the environmental justice movement in association with the 1960s civil rights movement (USEPA, 2011b).

Nurses have taken a leadership role in working to promote environmental justice (see Box 11.3). One example of a leadership program is the Luminary Project (2005), whose slogan is "nursing lighting the way to environmental health." The project is a collaborative effort of nursing workgroups and organizations and is funded by the Beldon Fund. The project's website is dedicated to spreading stories about nurses who are improving human health by improving the environment.

BOX 11.6 ETHICAL FORMATIONS: FUNDAMENTAL PRINCIPLES OF ENVIRONMENTAL JUSTICE

There are three fundamental environmental justice principles:

1. To avoid, minimize, or mitigate disproportionately high and adverse human health or environmental effects, including social and economic effects, on minority populations and low-income populations.
2. To ensure the full and fair participation by all potentially affected communities in the transportation decision-making process.
3. To prevent the denial of, reduction in, or significant delay in the receipt of benefits by minority populations and low-income populations.

Source: U.S. Department of Transportation: Federal Highway Administration. (2011). *Environment: The facts.* Retrieved from http://www.fhwa.dot.gov/environment/ejustice/facts/index.htm

Virtue Ethics: *Just Generosity*

To a [disciple] the Master said, "I fear you are doing more harm than good."
"Why?"
"Because you stress only one of the two imperatives of justice."
"Namely?"
"The poor have a right to bread."
"What's the other one?"
"The poor have a right to beauty."

—*Anthony De Mello,* One Minute Nonsense

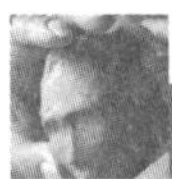

Ethical Reflections

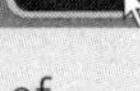

- Can you identify examples of environmental *injustice* in your geographic community? Describe them.
- Visit the Luminary Project website (http://www.theluminaryproject.org) and read some of the stories of nurse luminaries. Which stories do you find to be particularly interesting? Which stories do you believe convey particularly innovative actions?

Pieper (1966) proposed that "the subject of justice is the 'community'" (p. 70). Justice can be viewed in terms of what rights or resources should be accorded or distributed to persons or populations. However, there is another conception of justice that is communitarian in nature. This approach is based on virtue ethics and emphasizes the virtue of **just generosity**, which is a conception of justice that highlights human connections and not separateness. Indebtedness is the hallmark of this type of justice, and although the concept of justice as a stand-alone virtue is important to public health ethics, the combination of the virtue of justice with the virtue of generosity expands the scope of justice.

People are accustomed to thinking of justice in limited terms, and they are accustomed to separating the individual virtues of justice and generosity. Thinking and acting in terms of the comprehensive virtue of just generosity sometimes requires the use of one's moral imagination to envision "what could be." Whereas justice involves giving others what they are due, generosity involves giving to people from a source that is somehow personal. Fusion of the single virtues of justice and generosity into a combined, activated virtue is important for people in facilitating the development of flourishing communities, both communities as large as the global community and as small as families.

Cultivation of the virtue of just generosity is based on a person's motivation to actively participate in a community-centered network of giving and receiving. Persons, including nurses, who exhibit the virtue of just generosity do not give merely in proportion to what an individual receiver or community is perceived as being due, but instead they give to persons or communities based on the receivers' or communities' needs. The giver believes in and does more than dispassionately allocate or distribute resources. The person or group that exhibits just generosity gives from resources that in some way touch the giver(s) personally, which may not necessarily involve the giving of something that is material or tangible but often involves what might be called giving from the heart.

Salamon (2003), in her book, *Rambam's Ladder*, adapted the Jewish physician and philosopher Maimonides's (1135–1204) "ladder of charity" for contemporary use. Salamon's book provides a meditation on generosity and underscores that an awareness of the need for giving has become more important than ever in a post-9/11 world. Salamon's ladder of charity starts, as did Maimonides's ladder, with the bottom rung representing the least generous motivation for giving and progresses upward, with the top step being what Salamon proposed to be the highest form of giving. The eight steps of the ladder are as follows, beginning with the lowest:

1. Reluctance: To give begrudgingly.
2. Proportion: To give less to the poor than is proper, but to do so cheerfully.
3. Solicitation: To hand money to the poor after being asked.
4. Shame: To hand money to the poor before being asked, but risk making the recipient feel shame.
5. Boundaries: To give to someone you don't know, but allow your name to be known.
6. Corruption: To give to someone you know, but who doesn't know from whom he is receiving help. (For example, this occurs when people are concerned that the "middlemen" distributing the gifts are not trustworthy.)
7. Anonymity: To give to someone you don't know, and to do so anonymously.
8. Responsibility: At the top of the ladder is the gift of self-reliance. To hand someone a gift or a loan or to enter into a partnership with him or to find work for him so that he will never have to beg again. (Salamon, 2003, Introduction)

Public health nurses can use the ladder of charity as a gauge of the type of giving that occurs within communities while keeping their eyes focused on aiming for the top step of the ladder. Public health nurses usually do not directly give money or material resources to people; nurses' services to individuals, families, communities, and populations can be substituted for monetary or material giving in the steps of the ladder. Salamon (2003) herself recognized that monetary giving is not always the primary means of generosity. However, depending on their particular jobs, PH nurses sometimes are responsible for coordinating and distributing gifts and donations to populations.

Nurses might ask themselves whether they give begrudgingly during their work. Do they work from the motivation of a generous servant, hoping to affect the well-being of a population or community who will not know how the nurse's services have positively affected them and their health? Must individual and community recipients of the services of PH nurses directly ask for each of their specific needs to be met? Do nurses use their moral imagination and anticipate needs, reflecting and acting based on the "big picture" of "what could be" that may not be readily apparent to them unless they suspend their initial judgments? When the practice of just generosity is consistent with the top step of Maimonides's ladder, PH nurses enter into community partnerships and teach other people to be responsible for helping themselves and their communities, so that community members and, ultimately, whole communities, become self-reliant whenever possible.

Communicable Diseases

Public health advances in the 20th century dramatically decreased morbidity and mortality from infectious diseases in the United States; because of this progress, national health officials began to lose interest in funding and promoting research directed at infectious disease treatment and control (CDC, 2003). However, people in the government, healthcare systems, and the general public now realize that humanity's fight against infectious diseases is never ending (Markel, 2004). In her book about the global collapse of the public healthcare system, Garrett (2000) stated "we now live in comfortable ignorance about the health and well-being of people in faraway places. But in truth we are never very far away from the experiences of our forebears" (p. xii).

Societies are still tormented by diseases that have affected the public's health since ancient times, while the threat of new infections looms ominously in the future. "Together, malaria, tuberculosis and AIDS killed 5.7 million people in 2004, accounting for about one-tenth of the world's deaths" (World Health Organization [WHO], 2011b, para. 1). Some people in the United States try to avert their eyes from the global scourge of malaria, tuberculosis (TB), and AIDS, but due to media coverage of communicable disease threats such as pandemic influenza, it has become apparent that no one in the United States or elsewhere should feel safe from mass casualties involving infectious diseases. Public health nurses will be at the epicenter of the healthcare system if a highly contagious pandemic occurs, and they also must take a prominent role in current epidemics such as malaria, TB, and AIDS. The words of the poet John Donne (1962) provide a good representation of how infectious diseases that affect the global community are related to ethics in nursing:

> No man is an island, entire of itself; every man is a piece of the continent, a part of the main. If a clod be washed away by the sea, Europe is the less, as well as if a promontory were, as well as if a manor of thy friend's or of thine own were. Any man's death diminishes me, because I am involved in mankind; and therefore never send to know for whom the bell tolls; it tolls for thee. (p. 1107)

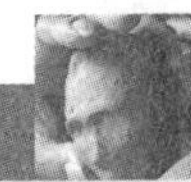

www Ethical Reflections

- Is being aware of the state of health care and epidemic diseases in poor countries a moral issue? Why or why not?
- Do you believe that there are enough resources to treat diseases in populations severely affected by health disparities? Explain.
- What can nurses do to become more aware of people's access to health care and how healthcare resources are distributed in poor countries? What can nurses do to try to improve healthcare access for people in poor countries that are far from the nurses' own home?

Paul Farmer (2001), a physician at Harvard Medical School who travels to central Haiti to work at the Clinique Bone Sauveur, advocated "we can no longer accept whatever we are told about 'limited resources'" (p. xxvi). Healthcare professionals must challenge the often-repeated line that resources are too limited to fund programs to treat epidemics. According to Farmer, "the wealth of the world has not dried up; it has simply become unavailable to those who need it most" (p. xxvi). He proposed that people must ask to be shown the data that support the truth of statements that there are fewer resources for public health than there were when effective therapies were not available to treat many diseases. "Our challenge, therefore, is not merely to draw attention to the widening outcome gap, but also to attack it, to dissect it, and to work with all our capacity to reduce this gap" (p. xxvi). Healthcare professionals and the public must make it clearly known that they are not willing to idly watch when the wealth of nations is being concentrated on limited populations and programs while, on a mass scale, people in other populations die of treatable diseases.

Malaria

Malaria, which means "bad air," has been a problem for humans for over 4,000 years (CDC, 2010). "In 2008, there were 247 million cases of malaria and nearly one million deaths—mostly among children living in Africa. In Africa a child dies every 45 seconds of malaria, the disease accounts for 20% of all childhood deaths" (WHO, 2010b, para. 2).

However, good news is on the horizon. Because of an enormous amount of money and collaborative efforts targeted toward malaria control programs, the burden of malaria is beginning to decrease (WHO, 2010c). From 2008 to 2010, more than 578 million people in sub-Saharan Africa were protected from malaria through the use of insecticide-treated mosquito nets. In 2009, 10% of the at-risk population (75 million people) was protected from malaria by having the inside of their homes sprayed with insecticide. "In Africa, a total of 11 countries showed a greater than 50% reduction in either confirmed malaria cases or malaria admissions and deaths over the past decade" (WHO, 2010c, para. 2); even with the good news, however, WHO officials warn the world community not to be complacent with the fight to eliminate malaria:

> While progress in reducing the burden of malaria has been remarkable, resurgences in cases were observed in parts of at least three African countries (Rwanda, Sao Tome and Principe, and Zambia). The reasons for these resurgences are not known with certainty but illustrate the fragility of malaria control and the need to maintain intervention coverage even if numbers of cases have been reduced substantially. (WHO, 2010c, para. 6)

To eliminate malaria, a variety of interdependent investments will be needed (WHO 2010e):

1. **Financial**: accurate costing of malaria control activities and analysis of malaria expenditures so that resources match requirements
2. **Logistics**: ensuring timely procurement of quality-assured commodities and improving supply chain management
3. **Human resources**: developing, sustaining, and supervising a skilled cadre of malaria staff (including vector control specialists) at national, district, and local levels
4. **Regulation**: strengthening quality control of commodities and services in both private and public sectors, including appropriate regulatory policies and enforcement mechanisms
5. **Diagnostics**: guaranteeing universal access to diagnostic confirmation of suspected malaria cases and ensuring quality assurance of malaria diagnostic services to sustain required laboratory skills
6. **Surveillance:** ensuring timely and accurate collection, reporting, and analysis of malaria cases as an integral part of national health management information systems; building response capacity based on malaria surveillance; and conducting routine monitoring of drug and insecticide resistance. (p. 2)

Partnerships among members of the global community who have resources to combat this deadly disease are still needed to help poor populations whose members are suffering and dying needlessly from malaria. It is morally incumbent upon PH nurses to understand the human and economic burden of malaria and to advocate for adequate prevention and treatment of this serious disease.

Tuberculosis

Tuberculosis (TB) primarily occurs among people living in poverty, and it killed 4,700 people per day (1.7 million people) in 2009 (WHO, 2010a). As with malaria, there is some good news in the rollback of TB; leaders in infectious disease control believe that, in 2004, the global incidence of TB hit its peak rate (WHO, 2010d).

Tuberculosis is airborne, and this makes the treatment of TB a major public health concern in terms of infected persons' infringement on the well-being of noninfected persons. Nonadherence to prescribed TB therapy is believed to occur in about one-third of the population with TB. The reasons that patients fail to follow their treatment regime usually relate to the social and psychological factors that led to their infection in the first place (Beauchamp & Childress, 2009). Unfortunately, healthcare professionals have no convenient and reliable way to know who will and who will not adhere to their TB treatment plan. People infected with TB who are unable or do not choose to adhere to recommended treatment present a moral problem. Freedom and autonomy should, of course, be supported whenever possible; however, when persons infected with active TB do not voluntarily adhere to treatment, it is ethically and legally obligatory to mandate treatment because of health threats to others. This means that one person's privacy and autonomy may be breached in deference to protecting the welfare of other people. The least restrictive means should be used to gain a TB-infected person's cooperation with treatment, but detention and quarantine are legal and ethical, if needed, to protect the public's safety (Beauchamp & Childress, 2009). This is a classic example of utilitarianism.

www Ethical Reflections

- Do you believe that the global burden of malaria is a moral issue? Defend your answer. On which ethical approach have you based your position? Explain.
- The use of DDT to prevent malaria has been controversial. Go to the Internet and locate evidence that supports and evidence that contradicts the benefits of using DDT. What is your position about this issue? If the precautionary principle is used in relation to the use of DDT, do you believe that it is ethical to use DDT to prevent the spread of malaria? Why or why not?

Directly observed therapy (DOT), in which persons are watched while taking their TB medications, is one means of ensuring that affected individuals adhere to their treatment regimen. The international community has responded to the problem of the spread of TB with coordinated efforts to control it through DOT. Beauchamp and Childress (2009) presented typical arguments for and against using DOT as a routine practice in the majority of active TB cases. Since most patients with active TB adhere to their treatment plan, critics of using DOT with all patients say that to do so would be "wasteful, inefficient, and gratuitously annoying" (p. 301). Using DOT with patients who adhere to their therapy also is not the least restrictive means of treating patients. On the other hand, advocates of the widespread use of DOT contend that not using DOT risks the escalation of the number of TB cases and costs, especially in regard to drug resistant forms of the disease.

The least problematic way to address the global burden of TB is to develop public policies to address the underlying causes of TB and patient nonadherence with treatment. Priority should be given to policies that protect a person's privacy and autonomy. The ethical issue that looms large when considering adherence or compliance with treatment is that "how a society ensures compliance often reflects its attitudes toward its vulnerable members" (Beauchamp & Childress, 2009, p. 301). Coercive approaches should be balanced with policies sensitive to the needs of persons with TB.

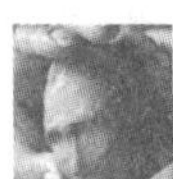

Ethical Reflections www

- Search the Internet and review the case of the American attorney, Andrew Speaker, who was infected with TB.
- List and discuss the ethical issues involved with Mr. Speaker's case.
- What ethical theories or approaches can be applied to the case? Explain. Consider different perspectives.
- What is your position about the ethics surrounding the case? Be sure to provide a clear position and support it. Include one or more ethical approaches as part of your justification.

HIV/AIDS

According to the Joint United Nations Programme on HIV/AIDS (UNAIDS, 2011) report for 2009, 33.3 million people are living with HIV, 2.6 million people were newly infected during 2009, and 1.8 million people died of AIDS-related causes. CDC-supported research published in 2011 revealed that the incidence of HIV cases in the United States essentially is stable, at about 50,000 per year (Prejean et al., 2011). However, there was one population that the researchers identified as having a significant increase in HIV incidence: black men between the ages of 13 and 29 who have sex with men. More than one-half of the new cases in the United States each year were among men who have sex with men. Norton (2010) reported a research study that may provide an explanation for the rise in HIV among young black men: social stigma. Researchers found that young black men generally have negative feelings about homosexuality and believe that it is wrong. "When the researchers looked at the men's reported rates of HIV testing, they found that those who regarded homosexuality as wrong were less likely to have ever been tested: 36 percent, versus 73 percent of those with a more favorable view of homosexuality" (para. 7). This means that even when a black man has sexual relations with another man, because of stigma, he might be more reluctant than members of other populations to be tested for HIV.

HIV Testing

In 2006, the CDC published major revisions to its HIV testing guidelines, and the new recommendations include routine HIV testing for patients in all healthcare settings. Because basic screening for treatable conditions is a common public health secondary prevention tool, it is believed that early identification of HIV infections will lead to better health outcomes. Also, risk-based screening is less effective now because the mix of people becoming infected with HIV is changing to persons who frequently are unaware of their high-risk status—racial and ethnic minorities, people less than 20 years of age, nonmetropolitan-area dwellers, and heterosexuals.

Major revisions in the CDC's (2006) guidelines are contained in Box 11.7. The CDC's position is unchanged in its continued advocacy for voluntary, noncoerced agreement for testing, for no testing without a patient's knowledge, and for access to clinical care and counseling for persons whose tests are positive. However, the

BOX 11.7 ETHICAL FORMATIONS: HIV TESTING GUIDELINES FROM THE CDC

Major revisions from previously published guidelines are as follows:

For patients in all healthcare settings

- HIV screening is recommended for patients in all healthcare settings after the patient is notified that testing will be performed unless the patient declines (opt-out screening).
- Persons at high risk for HIV infection should be screened for HIV at least annually.
- Separate written consent for HIV testing should not be required; general consent for medical care should be considered sufficient to encompass consent for HIV testing.
- Prevention counseling should not be required with HIV diagnostic testing or as part of HIV screening programs in healthcare settings.

For pregnant women

- HIV screening should be included in the routine panel of prenatal screening tests for all pregnant women.
- HIV screening is recommended after the patient is notified that testing will be performed unless the patient declines (opt-out screening).
- Separate written consent for HIV testing should not be required; general consent for medical care should be considered sufficient to encompass consent for HIV testing.
- Repeat screening in the third trimester is recommended in certain jurisdictions with elevated rates of HIV infection among pregnant women.

Source: Centers for Disease Control and Prevention. (2006). Revised recommendations for HIV testing of adults, adolescents, and pregnant women in health-care settings. *Morbidity and Mortality Weekly Report, 55*(RR14), 1–17. Retrieved from http://www.cdc.gov/mmwr/preview/mmwrhtml/rr5514a1.htm

CDC now advocates that screening should be provided in a manner similar to other diagnostic testing without special pretest counseling.

Even when it is voluntary, HIV testing carries with it certain risks and benefits. Since the emergence of HIV, a policy issue that has generated ethical concern is how to protect the public while respecting individual rights and privacy (Beauchamp & Childress, 2001). Psychological well-being and the opportunity to prevent future infection are among the benefits to people whose test results are negative. For people whose test results are positive, benefits include "closer medical follow-up, earlier use of antiretroviral agents, prophylaxis or other treatment of associated diseases, protection of loved ones, and a clearer sense of the future" (p. 298).

Good communication is an important skill for healthcare professionals who coordinate and order HIV testing. The effectiveness of health professionals' communication with patients can have a significant impact on the patients' health outcomes. Galanti (2008) presented one startling example illustrating a problem with "same language, different meaning" (see Box 11.8).

BOX 11.8 ETHICAL FORMATIONS: "SAME LANGUAGE, DIFFERENT MEANING"

Even American English can have different meanings for hearing and deaf people. While Kelly, a young gay male, was a patient in the hospital, blood was drawn for an HIV test. When the results came back, no interpreters for the deaf were available. Because Kelly was adept at reading lips, he was given the test results directly [by a nurse]. He was told that his results were positive, meaning, of course, that he was HIV positive. In deaf culture, however, "positive" means good and "negative" means bad. Kelly was relieved to hear that his test results were "positive": that meant he was *not* HIV positive! He went home and did not return for follow-up.

1. How could this situation have been handled better?
2. What signs might have alerted the nurse to the patient's mistaken interpretation of her message?

Source: Galanti, G.A. (2008). *Caring for patients from different cultures* (4th ed.). Philadelphia, PA: University of Pennsylvania Press, p. 28.

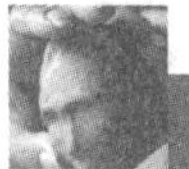

Ethical Reflections

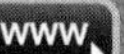

Imagine that you are a nurse participating in a research study with a pharmaceutical company that develops drugs to treat HIV/AIDS. You and your professional colleagues discuss that the experimental drug being researched seems to be causing severe adverse reactions in a few of the patients with AIDS and even may have caused one or two deaths. These findings have not been shared with anyone outside of the research team. The "line" that is delivered by the primary investigator is that AIDS patients already are at a high risk for having a shortened lifespan. He states that although the drug may cause adverse reactions in a few patients, overall he is hoping to achieve "the greatest good for the greatest number of patients." How do you feel about this position? Is it ethical? Why or why not? What would you do if you were helping to conduct this research?

People who are seronegative have no significant risks from testing; however, the psychological and social risks are significant for people who are seropositive (Beauchamp & Childress, 2001). People who are HIV positive are at a high risk psychologically for anxiety, depression, and suicide and are at a high risk socially for "stigmatization, discrimination, and breaches of confidentiality" (Beauchamp & Childress, 2001, p. 299). These common risks sometimes are compounded by a patient's cultural heritage as illustrated with another example from Galanti (2008) (see Box 11.9). It is the ethical responsibility of healthcare professionals to try to minimize the risks to these individuals. Participating in counseling, community education, and social and political activism are ways that PH nurses can play an important role in minimizing the risk of HIV infection among populations served and in minimizing the risk of negative effects on people who undergo HIV testing.

Exceptions to voluntary consent for HIV testing include situations in which there has been significant occupational exposure (e.g., to nurses, emergency medical technicians, or firefighters) and the person whose HIV status is in question refuses testing. Other exceptions are prior to organ transplant donation, when a coroner needs to determine cause of death, and when testing is needed for emergency diagnostic purposes when the patient is unable to consent and a surrogate is not available (Dempski, 2009).

BOX 11.9 ETHICAL FORMATIONS: STIGMA AND HIV

Juan Vega [did not have a] happy outcome when a family member was used to interpret a diagnosis of HIV and a detailed explanation of the disease process and prognosis. The family member left the hospital immediately after interpreting and never returned. Mr. Vega's family, who had been very supportive of him since he had become ill, abandoned him when they were given the details through the family interpreter. After this unfortunate incident, the staff took time to locate a professional interpreter when the patient did not speak English.

1. What might nurses and other healthcare professionals do to help Mr. Vega with his problem?
2. What ethical issues, concepts, and approaches relate to this case? Explain.

Source: Galanti, G.A. (2008). *Caring for patients from different cultures* (4th ed.). Philadelphia, PA: University of Pennsylvania Press, p. 39.

Confidentiality

Confidentiality and the duty to warn were discussed in Chapter 10 and have similar applications in ethical relationships with persons infected with HIV. Persons who know or suspect that they have HIV sometimes avoid testing or treatment because of fears about exposure of lifestyle, including sexual practices or drug use; discrimination and stigmatization; and loss of relationships (Beauchamp & Childress, 2001; Chenneville, 2003). As a general rule, a person's HIV status is confidential information (Dempski, 2009). HIV status may be disclosed when persons or their proxies provide written authorization to do so and when healthcare providers have a need to know, such as workers at a coroner's office or the healthcare staff of a correctional facility.

Statutory laws in each state must be consulted for directions regarding the duty to warn known sexual partners about possible risk of exposure from individuals with HIV. Before a person's HIV status is disclosed to a known partner or partners, attempts should be made to encourage HIV-positive persons to self-disclose to other people who are at risk of infection due to their seropositive status. Newly diagnosed HIV-positive persons need to be informed that health department personnel may contact them to voluntarily discuss partner notification (CDC, 2006). Professionals working at health departments should be available to help patients notify sexual partners and to provide HIV counseling and testing while keeping the patient's name confidential. "In the final analysis, the health professional is expected to weigh the likelihood of harm to other parties against his or her duty to keep confidentiality and act accordingly" (Fry & Veatch, 2006, p. 305). Nurses also should seek legal guidance to help reconcile ethical dilemmas involving a duty to warn and HIV (Dempski, 2009).

Chenneville (2003) proposed a decision-making model that takes into consideration the premises contained within the Tarasoff legal case (see Chapter 10) as well as healthcare ethics that focuses on the best interest of the person who is seropositive. The first step in Chenneville's model is to determine whether disclosure is warranted. Assess the foreseeability of harm and the identifiability of the victim. Questions to consider when determining foreseeability of harm are included in Box 11.10. Chenneville's second step is to refer to professional ethical guidelines, and the final step is to refer to state guidelines (pp. 199–200).

Beauchamp and Childress (2009) presented a decision-making chart that can be helpful in considering when it is justified to breach patients' confidentiality in regard to their HIV-positive status (see Box 11.11). If there is a high probability of harm to another person and the magnitude or seriousness of the harm is great (i.e., category 1), there may be good justification for infringing on a patient's right to confidentiality. When using this chart, the justification lessens as the circumstances of a case move toward a category 4. Although the chart provides guidance, making real-life decisions in practice can be difficult and fraught with uncertainty. It can be problematic to try to fit ethical decisions being made in the swampy low ground (see Chapter 1) into an algorithm. Lo (2009) suggested five criteria similar to the criteria outlined by Beauchamp and Childress (2009) that can be used to decide whether to override a patient's confidentiality (see Box 11.12).

BOX 11.10 ETHICAL FORMATIONS: QUESTIONS TO ASSESS FORESEEABILITY OF HARM

- Does the client use condoms?
- Is the client impulsive? Aggressive? Submissive?
- Does the client use substances (e.g., alcohol) that decrease inhibitions?
- Is the client afraid to disclose HIV status because of fear of rejection, discrimination, and so forth?
- Is the client intentionally trying to harm others?

Source: Chenneville, T. (2003). HIV, confidentiality, and duty to protect: A decision-making model. In D. N. Bersoff (Ed.), *Ethical conflicts in psychology* (3rd ed.) (pp. 198–202). Washington, DC: American Psychological Association, p. 199.

BOX 11.11 ETHICAL FORMATIONS: JUSTIFYING INFRINGEMENTS OF CONFIDENTIALITY

	Magnitude of Harm	
Probability of Harm	*Major*	*Minor*
High	1	2
Low	3	4

Source: Beauchamp, T. L., & Childress, J. F. (2009). *Principles of biomedical ethics* (6th ed.). New York, NY: Oxford University Press, p. 307.

BOX 11.12 ETHICAL FORMATIONS: CRITERIA THAT WARRANT OVERRIDING CONFIDENTIALITY

- The potential harm to third parties is serious
- The likelihood of harm is high
- No alternative for warning or protecting those at risk exists
- Breaching confidentiality will prevent harm
- Harm to the patient is minimized and acceptable

Source: Lo, B. (2009). *Resolving ethical dilemmas: A guide for clinicians* (4th ed.). Philadelphia, PA: Wolters Kluwer, p. 44.

The Duty to Provide Care

In accepting their professional nursing role, nurses make a contract or covenant with the public to provide certain services. There are only a few situations in which nurses ethically are permitted to refuse care to individuals with HIV and these are based on the patient being a danger to the nurse. Each healthcare institution should have policies that nurses can refer to for guidance in determining when concerns about the risks of care are justified in allowing nurses to refuse to provide care to patients infected with HIV. One commonly accepted example or justification for refusal is when a nurse is pregnant. Patients with HIV may have concomitant infections, such as cytomegalovirus, that may put a fetus at risk. When patients with HIV are considered to pose a significant risk to nurses because of the patients' impaired judgment or altered mental status, security should be provided for all healthcare workers who are at risk. Patients should not be denied care based only on their HIV-positive status. In such cases, transfer of patients with HIV to other healthcare providers must be in the patients' best interest (Dempski, 2009).

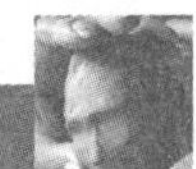

www Ethical Reflections

- Read your state's laws regarding the duty to warn known sexual partners of individuals with HIV. Outline these laws.
- Do you agree or disagree with the ethics of these laws? Explain.
- What are the ethical principles or approaches that are reflected in the laws?
- Your patient is a 30-year-old married man with two young children. In the clinic where you work, he was just diagnosed with HIV. He immediately tells you and the physician that he does not plan to tell his wife about his HIV-positive status. He says that he is afraid that his wife will leave him, that he will lose his friends, and that he may lose his job.
  - What do you do in the above situation?
  - What do you need to know?
  - Who might provide guidance for you and the patient's physician?

Pandemic Influenza

Pandemics of influenza are considered to be rare but consistently recurring events (WHO, 2005). During the 1900s, three influenza pandemics occurred—in 1918, 1957, and 1968. The 1918 pandemic was one of the deadliest disease events that ever occurred, with approximately 40–50 million people dying worldwide during the pandemic. When new influenza viruses emerge and spread rapidly among the global population, the human immune system is not prepared to combat the new infection. The lack of immunity to a new influenza virus can result in many deaths, just as it did in 1918.

Although the pandemic did not become as serious and as deadly as some people feared, the WHO declared a pandemic in 2009 when a novel H1N1 influenza virus surfaced. The U.S. public closely watched the events of the pandemic unfold to see how well the government handled the crisis. After reviewing the events, the United States Government Accountability Office (GAO, 2011) identified key issues related to the government's response to the 2009 H1N1 pandemic. The report indicated that: (1) prior planning and funding to prepare for a potential H5N1 avian influenza threat was beneficial during the H1N1 pandemic; (2) the number of available vaccine doses did not meet the expectations set by the government, and as a result, the government's credibility was hurt; (3) a mandate for a 100-dose minimum vaccine order was problematic; (4) the CDC generally was rated well in terms of communication with the public, but communication fell short with non-English speaking people; and (5) medicines and supplies from the Strategic National Stockpile were sufficient to meet goals but disparities were identified between the materials ordered and received and problems were identified with long-term storage of materials.

One key problem that was expected during the 2009 pandemic, and remains a serious problem with other potential influenza pandemics, involves the time needed to produce a vaccine after a pandemic-type influenza virus first appears. The novel H1N1 virus first was identified in the United States on April 15, 2009, when a 10-year-old patient in California was tested as part of a clinical study (CDC, 2010a). However, the first vaccine for the pandemic was not distributed until October 5, 2009 (Cox, 2011). This means that the public had no vaccine protection from the pandemic virus for about 6 months after the virus first appeared. Healthcare professionals who work directly with people who are ill with the flu also were left without vaccine protection during the period from April to October. Fortunately, the H1N1 pandemic was not particularly deadly; however, during a pandemic with a high case-fatality rate, such as a pandemic caused by the avian H5N1 influenza virus, which as of August 2011 had a case fatality rate of 59% (WHO, 2011a), the lives of healthcare professionals likely would be at risk, especially before a vaccine is available. If the avian H5N1 virus in Asia mutates to the point that it becomes easily transmissible from human-to-human, nurses would have to decide if they are willing to risk their lives and the lives of their families by exposing themselves to patients and coworkers who are ill with the H5N1 virus. According to a Homeland Security Council (2006) report:

> The Federal Government recommends that government entities and the private sector plan with the assumption that up to 40 percent of their staff may be absent for periods of about 2 weeks at the height of a pandemic wave, with lower levels of staff absent for a few weeks on either side of the peak. Absenteeism will increase not only because of personal illness or incapacitation but also because employees may be caring for ill family members, under voluntary home quarantine due to an ill household member, minding children dismissed from school, following public health guidance, or simply staying at home out of safety concerns. (p. 13)

In addition to the problem of not having early access to a reliable vaccine, when the next serious influenza pandemic occurs, healthcare professionals, including PH nurses, will be faced with many other ethical issues and decisions. Among these issues will be a need to make decisions about how to fairly distribute vaccines and antiviral medications and how to fairly decide about restricting personal freedoms (CDC, 2007a). The CDC's (2007a) pandemic influenza document outlines specific guidelines to address ethical considerations in the management of pandemic influenza. The following guidelines are contained within this document:

- Identification of clear overall goals for pandemic influenza (p. 2): Goals are different than in interpandemic years. During a pandemic, the goal is "preserving the functioning of society" (p. 3) rather than protecting people who are at the most serious risk from being harmed by influenza, such as elders and young children.
- A commitment to transparency throughout the pandemic influenza planning and response process (p. 3): Language used in explaining reasons for decisions must be clear, the basis for decisions must be open for review, and the process must reflect a respect for persons and involved communities.
- Public engagement and involvement are essential to build public will and trust and should be evidenced throughout the planning and response process (p. 3): The public is treated as a partner with the influenza experts. Vulnerable and marginalized people need to be included in related processes.
- Public health officials have a responsibility to maximize preparedness in order to minimize the need to make allocation decisions later (p. 3): Examples "include shortening the time for virus recognition or vaccine production, increasing the capacity to produce vaccines or antivirals, and increasing the supplies of antivirals" (pp. 3–4).
- Sound guidelines should be based on the best available scientific evidence (p. 4): Processes and actions should be evidence based whenever possible. However, some processes and action may need to be based on evidence-informed data, which is a bit less rigorous.

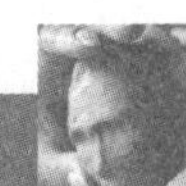

WWW **Ethical Reflections**

- If you were a PH nurse working during a severe flu pandemic before a vaccine is available, would you report to your job at the local health department or stay home with your family? If you were a direct-patient-care hospital nurse working during a severe flu pandemic before a vaccine is available, would you report to your job or stay home with your family? Describe your concerns and issues for consideration in your decision making for both situations. Explain the ethical rationale for your decisions.
- What guidance does the ANA and other professional nursing organizations provide to answer the above questions? Search for information and explain.
- What ethical principles and approaches underlie your decision making in the above situations? Explain your analysis.
- During a nonpandemic year, do you believe that it is ethical and should be legal for administrators of a healthcare organization to mandate that their nurse employees receive the annual influenza vaccine? Support your answer using an ethical basis.

- The pandemic planning process acknowledges the importance of working with and learning from preparedness efforts globally (p. 4): This guideline is not based on merely benefitting U.S. citizens but rather on maximizing the common good of the global community.
- Balancing of individual liberty and community interests (p. 4): During a pandemic, usual individual liberties that are highly valued in our society may need to be suspended. If suspending liberties is necessary, care needs to be taken to use the least restrictive policies, to ensure "that restrictions are necessary and proportional to the need for protection" (p. 5), and to support people who are affected by the restrictions.
- Diversity in ethical decision making (p. 5): Historically, groups of people have been abused "in the name of the public good" (p. 5). During pandemic influenza, a variety of public voices must be included in planning and implementation processes.
- Fair process approach (procedural justice) (p. 5): Procedures must be well designed, transparent, include consistent standards, and be managed by people who are impartial, neutral, and accountable so that they lead to fair outcomes.

See Box 11.13 for a reproduction of the CDC's (2007b) *Planning and Responding to Pandemic Influenza: Ethical Considerations Checklist.*

On July 1, 2011, the CDC published a document outlining ethical guidelines for allocating scarce ventilator resources during a severe pandemic. This document is intended to be a supplement to the 2007 document discussed above that addresses ethical issues surrounding the distribution of scarce resources, especially vaccines and antiviral medications, and the need for social distancing and limitations on personal liberties. Ethical questions arise about how to allocate mechanical ventilators "when there is a substantial extreme mismatch between patient need and available resources" (p. 7). The CDC recommended that the focus should shift "from individual patient-focused clinical care to a population-oriented public health approach intended to provide the best possible outcomes for a large cohort of critical care patients" (p. 7). Once triage is begun in regard to allocating mechanical ventilators, designated individuals must decide how to distribute these scarce resources.

Whereas the recommendations in the CDC's 2007 pandemic influenza document focused on giving priority to people who will keep society functioning during a pandemic, the 2011 document reflects a different philosophy for decision making about allocating scarce mechanical ventilators. People whose jobs are to keep society functioning might be kept on the job longer if they are given an effective influenza vaccine or prophylactic antiviral drugs during a serious pandemic. Both of these interventions are aimed at keeping people healthy. However, people need a mechanical ventilator when they already are infected with a pandemic influenza

BOX 11.13 ETHICAL FORMATIONS: PLANNING AND RESPONDING TO PANDEMIC INFLUENZA: ETHICAL CONSIDERATIONS CHECKLIST

This checklist should be used by public health officials when developing or approving plans that will have a substantive impact on policy, practice, or the public. Not every question may be applicable in every situation, but every question should be considered. The checklist is intended to enhance ethical decision making and is not meant to be used for official reporting or accountability purposes.

General Ethical Considerations

Yes No

- Have clear overall goals for pandemic influenza planning been identified?
- Have the rules that will govern public health decision making during a pandemic been determined and clearly articulated in advance of the need for decision making?
- Have public health response decisions been made in a clear, open, and transparent manner?
- Have those who will be affected by the public health measures been provided with timely information and given the opportunity to provide input into decision making?
- Are decisions being made based on the best available scientific evidence?
- Have the least restrictive public health measures necessary to protect the common good been used?
- Are decisions about protecting the common good being balanced with protecting the rights of individuals?
- Have efforts been made to minimize the negative impacts of the public health measures?
- Have the public health response measures anticipated and respected the diverse values, beliefs, and cultures in the community?
- Has a process been established to revise or correct decisions to address new information?
- Have efforts been made to acknowledge and respond to public suspicion and distrust of local, state, or federal government decisions?
- Have state and local authorities had adequate opportunity to have input into decision making?
- Have efforts been made to work with and learn from global preparedness and response efforts?

Ethical Issues Relating to Data Collection

Yes No

- Is the data collection necessary to respond to the public health emergency?
- Has use of data for non-public-health response purposes (such as research) been justified based on the scientific need for the information?
- Have measures been taken to protect the privacy and security of the data?
- If collecting information from people, has the need for the data collection been explained and consent obtained?
- If data collection involves research, has appropriate approval by an appropriate Institutional Review Board been obtained?

(*continues*)

BOX 11.13 ETHICAL FORMATIONS: PLANNING AND RESPONDING TO PANDEMIC INFLUENZA: ETHICAL CONSIDERATIONS CHECKLIST (continued)

Ethical Issues Relating to Liberty-Limiting Measures

Yes No

- Are the proposed liberty-limiting measures considered voluntary?
- Has the imposition of quarantine or other liberty-limiting measures been balanced with protection of individual rights?
- Have steps been taken to protect affected individuals' privacy?
- Have steps been taken to protect affected individuals against stigmatization or long-term psychological impact?
- Have steps been taken to minimize an unequal burden being placed on specific individuals or groups?
- Have restrictions on personal freedom been equitably applied?
- Has the justification behind the liberty-limiting measures been fully articulated in language appropriate for the intended audience?
- Is there clear scientific evidence of person-to-person spread of disease that would indicate the need for liberty-limiting measures?
- Is the liberty-limiting measure being proposed the least restrictive measure?
- Is the liberty-limiting measure proportional to the goal of achieving disease control?
- Have steps been taken to provide necessary support services for those affected by the liberty-limiting measure?
- Have measures been put in place to ensure that persons under quarantine or isolation are not placed at increased risk?
- Have plans been developed to monitor the onset of symptoms among those who are quarantined?
- Has an appeals process for those affected by the liberty-limiting measures been established?

Ethical Issues Relating to Allocation of Scarce Resources

Yes No

- Have relevant stakeholders been engaged in determining what criteria should be used to make resource allocation decisions?
- Have decisions about allocation of resources been made using a fair and equitable process?
- Has the reasoning behind allocation choices been fully articulated in language appropriate for the intended audience?
- Have the values and principles justifying these decisions been identified and made available for examination?
- Do the allocation plans specify what goods are involved, who will make decisions about prioritization and distribution, who will be eligible to receive the scarce resources, and what relevant criteria will be used to prioritize who will and will not receive resources?

Source: This checklist is based on the document *Ethical Guidelines in Pandemic Influenza*, developed by the Ethics Subcommittee of the Advisory Committee to the Director, Centers for Disease Control and Prevention. Retrieved fromhttp://www.cdc.gov/od/science/phethics/panFlu_Ethic_Guidelines.pdf

virus. This means that these persons already would be "off the job." It is a key assumption of experts that a serious pandemic would occur in waves, separated by weeks or months with no significant influenza disease. It is unlikely that a person with influenza who needs ventilator support would be able to recover sufficiently to go back to work within any one wave of the pandemic. Therefore, there is no justifiable reason to give these persons priority merely based on their role in keeping society functioning. Priorities need to be organized around giving ventilator resources to the people "who are *most likely to recover* after receiving them" (p. 9). It is worth noting that an available and effective vaccine currently is not expected until the second influenza wave.

So, is there a clear answer about how to ethically distribute mechanical ventilators during a severe pandemic? The CDC staff who developed the 2011 document said "no." As indicated in the document, at best the CDC has offered only "a conceptual framework to assist the planning process" (p. 3). The scope of the document is too big to adequately be covered in this chapter, but Box 11.14 provides an overview of some of the principles that were discussed as possibilities for guiding ventilator allocation.

Other issues and questions that need to be considered when addressing mechanical ventilator allocation during a severe influenza pandemic include (CDC, 2011):

- Who should make decisions about distributing resources?
- Should uniform criteria across geographic areas be used or should local flexibility be the norm?
- How can public health workers engage local communities in decision making and the triage process?
- Who clarifies the roles of healthcare professionals during public health emergencies? How will nurses and physicians be protected from tort liability from actions that they took during an emergency?
- If, based on their work, healthcare professionals become severely ill from the flu, should they be given priority for ventilator resources because they faced additional risks by helping patients?
- What are the special needs of children?
- How will decisions be made to remove patients from a ventilator?

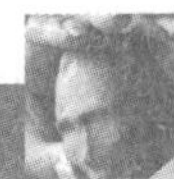

www Ethical Reflections

- The people who developed the CDC document about ethical guidelines during an influenza pandemic proposed that preserving the functioning of society needs to be prioritized above protecting people who are most at risk for developing the flu. If this guideline was used, who do you believe would be highly prioritized to receive a flu vaccine when it is available? Do you believe that this guideline is ethical? Why or why not?
- Discuss specific procedures that would be consistent with a "fair process approach" (procedural justice).
- Who (individuals or agencies) should decide about the priorities of distributing scarce resources during an influenza pandemic?
- How might governments act in unethical ways during a flu pandemic?
- When are limitations on personal autonomy ethically justified during an influenza pandemic?
- How could a PH nurse act as a community advocate during an influenza pandemic?

BOX 11.14 ETHICAL FORMATIONS: CONSIDERATIONS FOR ALLOCATING VENTILATOR SUPPORT DURING A MAJOR INFLUENZA PANDEMIC

- Respect for persons and their autonomy: "During a severe influenza pandemic, public health mandates may override patient autonomy. Patients still must be treated with dignity and compassion" (p. 10).
- Beneficence: Providers must balance obligations for doing good for individual patients while acting according to the good of a whole population. Individual patients need to receive palliative care, when appropriate, and should not be abandoned.
- Justice: Distribution of resources should be fair and "should not exacerbate existing disparities in health outcomes" (p. 10). Procedural justice is required.
- Maximizing net benefits: Maximizing "the number of people who survive to hospital discharge" (p. 12). This consideration can be broken down further into maximizing the number of lives saved, maximizing years of life saved, or maximizing adjusted years of life saved. The authors of the CDC document contended "that ethically, allocating scarce resources during a severe pandemic by only considering chances of survival to hospital discharge is insufficient because it omits other important ethical considerations" (p. 14).
- Social worth: There are two primary ways to approach a social worth criterion: broad social value and instrumental value or the multiplier effect. The determination when considering broad social value is "whether an individual's past and future contributions to society's goals merit prioritization for scarce resources" (p. 14). "Instrumental value refers to an individual's ability to carry out a specific function that is viewed as essential to prevent social disintegration or a great number of deaths" (p. 14). Proponents believe that using instrumental value as a criterion for allocating resources is ethical because it achieves a "multiplier effect." That is, if key people in a society are protected or saved, they will in turn save more lives through their work. This is the criterion recommended by the CDC for allocating vaccine doses and antiviral medications during a serious influenza pandemic. However, as mentioned previously, it is believed that using this criterion will not provide much benefit when deciding about allocating mechanical ventilators.
- The life cycle principle: Using this principle means that younger people are given priority over old people. It is debatable whether using this principle is discriminatory or egalitarian.
- Fair chances versus maximization of best outcomes: This criterion supports giving ventilators to people with the best chance of survival over people who have a lower probability "but still [have] significant chance of survival" (p. 16).
- A composite priority score: Combining several principles into an allocation system that can be used to compute a score to assign priority.

Source: Centers for Disease Control and Prevention, Ethics Subcommittee of the Advisory Committee to the Director, Ventilator Document Workgroup. (2011). *Ethical considerations for decision making regarding allocation of mechanical ventilators during a severe influenza pandemic or other public health emergency.* Retrieved from http://www.cdc.gov/od/science/integrity/phethics/docs/Vent_Document_Final_Version.pdf

As per the CDC's (2011) ethics document, the roles of clinical care and triage should be separated. It was emphasized that guidelines and procedures should be in place prior to an emergency situation. A triage expert should be identified who has senior status at the institution where he or she will make decisions. The expert should be someone who is respected by the staff, has relevant clinical experience, and has the authority to carry out his or her decisions. A team of at least three members should be assembled to help the triage expert. The CDC committee that authored the document proposed, "the presumption should be to follow uniform guidelines in the interest of fairness, consistency, and coordination of efforts" (p. 18). However, there should be enough flexibility for local changes that meet the needs of any one institution or community. Communities are more likely to be engaged in the process when messages are consistent, when marginalized and vulnerable groups receive special attention, and when spokespeople are chosen who are best heard by the target community.

Depending on the characteristics of the pandemic influenza strain, children may have a high susceptibility to the virus and a greater need for ventilation resources. Since all ventilator equipment that is suitable for adults is not suitable for children, and since professionals who normally care for adults may not be comfortable caring for children, prepandemic activity is very important to assess and secure resources for children (CDC, 2011).

Decisions surrounding palliative care and withdrawing mechanical ventilator support from patients are likely to present significant ethical distress for physicians and nurses during a severe influenza pandemic. Decision-making procedures should be established prior to being needed in order to ensure that decisions to remove patients from ventilators are ethical. Respectful and compassionate palliative care should be provided to patients with respiratory failure who do not receive mechanical ventilation or who have ventilator support withdrawn based on an allocation system. During a crisis situation involving a scarcity of ventilators (demand exceeding supply), elective surgeries usually are delayed and patients whose condition is improving are weaned from ventilators. However, these strategies may not be enough. According to the CDC (2011), it may become necessary to remove patients from ventilators without obtaining consent. The following information is taken directly from the CDC's document regarding ethical care involving ventilator support during a pandemic:

> To achieve the public health goal of minimizing the number of preventable deaths during a severe pandemic emergency, states and hospitals need to address the issue of removing from ventilators patients with respiratory failure whose prognosis has significantly worsened in order to provide access to patients with a better prognosis. . . . Policies for withdrawal of patients from ventilators need to be the least restrictive possible—i.e., withdrawing of ventilation without requiring assent of patient or surrogate continues only as long as the shortage of ICU resources continues. . . . Patients

who are removed from mechanical ventilation and their families or surrogates, like patients with respiratory failure who are not placed on mechanical ventilation, should be notified this will occur, given a chance to say good-byes and complete religious rituals, and provided compassionate palliative care. (p. 21)

Terrorism and Disasters

The great lesson of September 11 is that we are all connected. Either we are all safe or none of us is safe. Either we are all free of fear or none of us is.

—*M. Pipher, 2002,* The Middle of Everywhere, *p. xiii*

The terrorist attacks on September 11, 2001, and the anthrax-laced letters that followed this event, highlighted the possible dangers of terrorist-related infectious diseases invading society (Farmer, 2001). Farmer proposed that

> investing in robust public health infrastructures, and in global health equity in general, remains our best means of being prepared for—and perhaps even preventing—bioterrorism. Indeed, this was the refrain of several of our best public health leaders during the taxing investigations of these [anthrax] attacks. (p. xi)

Ethics-related guidance for PH nurses during any type of terrorism attack or before, during, or after natural or human-made disasters can be referred back to a variety of ethical approaches, such as social justice (fair distribution of resources), communitarian ethics (acting to facilitate the common good for communities), utilitarianism (considering actions that produce the greatest good for the greatest number of people), virtue ethics (having good character and being concerned about the common good), deontology (acting according to one's duty), and ethical principlism (applying rule-based principles, such as respect for autonomy, beneficence, nonmaleficence, and justice). During disasters, public health professionals must make critical decisions about how to triage scarce resources and everyday personal rights—health care, including first aid; food and water; medications and immunizations; warmth and housing; protection from harmful environmental elements; and the individual freedom to travel and mingle with other people. Because of the major impact that public health actions can have on human suffering and well-being, the decisions made by public health professionals during disasters are inherently ethical in nature.

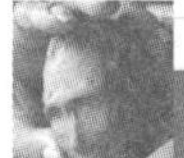

Ethical Reflections

- How does the allocation of scarce healthcare resources differ when distributing vaccines and antiviral medications and when allocating ventilator resources during a severe influenza pandemic?
- Do you believe that the allocation positions included in the two CDC documents discussed in this section of the chapter are ethical? Support your position.
- How are the principles of respect for autonomy, beneficence, nonmaleficence, and justice relevant to the ethical distribution of resources during a severe influenza pandemic?
- What ethical approaches might help healthcare professionals manage moral distress during a severe pandemic? Explain.

Generally, in terrorism and natural disasters, military triage is used rather than traditional medical or emergency room triage. Usual emergency room triage rules are focused on prioritizing patients who are the sickest or most gravely injured, even those whose lives may not be salvageable. In military triage, medical need is considered, but decisions are balanced with consideration of the principle of social utility (Campbell, Hart, & Norton, 2007). When managing emergency care in the battlefield, priority is given to soldiers who can quickly be returned to the battlefield to continue the fight. This approach to triage provides a social benefit to the whole population of soldiers in a given area. Ultimately, resources are allocated to provide the greatest benefit to the greatest number of people.

Another important element in ethics and public health care during disaster situations is trust. Members of society expect healthcare professionals, especially public health professionals, to be trustworthy, as well as competent, while carrying out their roles during disasters. "Public health agencies [and public health professionals] cannot function well in the absence of public trust" (Public Health Leadership Society, 2004, p. 4). People should be able to trust public health professionals to act according to the public's best interest during a disaster. Actions to achieve the common good and good outcomes for the whole community must be balanced with actions directed at caring for the needs of individuals. Each community member has a personal story and each person's life narrative is important. Equanimity—evenness of temperament—is a good virtue for nurses to have during a disaster. Thich Nhat Hanh's story about Vietnamese boat people from Chapter 8 also is very relevant to ethical nursing care during disasters (see Box 8.6).

Although standards of nursing practice may need to be altered during a disaster situation, a nurse's ethics should not be compromised during a disaster. At the point of a disaster is not the time for nurses to begin pondering and sorting out their ethical philosophies. The 5 R's Approach to ethical nursing practice (see Chapter 2) provides a preevent guide for nurses to prepare to act ethically under any sudden and stressful situation, including situations such as those that occur before, during, and after disasters.

www Ethical Reflections

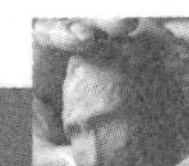

- Nurses are likely to be presented with ethical dilemmas during disaster situations. Review the definition of an ethical dilemma in Chapter 2. Should nurses expect to receive or know clear and certain answers to questions arising from ethically laden situations during a disaster? Why or why not?
- What can nurses do to best prepare themselves to navigate ethical dilemmas before, during, and after disaster situations? Explain.
- Consider a natural disaster situation such as the one that occurred after Hurricane Katrina. Identify specific situations in which nurses may have to make ethical decisions when providing disaster care to a community. Include opportunities that are obvious as well as indistinct opportunities. What process would you use to answer the associated ethical questions?
- Do you believe that public health nurses and acute care nurses face similar or different ethical dilemmas during a disaster? Explain and provide examples.

Genomics

In 2003, the Institute of Medicine (as cited in ANA, 2007) outlined eight new domains of public health practice. In addition to the content area of ethics, another of the eight domains is genomics. The Human Genome Project (HGP) spanned 13 years and was a joint project overseen by the U.S. Department of Energy (DOE) and the National Institutes of Health (U.S. DOE Office of Science, 2006b). The project was completed in 2003, but a full analysis of the data obtained will require many years of work. The goals of the HGP were to:

- Identify all the approximately 20,000–25,000 genes in human DNA
- Determine the sequences of the 3 billion chemical base pairs that make up human DNA
- Store this information in databases
- Improve tools for data analysis
- Transfer related technologies to the private sector
- Address the ethical, legal, and social issues that may arise from the project (para. 2)

Three to five percent of the HGP budget was allocated to studying ethical, legal, and social issues (ELSI) (U.S. DOE Office of Science, 2006a). Some of the ELSI identified include the fair use of information obtained from genetic testing; the maintenance of informational privacy and confidentiality; stigmatization due to genetic differences among people; a number of reproductive issues, such as the impact of genetic information on reproductive decision making and reproductive rights; clinical issues, such as education and implementation of quality standards; uncertainty in regard to gene testing when multiple genes or gene–environment interactions are involved; considerations of whether behaviors occur according to free will or are determined according to genetic makeup; the safe use of genetically modified foods and microbes; and how property rights should be handled in regard to the commercialization of products. The HGP has opened up a wide array of issues about which all health professionals, including PH nurses, will continually need to become more familiar. However, many people in society still are not sure if the HGP has opened a Pandora's box. Box 11.15 contains some of the questions directly cited from the ELSI study. See Box 11.16 for stories about ethical dilemmas in genetics.

Public Health Nursing: Contributing to Building the World

Because PH nursing is population focused, PH nurses often have opportunities to improve the welfare of many people. Public health nurses work with members of populations as equal partners and they collaborate with a variety of people to promote and protect the public's health (ANA, 2007). Participating in service learning experiences and adopting a philosophy of servant leadership are two ways to ground nursing practice in the principles of PHN.

BOX 11.15 ETHICAL FORMATIONS: QUESTIONS GENERATED BY THE ELSI STUDY

Gather reliable data and generate informed positions that answer the following questions. Engage in a debate with your colleagues about differing positions and provide examples.

Societal Concerns Arising from the New Genetics

Fairness in the use of genetic information by insurers, employers, courts, schools, adoption agencies, and the military, among others.
Who should have access to personal genetic information, and how will it be used?

Privacy and confidentiality of genetic information.
Who owns and controls genetic information?

Psychological impact and stigmatization due to an individual's genetic differences.
How does personal genetic information affect an individual and society's perceptions of that individual? How does genomic information affect members of minority communities?

Reproductive issues including adequate informed consent for complex and potentially controversial procedures, use of genetic information in reproductive decision making, and reproductive rights.
Do healthcare personnel properly counsel parents about the risks and limitations of genetic technology? How reliable and useful is fetal genetic testing? What are the larger societal issues raised by new reproductive technologies?

Clinical issues including the education of doctors and other health service providers, patients, and the general public in genetic capabilities, scientific limitations, and social risks, and implementation of standards and quality-control measures in testing procedures.
How will genetic tests be evaluated and regulated for accuracy, reliability, and utility? (Currently, there is little regulation at the federal level.) How do we prepare healthcare professionals for the new genetics? How do we prepare the public to make informed choices? How do we as a society balance current scientific limitations and social risk with long-term benefits?

Uncertainties associated with gene tests for susceptibilities and complex conditions (e.g., heart disease) linked to multiple genes and gene–environment interactions.
Should testing be performed when no treatment is available? Should parents have the right to have their minor children tested for adult-onset diseases? Are genetic tests reliable and interpretable by the medical community?

Conceptual and philosophical implications regarding human responsibility, free will versus genetic determinism, and concepts of health and disease.
Do people's genes make them behave in a particular way? Can people always control their behavior? What is considered acceptable diversity? Where is the line between medical treatment and enhancement?

BOX 11.16 ETHICAL FORMATIONS: ETHICS AND GENETICS

Genetic research raises ethical and moral questions that the public, researchers, and policymakers must consider. [These] are stories about some of the ethical dilemmas that people are now facing every day. As you read each story, think about your reaction.

Prenatal Testing

A couple has one child with a severe genetic disease. They are thinking of having a second child. The doctor tells them that it has recently become possible to test an unborn child for this disease.

- Would you want to know?
- If you wanted advice, with whom would you talk?
- Should insurance companies or the government require you to have an unborn child tested to reduce healthcare costs?
- Who should have access to the results of the test, if you do get tested?

Adult Testing

Your family has a history of Huntington's disease, a genetic disease that causes a long and painful decline. Because a person doesn't develop any symptoms of Huntington's Disease until adulthood, you are uncertain if you have inherited the disease. A reliable genetic test for Huntington's disease is available, but there is no effective cure or treatment for the disease.

- Would you want to be tested? Should you be required to be tested?
- If you have the genetic mutation that causes the disease, will you choose to have children?
- To whom would you tell the results of your test? How would your family and friends react?

Discrimination

You have just received the results of a genetic test for the presence of a breast cancer mutation and discovered that you have the mutation. Now you fear the possibility of disease—and discrimination.

- Who should have access to this information? Your family, your insurance company, your employer?
- The U.S. Equal Employment Opportunity Commission finds that people carrying abnormal genes are protected from job discrimination under the Americans with Disabilities Act. Still, will your employer try to fire you?
- Will your insurance company drop you? As genetic testing becomes more sophisticated, every person likely will be found to carry genes that could predispose him/her to disease. Should potential genetic diseases be considered "preexisting conditions"?
- If a genetic disease is known to be common among a certain ethnic group, should this information be used to justify job or insurance discrimination?
- Will the possibility of disease motivate you to take better care of yourself? How can your environment affect your susceptibility to disease?

(*continues*)

BOX 11.16 ETHICAL FORMATIONS: ETHICS AND GENETICS (continued)

Designing Your Children

Our increasing ability to manipulate genes raises the promise of treating or curing genetic diseases. These same tools could be used to enhance other traits such as height, weight, and intelligence.

- If you could design your "perfect" baby, would you?
- In the next several decades, will our concept of "normal" become more narrow?
- Will we see baldness, freckles, and shyness as "genetic diseases" to be cured?

Gene Therapy

Although the effectiveness of gene therapy has yet to be proven, some people imagine a time when many diseases will be treated this way.

- Who will have access to gene therapy? Will we create a genetic underclass of people who cannot afford it? Or will universal access give all people equal potential to live longer and more productive lives?
- Is gene therapy different from drug treatments, surgery, or organ transplants?
- Who should set national ethical standards for gene therapy? Politicians, insurance companies, physicians, the public?

Source: Stetten, D. (n.d.). *A revolution in genetics: Human genetics and medical research: Ethics and genetics.* Retrieved from http://history.nih.gov/exhibits/genetics/sect6f.htm

Service Learning

Service learning is "academic experiences in which students engage both in social action and in reflection on their experiences in performing that action" (Piliavin, 2003, p. 235). Service learning is ideally suited for supporting the moral development of PH nursing students. Kaye (2004) defined service learning as "a teaching method where guided or classroom learning is deepened through service to others in a process that provides structured time for reflection on the service experience and demonstration of the skills and knowledge acquired" (p. 7). Service learning is a means for students and teachers to work with community leaders and agencies in collaboratively identifying and working toward a common good. All participants, including teachers, agency administrators, and staff, learn from the students during their interactions with them while the students benefit from developing increased community awareness. In service learning, "community develops and builds through interaction, reciprocal relationships, and knowledge of people, places, organizations, governments, and systems" (Kaye, 2004, p. 8).

Service usually is focused on direct or indirect services, advocacy, or research (Kaye, 2004). In direct services, person-to-person interactions occur between students and the recipients of the students' work. Direct services may be aimed at students developing a broader awareness of the needs and issues of varying cultures, populations, or age groups while providing a needed service to a population—for example, providing a service to people with AIDS who are living at a specific AIDS hospice, to people who are staying at a particular homeless shelter, or to elderly persons who attend a specific day care center. A whole community or the environment is the focus of indirect service learning interventions, such as activities aimed at helping to organize and implement a community-wide health education program about safe sex or organizing an effort to decrease pollution of a local waterway. Advocacy—which is a key role of PH nursing—combined with service learning involves creating and supporting change in communities to benefit people in the community. Advocacy includes grassroots societal and political activism, such as working to educate a city council about the unmet needs of people with AIDS in the city. Service learning provides an excellent opportunity for students to become involved in community research. Students can participate in developing and conducting surveys and gathering, analyzing, and reporting data regarding issues of public health concern.

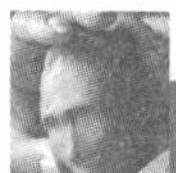

Ethical Reflections

- Conduct a literature review about service learning in nursing. Develop suggestions for service learning experiences that focus on each of the following: direct services, indirect services, advocacy, and research.
- Explain why service learning is related to ethics in PH nursing.

Students' reflections on service learning experiences are an integral and defining part of service learning. It is in this area that the students' moral imaginations and the development of intelligent habits are cultivated. Reflection helps service learners to consider the "big picture" in working for the good of communities. Reflective experiences can be guided through activities such as journal writing or teacher-led group discussions and processing of experiences. Service learners may benefit from thinking in terms of the intersecting human narratives that exist among themselves, their community collaborators, and the recipients of their services.

Servant Leadership

In the late 1960s and early 1970s, Robert Greenleaf (2002) was one of several businesspeople who developed and articulated the concept of servant leadership in management. Greenleaf developed the idea of servant leadership after reading the book *The Journey to the East,* written by Herman Hesse (1956). Hesse's book relates a story about a servant named Leo who is on a journey to the East with a group of men, members of a mysterious league, who are on a mission to find spiritual renewal. Leo brings the group together as a community with his spirit and songs. When Leo decides to leave the group, the small community becomes dysfunctional and disbands. Later, one of the journeymen discovers that, unknown to the journeymen, Leo was really the head of the league that had sponsored their original journey.

Leo was a noble leader who had chosen the role of a servant, a servant whose leadership was of the utmost importance to the sense of community of the journeying group. Greenleaf (2002) proposed that Hesse's story clearly exemplifies a servant leader through the portrayal of Leo. He suggested "the great leader is seen as servant first, and that simple fact is the key to his [or her] greatness" (p. 21). In the story, even while Leo was directly in the role of the leader of his league, he viewed himself first and foremost as a servant (see Box 11.17).

Servant leaders see themselves first as servants, and at some later point in time make the choice to lead while serving. People who are more concerned with leading before serving often are motivated by a desire for power or to obtain material possessions, although a strong concurrent secondary motivation to serve is possible. Greenleaf (2002) explained how to distinguish between a servant-first leader and a leader who views service as a secondary or lower priority:

> The difference manifests itself in the care taken by the servant-first [leader] to make sure that other people's highest priority needs are being served. The best test, and difficult to administer, is this: Do those served grow as persons? Do they, while being served, become healthier, wiser, freer, more autonomous, more likely themselves to become servants? And, what is the effect on the least privileged in society? Will they benefit or at least not be further deprived? (p. 27)

When thinking about servant leadership, it is important to note that the role of the servant follower is as important as that of the servant leader. If there are no servant followers, or seekers, great leaders are not recognized because there is no one with the awareness to recognize them. "If one is servant, leader or follower, one is always searching, listening, expecting that a better wheel for these times is in the making" (Greenleaf, 2002, p. 24).

Covey (2002) defined servant leadership as being consistent with moral authority and proposed that servant leaders and servant followers are, in reality,

BOX 11.17 ETHICAL FORMATIONS: THE NATURE OF SERVICE

During a Midwestern storm of rain, hail, lightning, and thunder, my mother stopped at the grocery store and asked me to run in for a loaf of bread. As I prepared to get out of the car, I noticed little Janie running down the street. She wore her usual tattered clothes, and her bald head, the result of some condition unknown to me, was unprotected from the hail. Many of our schoolmates teased her, judging her as inferior because of her poverty and appearance. I jumped out of the car and gave her my raincoat. She put it over her head and continued running. I remember thinking, "I am here to help others." I was ten years old.

Source: Trout, S. S. (1997). *Born to serve: The evolution of the soul through service.* Alexandria, VA: Three Roses Press, p. 13.

BOX 11.18 ETHICAL FORMATIONS: "ALL ARE SIGNIFICANT"

During my second year of nursing school, our professor gave us a quiz. I breezed through the questions until I read the last one. "What is the first name of the woman who cleans the school?" Surely this was a joke. I had seen the cleaning woman several times but how would I know her name? I handed in my paper, leaving the last question blank. Before the class ended, one student asked if the last question would count toward our grade. "Absolutely," the professor said. "In your careers, you will meet many people—all are significant. They deserve your attention and care. Even if all you do is smile and say hello." I have never forgotten that lesson. I also learned her name was Dorothy.

Source: Covey, S. (2002). Foreword. In R. K. Greenleaf, *Servant leadership: A journey into the nature of legitimate power and greatness* (25th ed.) (pp. 1–13). New York, NY: Paulist Press, p. 10.

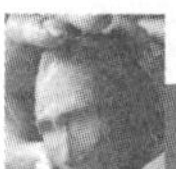

Ethical Reflections

- Reflect and write a narrative about why you want(ed) to become a nurse.
- Was (is) your primary motivation the desire to be a servant or a leader? Has your perception of the servant/leadership role changed over time? How?
- Consider several different work settings and jobs for PH nurses. Describe how you could be a servant leader in each of these settings and jobs.
- Box 11.19 contains examples from the ANA's (2001) *Code of Ethics for Nurses with Interpretive Statements.* How are these examples relevant to PH nursing?
- What other provisions and statements in the ANA's *Code of Ethics for Nurses* are particularly pertinent to PH nursing [see Appendix A]? Discuss these provisions and provide examples of how they apply to nursing practice.

both followers, because both are following the truth. Moral authority was described in terms of conscience and includes four dimensions:

1. Sacrifice is the heart of moral authority or conscience. Sacrifice involves an elevated recognition of one's small, peaceful inner voice while subduing the selfish voice of one's ego.
2. Being inspired to become involved with a cause that is worth one's commitment to it. A worthy cause inspires people to change their "question from asking what is it we want to what is being asked of us" (Covey, 2002, p. 7). One's conscience is expanded and becomes a factor of great influence in one's life.
3. The inseparableness of any ends and means. Moral leaders do not use unethical means to reach ends; as the philosopher Kant advocated for moral behavior, servant leaders always must treat others as ends in themselves, never as a means to an end.
4. The importance of relationships is enlivened through the development of conscience. "Conscience transforms passion into compassion" (Covey, 2002, p. 9). Living according to one's conscience emphasizes the reality of the interdependence of people and relationships. In relation to this fourth dimension of moral authority, Covey conveyed a story told by a nursing student, JoAnn C. Jones (see Box 11.18).

BOX 11.19 ETHICAL FORMATIONS: *CODE OF ETHICS FOR NURSES*

- Individuals are interdependent members of the community (1.4, p. 9).
- The nurse recognizes that there are situations in which the right to individual self-determination may be outweighed or limited by the rights, health, and welfare of others, particularly in relation to public health considerations (1.4, p. 9).
- Nurses, individually and collectively, have a responsibility to be knowledgeable about the health status of the community and existing threats to health and safety (8.2, p. 24).
- Nurses can work individually as citizens or collectively through political action to bring about social change (9.4, p. 25).

KEY POINTS

- Members of a community have a shared interest in a common good.
- Communities are moral in nature.
- The epicenter of communitarian ethics is the community, rather than the individual perspective of any one person.
- There are a number of ethical theories and approaches that are useful in PH nursing. Nurses need to understand different ethical approaches and develop an ethical philosophy before a crisis or stressful situation arises.
- It is a moral choice when people decide how they choose to distribute societal benefits and burdens among the members of communities.
- Healthcare disparities often are associated with race, ethnicity, and economic status.
- Humans will not achieve true moral progress until people perceive the suffering of others who are not personally known to them as important in their daily lives.
- Pandemics and disasters may require different priority setting than happens during everyday health care. Nurses should be familiar with policies and guidelines before they are faced with providing care during a pandemic or disaster.
- The human genome project has generated a plethora of ethical questions that will need to be answered by members of the global community.
- Servant leaders view themselves as servants first and leaders second.

Situations for Reflection

Discuss the following situations and apply ethical theories and approaches discussed in this chapter and other chapters of the book. As needed, search the Internet for more information. What theories or approaches are applicable in each situation? Could more than one approach be useful? What do you believe are the most ethical actions or positions in these situations? List and discuss as many relevant issues and considerations as possible. What additional information might you need to make your decisions? Specifically, how and where would you obtain this information?

1. You are a school nurse in Mississippi. A mother does not want her school-aged child immunized for chicken pox before entering the school where you work. The child was not previously immunized and has not had chicken pox.
2. During your public health class, you study the problem of malaria around the world and realize that even though malaria is no longer endemic in the United States, it could again become a problem at some point. Even though this is so, you realize that the people bearing the burden of malaria today are in poor countries and not in the United States. You talk with your friend about your concern for the many people sick and dying from malaria. You know that malaria is associated with a cycle of poverty. Sick children cannot attend school regularly and sick adults cannot work. Your friend says, "This is sad, but we have enough problems in the United States to be concerned about. I am not going to worry about people and diseases in other countries that don't affect us."
3. Your rich friend who owns a very successful small business and has health insurance tells you that he does not believe that it is his responsibility to provide health insurance for his employees.
4. You are the tuberculosis (TB) nurse at the county health department. You regularly make home visits for directly observed therapy (DOT) for a woman with TB. The woman is frequently not home when she knows that you are coming to her house.
5. You are a nurse working at the county health department. You learn that a rich developer is planning to build low-income housing on an old landfill that was used by a chemical company. The developer stated that there is no evidence that chemicals at the landfill will harm anyone.
6. You are a nurse working at the county health department. An influenza pandemic has been declared. When the vaccine is available, you have access to it at your clinic. However, you have been given a procedure to follow regarding how to prioritize who receives the vaccine. Your sister is not among the priority categories, yet she wants the vaccine.
7. You are an elementary school nurse. Many of the children at the school are ethnic minorities living in single-parent families. The population of

children at the school has a high incidence of health-related problems as compared to the children at the private school where your nurse friend works. You frequently are frustrated because you do not see the children's mothers trying to break their cycle of poverty. You love the children that you care for but you consider quitting your job.

8. While working as an occupational health nurse at a microwave popcorn factory, it seems to you that a high number of employees have respiratory disorders. You wonder if the employees' exposure to the flavoring ingredient, diacetyl, which is heated in the factory to add the popcorn's buttery taste, might be the problem. You tell your supervisor about your suspicions, and your supervisor tells you that it would cost too much money to reduce exposure to diacetyl. He also says that there is no proof that diacetyl exposure in popcorn factories negatively affects human lungs.
9. Your nonsmoker friend tells you that she is angry because she has to pay healthcare costs for tobacco users. She states that tobacco use is one of the leading causes of diseases requiring major expenditures of healthcare dollars and that the smoking-related expenditures cause her cost of health care to rise. She complains that smokers are "choosing their own health" and should not receive federally funded health care through Medicare and Medicaid programs.
10. You are an elementary school nurse. You are informed that the school cafeteria will begin including food from cloned animals. This type of food has not been tested exhaustively by the FDA. The school superintendent does not want to publicize the addition of the new food sources at the school.

References

American Nurses Association. (2001). *Code of ethics for nurses with interpretive statements.* Silver Spring, MD: Author.

American Nurses Association. (2007). *Public health nursing: Scope and standards of practice.* Silver Spring, MD: Author.

American Public Health Association: Public Health Nursing Section. (2006). *Environmental health principles for public health nursing.* Retrieved from http://www.apha.org/membergroups/newsletters/sectionnewsletters/public_nur/winter06/2550.htm

American Public Health Association: Public Health Nursing Section. (2011). *Public health nursing.* Retrieved from http://www.apha.org/membergroups/sections/aphasections/phn/

Beauchamp, D. (1999). Public health as social justice. In D. E. Beauchamp & B. Steinbock (Eds.), *New ethics for the public's health* (pp. 101–109). New York, NY: Oxford University Press.

Beauchamp, T. L., & Childress, J. F. (2001). *Principles of biomedical ethics* (5th ed.). New York, NY: Oxford University Press.

Beauchamp, T. L., & Childress, J. F. (2009). *Principles of biomedical ethics* (6th ed.). New York, NY: Oxford University Press.

Berkowitz, B., Dahl, J., Guirl, K., Kostelecky, B., McNeil, C., & Upenieks, V. (2001). *Public health nursing leadership: A guide to managing the core functions.* Washington, DC: American Nurses Publishing.

Campbell, A. T., Hart, K. D., & Norton, S. A. (2007). Legal and ethical issues in disaster response. In T. G. Veenema (Ed.), *Disaster nursing and emergency preparedness for chemical, biological, and radiological terrorism and other hazards* (2nd ed.) (pp. 100–116). New York, NY: Springer.

Centers for Disease Control and Prevention. (2003). Achievements in public health, 1900–1999: Control of infectious diseases. In P. R. Lee & C. L. Estes (Eds.), *The nation's health* (7th ed.) (pp. 31–37). Sudbury, MA: Jones and Bartlett.

Centers for Disease Control and Prevention. (2006). Revised recommendations for HIV testing of adults, adolescents, and pregnant women in health-care settings. *Morbidity and Mortality Weekly Report, 55*(RR14), 1–17. Retrieved from http://www.cdc.gov/mmwr/preview/mmwrhtml/rr5514a1.htm

Centers for Disease Control and Prevention. (2009). *Eliminating racial & ethnic health disparities.* Retrieved from http://www.cdc.gov/omhd/About/disparities.htm

Centers for Disease Control and Prevention. (2010). *The history of malaria, an ancient disease.* Retrieved from http://www.cdc.gov/malaria/about/history/

Centers for Disease Control and Prevention, Ethics Subcommittee of the Advisory Committee to the Director. (2007a). *Ethical guidelines in pandemic influenza.* Retrieved from http://www.cdc.gov/od/science/integrity/phethics/panFlu_Ethic_Guidelines.pdf

Centers for Disease Control and Prevention, Ethics Subcommittee of the Advisory Committee to the Director. (2007b). *Planning and Responding to Pandemic Influenza:* Ethical Considerations Checklist. Retrieved from http://www.cdc.gov/od/science/integrity/phethics/guidelinesPanFlu.htm

Centers for Disease Control and Prevention, Ethics Subcommittee of the Advisory Committee to the Director, Ventilator Document Workgroup. (2011). *Ethical considerations for decision making regarding allocation of mechanical ventilators during a severe influenza pandemic or other public health emgergency.* Retrieved from http://www.cdc.gov/od/science/integrity/phethics/docs/Vent_Document_Final_Version.pdf

Chenneville, T. (2003). HIV, confidentiality, and duty to protect: A decision-making model. In D. N. Bersoff (Ed.), *Ethical conflicts in psychology* (3rd ed.) (pp. 198–202). Washington, DC: American Psychological Association.

Cox, N. (2011). *Pandemic influenza vaccines: Lessons learned from the H1N1 influenza pandemic.* Retrieved from http://www.who.int/influenza_vaccines_plan/resources/cox.pdf

Covey, S. (2002). Foreword. In R. K. Greenleaf, *Servant leadership: A journey into the nature of legitimate power and greatness* (25th ed.) (pp. 1–13). New York, NY: Paulist Press.

De Mello, A. (1992). *One minute nonsense.* Chicago, IL: Loyola University.

Dempski, K. (2009). Clients with AIDS and HIV testing. In S. J. Westrick & K. Dempski (Eds.), *Essentials of Nursing Law and Ethics* (pp. 110–113). Sudbury, MA: Jones and Bartlett.

De Saint-Exupery, A. (2002). *A guide for grown-ups: Essential wisdom from the collected works of Antoine De Saint-Exupery.* San Diego, CA: Harcourt.

Donne, J. (1962). Meditation 17. In *Norton Anthology of English Literature* (Vol. 1, 5th ed.). New York, NY: W. W. Norton.

Einstein, A. (1930). *What I believe.* Retrieved from http://home.earthlink.net/~johnrpenner/Articles/Einstein3.html

Farmer, P. (2001). *Infections and inequalities: The modern plagues* (Updated). Berkeley, CA: University of California Press.

Forsey, H. (1993). *Circles of strength: Community alternatives to alienation.* Philadelphia, PA: New Society.

Friis, R. H. (2007). *Essentials of environmental health.* Sudbury, MA: Jones and Bartlett.
Fry, S. T., & Veatch, R. M. (2006). *Case studies in nursing ethics* (3rd ed.). Sudbury, MA: Jones and Bartlett.
Galanti, G. A. (2008). *Caring for patients from different cultures* (4th ed.). Philadelphia, PA: University of Pennsylvania Press.
Garrett, L. (2000). *Betrayal of trust: The collapse of global public health.* New York, NY: Hyperion.
Greenleaf, R. (2002). *Servant leadership: A journey into the nature of legitimate power and greatness* (25th ed.) (L. C. Spears, Ed.), New York, NY: Paulist Press.
Hesse, H. (1956). *The journey to the east.* New York, NY: Picador.
Homeland Security Council. (2006). *National strategy for pandemic influenza implementation plan.* McLean, VA: International Medical Publishing.
Joint United Nations Programme on HIV/AIDS [UNAIDS]. (2011). *UNAIDS homepage.* Retrieved from http://www.unaids.org/en/
Kaye, C. B. (2004). *The complete guide to service learning: Proven, practical ways to engage students in civic responsibility, academic curriculum, and social action.* Minneapolis, MN: Free Spirit.
Kriebel, D., Tickner, J., & Crumbley, C. (2003). *Appropriate science: Evaluating environmental risks for a sustainable world.* Retrieved from http://www.uml.edu/com/CITA/Kriebel.pdf
Kush, C. (2004). *The one-hour activist: The 15 most powerful actions you can take to fight for the issues and candidates you care about.* San Francisco, CA: Jossey-Bass.
Lo, B. (2009). *Resolving ethical dilemmas: A guide for clinicians* (4th ed.). Philadelphia, PA: Wolters Kluwer.
The Luminary Project. (2005). *About the project.* Retrieved from http://www.theluminaryproject.org/article.php?id=42
Lundberg, K. (2005). An anthropologist's analysis. In B. C. White & J. A. Zimbelman (Eds.), *Moral dilemmas in community health care: Cases and commentaries* (pp. 152–155). New York, NY: Pearson Education.
MacIntyre, A. (1984). *After virtue: A study of moral theory* (2nd ed.). Notre Dame, IN: University of Notre Dame.
Markel, H. (2004). *When germs travel: Six major epidemics that have invaded America since 1900 and the fears they have unleashed.* New York, NY: Pantheon.
Minkler, M., & Pies, C. (2002). Ethical issues in community organization and community participation. In M. Minkler (Ed.), *Community organizing & community building for health* (pp. 120–138). New Brunswick, NJ: Rutgers University Press.
Norton, A. (2010). *Is homophobia a factor in HIV racial gap?* Retrieved from http://uk.reuters.com/article/2010/10/15/us-homophobia-gap-idUSTRE69E5BN20101015
Nussbaum, M. (2004). Compassion and terror. In L. P. Pojman (Ed.), *The moral life: An introductory reader in ethics and literature* (2nd ed.) (pp. 937–961). New York, NY: Oxford University Press.
Pieper, J. (1966). *The four cardinal virtues.* Notre Dame, IN: University of Notre Dame.
Piliavin, J. A. (2003). Doing well by doing good: Benefits for the benefactor. In C. L. M. Keyes & J. Haidt (Eds.), *Flourishing: Positive psychology and the life well-lived* (pp. 227–247). Washington, DC: American Psychological Association.
Pipher, M. (2002). *The middle of everywhere: Helping refugees enter the American community.* Orlando, FL: Harcourt.

Prejean, J., Song, R., Hernandez, A., Ziebell, R., Green, T., Walker, F., Hall, H. I. (2011). Estimated HIV incidence in the United States, 2006–2009. *PloS ONE, 6*(8), 1–13. doi: 10.1371/journal.pone.0017502

Public Health Leadership Society. (2002). *Principles of the ethical practice of public health.* Retrieved from http://www.apha.org/NR/rdonlyres/1CED3CEA-287E-4185-9CBD-BD405FC60856/0/ethicsbrochure.pdf

Public Health Leadership Society. (2004). *Skills for the ethical practice of public health.* Retrieved from http://phls.org/CMSuploads/Skills-for-the-Ethical-Practice-of-Public-Health-68547.pdf

Raffensperger, C., & Myers, C. (2001). Ethics for survival. *The Networker, 6*(1). Retrieved from http://www.mindfully.org/Sustainability/Ethics-For-Survival.htm

Riegelman, R. (2010). *Public health 101: Healthy people-healthy populations.* Sudbury, MA: Jones and Bartlett.

Salamon, J. (2003). *Rambam's ladder: A meditation on generosity and why it is necessary to give.* New York, NY: Workman.

Science and Environmental Health Network. (1998). *Precautionary principle: Wingspread statement.* Retrieved from http://www.sehn.org/wing.html

Science and Environmental Health Network. (2011). *Precautionary principle: FAQs.* Retrieved from http://www.sehn.org/ppfaqs.html

Sherwin, S. (1992). *No longer patient: Feminist ethics & health care.* Philadelphia, PA: Temple University.

Trout, S. S. (1997). *Born to serve: The evolution of the soul through service.* Alexandria, VA: Three Roses Press.

U.S. Department of Energy, Office of Science. (2006a). *Ethical, legal, and social issues.* Retrieved from http://www.ornl.gov/sci/techresources/Human_Genome/elsi/elsi.shtml

U.S. Department of Energy, Office of Science. (2006b). *Human genome project information.* Retrieved from http://www.ornl.gov/sci/techresources/Human_Genome/home.shtml

U.S. Department of Health and Human Services. (2011). *HealthyPeople.gov: About healthy people.* Retrieved from http://www.healthypeople.gov/2020/about/default.aspx

U.S. Environmental Protection Agency. (2011a). *Environmental justice.* Retrieved from http://www.epa.gov/environmentaljustice/

U.S. Environmental Protection Agency. (2011b). *Environmental justice: Basic information: Background.* Retrieved from http://www.epa.gov/environmentaljustice/basics/ejbackground.html

U.S. Government Accountability Office. (2011). Influenza pandemic: Lessons from the H1N1 pandemic should be incorporated in to future planning. Retrieved from http://www.gao.gov/new.items/d11632.pdf

Wheatley, M. (2002). *Turning to one another.* San Francisco, CA: Berrett-Koehler.

Wildes, K. M. (2000). *Moral acquaintances: Methodology in bioethics.* Notre Dame, IN: University of Notre Dame.

World Health Organization. (2005). *Ten things you need to know about pandemic influenza.* Retrieved from http://www.who.int/csr/disease/influenza/pandemic10things/en/

World Health Organization. (2010a). *2010/2011 tuberculosis global facts.* Retrieved from http://www.who.int/tb/publications/2010/factsheet_tb_2010_rev21feb11.pdf

World Health Organization. (2010b). *Malaria.* Retrieved from http://www.who.int/mediacentre/factsheets/fs094/en/index.html

World Health Organization. (2010c). *Malaria report shows rapid progress towards international targets.* Retrieved from http://www.who.int/mediacentre/news/releases/2010/malaria_report_20101214/en/index.html

World Health Organization. (2010d). *Tuberculosis*. Retrieved from http://www.who.int/mediacentre/factsheets/fs104/en/

World Health Organization. (2010e). *WHO global malaria programme. Q & A on malaria elimination and eradication*. Retrieved from http://www.who.int/malaria/elimination/WHOGMP_elimination_qa.pdf

World Health Organization. (2011a). *Cumulative number of confirmed human cases of avian influenza A/(H5N1) reported to WHO*. Retrieved from http://www.who.int/csr/disease/avian_influenza/country/cases_table_2011_08_02/en/index.html

World Health Organization. (2011b). *Strategic planning and innovation*. Retrieved from http://www.who.int/spi/en/

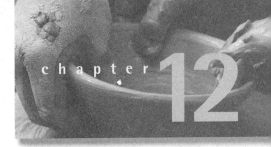

chapter 12

Ethics in Organizations and Leadership

Janie B. Butts

Just about every action we take has ethical implications.

—RITVO, OHLSEN, AND HOLLAND, 2004, P. 28

OBJECTIVES

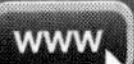

After reading this chapter, the reader should be able to:

1. Compare the definitions of organizational ethics and the ethic of an organization.
2. Discuss the significance of organizations being characterized as a good citizen in the community and society.
3. Explore the ethical dimensions that shape the ethical climate and culture of an organization.
4. Examine the definition and characteristics of organizational trust and integrity.
5. Identify the common unethical and illegal behaviors that people sometimes exhibit in organizations.
6. Discuss Jennings's seven signs of organizational ethical collapse.
7. Briefly explore the history of compliance programs and officers in healthcare organizations.
8. Contrast the types of occupational fraud and abuse.
9. Evaluate the cases presented in this chapter regarding conflicts of interest and health care fraud.

10. Define an ethical leader.
11. Differentiate the three types of leadership theories that are presented in this chapter.
12. Discuss the ethical challenges of a nurse leader and the ways to use power for leader success.

Organizational Ethics

An **organization** is defined as a group of two or more people that intentionally strives to accomplish a shared set of goals that are consistent with the organization's purpose and conduct. An organization is sometimes compared to a person because it functions as a moral agent that can be held accountable for its actions. Organizational ethics focuses "on the choices of the individual *and* the organization" (Boyle, DuBose, Ellingson, Guinn, & McCurdy, 2001, p. 16).

Organizational Culture and the Ethical Climate

Organizational culture refers to an organization's past and current shared assumptions, experiences, and philosophy, much like a tribe with its own "language, stories, beliefs, assumptions, ceremonies, and power structures" (Johnson, 2012, p. 319). Daft (2004) presented several types of organizational cultures and indicated that every culture has a potential to be successful (see Box 12.1). No matter which culture is promoted by the organization's leaders, the culture needs to fit with its strategy and environment.

The term **organizational ethics** is a broad concept that includes not only culture, but also the processes, outcomes, and character and denotes "a way of acting, not a code of principles . . . [and] is at the heart, pumping blood that perfuses the entire organization with a common sense of purpose and a shared set of values" (Pearson, Sabin, & Emanuel, 2003, p. 42). The **ethic of an organization** refers to an organization's attempt to define its mission and values, recognize values that could cause tension, seek best solutions to these tensions, and manage the operations to maintain its values. The ethics process serves as a mechanism for organizations to address ethical issues regarding financial, business, and management decisions. Organizations are systems, which means that an organization consists of highly integrated parts or groups to accomplish shared goals. An **open system**, such as a healthcare organization, focuses on external relationships, which places the organization within a larger context or environment (Boyle et al., 2001).

An **organizational citizenship** represents what society and communities expect from open systems (Johnson, 2007). The expectations are part of establishing and maintaining those external relationships, including those with suppliers, regulatory bodies, customers, allies, competitors, communities, and society as a whole.

BOX 12.1 ETHICAL FORMATIONS: DAFT'S TYPES OF ORGANIZATIONAL CULTURES (2004)

1. **Adaptability culture**: The focus is on the external environment where innovation, creativity, risk taking, flexibility, and change are the key elements for success. This type of organization creates change in a proactive way in an effort to anticipate responses and problems. Examples that Daft gave are e-commerce companies such as Amazon.com and Buy.com, which are required to change quickly in anticipation of customer needs.
2. **Mission culture**: The vision and goals are clearly focused on a high level of competitiveness and profit-making strategies. In this type of culture, executives and managers strongly communicate a strategic plan for the organization's employees and expect high productivity, performance goals, and fringe benefits for goal attainment. An example of a mission culture that Daft gave was PepsiCo.
3. **Clan culture:** The focus is on employee needs and the strategies in which employees can engage for high performance. Key values in this culture consist of leaders taking care of their employees and making sure they have appropriate avenues to satisfaction and productivity. Responsibility and ownership are other key values in this type of culture. Rapid change occurs in this environment because of changing expectations from the external environment. One example that Daft gave is the MTW Corporation, which sells Web-based software and provides consultation to state governments and the insurance industry.
4. **Bureaucratic culture**: The focus is primarily on the internal environment, where stability is a mainstay. Leaders develop and carry out scrupulous and detailed plans in a cautious and stable environment with slow-paced change. In this environment, personal engagement and involvement are not cultivated; instead, there is a high level of consistency, conformity, efficiency, and integration. Because of the inflexibility of this culture, many organizations are forced to change to a different, more adaptable culture. One successful organization that Daft offered as an example is the Pacific Edge Software company, run by a husband-and-wife team, which thrives on order, discipline, and control.

Source: Adapted from Daft, R. L. (2004). *Organizational theory and design* (8th ed., pp. 367–370). Mason, OH: South-Western.

For an organization to be characterized as **being a good citizen**, it must anticipate ethical issues or conflicts in external relationships and then engage in dialogue and activities to manage those concerns.

Even though the term "organizational ethics" often refers to an organization's image, people who work in the organizations are the ones who behave ethically or unethically and therefore shape the ambiance and character of the organization. Refer to Box 12.2 for a list of unethical and illegal behaviors in which one could engage within organizations; the list is not exhaustive, but consists of the more common behaviors. Many unethical behaviors of organizations are also illegal, so sometimes the lines between ethical and legal behaviors are blurred.

The ethical climate, which plays a large role in shaping the culture, is formed by the way the organization responds to the ethical issues and challenges. The **ethical**

BOX 12.2 ETHICAL FORMATIONS: TYPICAL UNETHICAL OR ILLEGAL BEHAVIORS IN ORGANIZATIONS

- Occupational fraud and abuse, including conflicts of interest and health care fraud
- Greediness
- Engaging in covert operations
- Producing misleading services
- Reneging or cheating on negotiated terms
- Creating fuzzy policies that can cause others to lie to get the job done
- Showing overconfidence in self-judgment
- Disloyalty
- Exhibiting poor quality in performance and apathy in goal attainment
- Engaging in humiliating and stereotyping tactics
- Engaging in bigotry, sexism, racism, or showing favoritism
- Suppressing rights such as freedom of speech and choice
- Obeying authority in a mindless routine
- Promoting people who are destructive go-getters, yet seem to outrun mistakes
- Price fixing as the standard
- Not speaking up when unethical practices become evident
- Stepping on others to climb the promotion ladder
- Sacrificing innocent people and blaming others to get the job done
- Knowingly exaggerating the advantages of a plan to gather support
- Failing to cooperate with others
- Lying for the sake of business
- Failing to take responsibility for injurious practices
- Abusing organizational perks
- Corrupting the public process through legal means
- Obstructing or stalling actions and processes
- Dithering
- Inefficiency

Source: Boyle, P. J., DuBose, E. R., Ellingson, S. J., Guinn, D. E., & McCurdy, D. B. (2001). Organizational ethics in health care: Principles, cases, and practical solutions (pp. 19–20). San Francisco, CA: Jossey-Bass/John Wiley & Sons.

climate is defined as the organizational members' shared perceptions of their values related to how ethical decisions are made on the issues of power, trust, and human interactions (Johnson, 2012). Numerous researchers have studied the idea of an ethical climate, but Victor and Cullen (1987) were first to discover and then reconfirm that organizations can have a combination of one or more of these five dimensions of ethical climates:

- Caring—interested in team values and goals, well-being of others, and friendships
- Law and code—guided by professional codes of conduct

- Rules—strict adherence to policies and procedures
- Instrumental—focused on self-interest and company profits
- Independence—focused on personal moral beliefs and decision making

The instrumental climate manifests from self-interest gains and profits within organizations and poses more serious ethical problems than any of the other ethical climates (Johnson, 2012).

Organizational Integrity and Trust

Organizational integrity generally means that good and right behavior in the relationships is found across the whole system (Brown, 2006). **Integrity** as a whole is equated with:

- Keeping consistency between what an organization does and what it says.
- Maintaining mindfulness of relationships with others.
- Listening and including all voices, whether disagreeable or not, in everyday business practices.
- Having a collective worthwhile purpose.

Most all of the major relationships transpire within five dimensions of organizational life: cultural, interpersonal, organizational, social, and natural. Integrity and trust go hand-in-hand; organizations and leaders with integrity are also trustworthy.

Trust is a multifaceted virtue that serves as an umbrella over the key values in organizations. Shore (2007) stated that **organizational trust** is the essential ingredient, what he labeled as the lubricant, that facilitates everyday business and interactions. People can trust other people to follow through on their work and commitments just as people in the community can depend on organizations to uphold their words and promises. **Fiduciary relationships** hold a high value in organizations because these relationships represent a formal duty to another or others imposed by loyalty, commitment, and organizational structure, which means that people place trust in others to carry out activities related to their position with morally good judgment.

Williams (2006) emphasized that trust can thrive in organizations only when the key element of fairness exists. Victor and Cullen's (1987) descriptions of the cultures of caring, law and code, and rule enable the achievement of fairness and justice. Practicing the virtue of justice promotes fair distribution of resources (of any type) among the individuals within the organizations and in the external community. According to Gutmann (1995), an organization must practice and sustain two principles so that the community it serves can have a sense of fairness: (1) nondiscrimination in the moral standing of each person, and (2) nonrepression, so that each person has a deliberate voice if they so choose. Without those principles, an organization's trust and justice will be questioned.

The ethic of the organization defines the mission and values. Some of those values are teamwork, community, achievement, competence, knowledge, innovation, having fun, valuing diversity, and encouraging others. Organizations need to define their values operationally, and likewise must define their ethical practices in writing and in verbal communication. Jack Welch, past chairman and CEO of General Electric, once said: "Good business leaders create a vision, articulate the vision, passionately own the vision, and relentlessly drive it to completion" (as cited in Kovanic & Johnson, 2004, p. 101).

As evidenced in many corporate scandals, trust in organizations has been eroding for years, such that it is now at an all-time low (Jennings, 2006; Shore, 2007). Healthcare organizations are similar. The rapid transformation in healthcare organizations has been a contributing factor in the erosion of trust. As organizations rapidly change to comply with regulatory standards, costs, the demands of internal and external stakeholders, and the needs of the populations they serve, the ethical questions that need to be answered have become more difficult to resolve. Abusive executive power and self-serving corporate decisions lead to unethical behaviors, which leave an air of mistrust within the organization and in the external community. Trust in organizations is an obscure concept that consists of a network of convoluted relationships, although researchers have found that trust critically matters in organizations for nurses and others healthcare personnel because:

- Trust promotes economic value within organizations.
- Trust increases strategic alliances, teamwork, and productivity.
- Nurses and other healthcare personnel experience a more positive practice environment as a result of trust.
- Nurses experience increased empowerment, autonomy, and overall job satisfaction because of organizational trust. (Kramer & Schmalenberg, 2002; Laschinger, Shamian, & Thomson, 2001; Williams, 2005)

A violation of trust in organizations will prompt verbalizations, such as angry and sarcastic remarks by personnel, especially if trust has been previously entrenched throughout the organizational levels (Williams, 2006). A violation of trust in organizations is generally illegal and less forgivable than in a personal relationship where trust historically exists between two people.

There are logical reasons for the way people perceive organizations. Untrustworthy leaders of organizations could have been engaging covertly in unethical or illegal behaviors for quite a long while, and if left unchecked, this will result in the ethical collapse of the organization.

Jennings's Seven Signs of Organizational Ethical Collapse

Jennings (2006) identified seven signs of ethical collapse and detailed how organizations can conduct business ethically and sustain its core values. The signs of collapse are the same whether the organization is for-profit or nonprofit, though there is some variation in the unethical activities. The signs are:

1. pressure to maintain numbers
2. fear and silence
3. "young 'uns and a bigger-than-life CEO"
4. weak board
5. conflicts
6. innovation like no other
7. goodness in some areas atones for evil in others

When these signs of ethical collapse are present, Jennings indicated that an organization is in profound trouble. An explanation of each sign follows.

Pressure to Maintain Numbers: The first and earliest sign that the organization is in trouble is an obsession to maintain numbers, as measured in quantifiable goals (Jennings, 2006). Numbers drive nonprofit and for-profit organizations.

Fear and Silence: In organizations about to collapse ethically, there is an air of fear, silence, and servility (Jennings, 2006). Organizations are on the road to ethical collapse when there is corruption and wrongdoing by administrators. Many times administrators prefer looking for gray ethical or legal areas so that they can manipulate or create confusion or vagueness in records, bookkeeping, and other areas in the hopes that they will conceal their behavior and not be caught. Even in the midst of an ethical meltdown, not many people challenge the workings of the organization for fear of being threatened, publicly shamed, dismissed, or demoted. Employees, as well as administrators, who have evidence of confusing, fuzzy bookkeeping or wrongdoing are silenced and sometimes bribed by those involved with the unethical, and perhaps illegal, conduct. Fear of not fitting in or being a team player is often a reason for employees' silence.

Young 'Uns and a Bigger-Than-Life CEO: The third sign of an ethical meltdown involves a CEO who is sometimes a generation or two older than the other members of the organization and is lavishly praised and held in high regard by the community and media (Jennings, 2006). To maintain this level of admiration, these CEOs surround themselves with extremely driven young people, sometimes their own sons or daughters, who vow loyalty to the CEO and the organization. The presence of a highly regarded CEO does not translate necessarily to organizational legal and ethical problems. However, when problems do exist or when employees see potential trouble coming, they or others hesitate to ask questions that could cause embarrassment to the bigger-than-life CEO. The sentiment is that "we don't ask questions."

Weak Board: A weak and inefficient institutional board of directors is the next sign of an organization on the edge of ethical collapse (Jennings, 2006). Several reasons for a weak board exist, alone or in combination. Sometimes, the board is composed of inexperienced members who are the CEO's cronies or are unwilling to confront the beloved CEO. The members may be inefficient and unreliable, such as not spending enough time prudently thinking about and interpreting the issues, not attending the meetings, and not fulfilling their obligations to the board. Weak board members often make decisions that are baseless and push the limits on ethical and legal matters.

Conflicts: Conflicts of interest can occur with the individual or organization or between the internal organization and the external community (Jennings, 2006). Executives or board members engaged in a conflict of interest must have used their position to benefit themselves in some way at the expense of the organization.

Innovation Like No Other: Organizations heading toward ethical collapse often have extremely high levels of innovation and achievement (Jennings, 2006). They are often successful, with unmatched performance that seems to defy the laws of gravity with unlimited gains and with the philosophy that they are above the law. Organizations with rapid, extreme success continuously seek new ways of keeping the success up, no matter what tactic has to be used. Eventually, as these successful organizations face strong competitors with higher quality and, in the case of healthcare organizations, better outcomes for patients while also maintaining a healthy financial bottom line, they are at risk of falling. However, Jennings (2006) emphasized that just because an organization has innovation and extreme success does not mean that it is on the verge of an ethical collapse. Some do collapse, but the collapse is linked to organizations never forming or practicing standards of ethical excellence that make up a healthy ethical climate.

Goodness in Some Areas Atones for Evil in Others: Some organizations and CEOs, especially of for-profit companies, are committed to the community, to public service, and to philanthropic activities, but sometimes this results in the philosophy that goodness in some areas (public philanthropy) atones for evil in others (unethical practices) (Jennings, 2006). Sometimes nonprofit organizations, when acting as a noble public servant, such as giving back to the community with an emphasis in environmentalism and human rights, also manifest the "good atoning for evil" philosophy, but Jennings contended that goodness in some areas will not overcome the improprieties in others.

Compliance and Ethics Programs

Today, the compliance officer is one of the most sought-after roles in a healthcare organization. This officer oversees and monitors regulatory requirements and internal policies because organizations, like individuals, are at risk for being found guilty of criminal conduct, such as felonies and some types of misdemeanors (Desio, 2010). A **compliance program** (also known as a risk-management program) is designed to "prevent unlawful conduct and to promote conformity with externally imposed regulations [and] provide a second component of background for organizational ethics" (Pearson et al., 2003, p. 28). During the 1980s, compliance programs became popular as a way for healthcare organizations to satisfy the mandate for addressing ethical and legal issues, primarily Medicare and Medicaid. Compliance programs were expanded in 1991 when officials in the U.S. Department of Justice created the U.S. Sentencing Guidelines to make consistent the sentencing process in federal courts (Pearson et al., 2003). The guidelines allowed for a reduction in penalties if a corporation had previously implemented the seven standards of compliance before the organization incurred a federal violation. The current sentencing guidelines include criteria for organizations and CEOs to implement best ethical practices (Desio, 2010). See best practices for effective compliance and ethics programs in Box 12.3. When these guidelines are implemented and consistently practiced as a whole, organizations are portrayed as a being a good citizen.

From the ethical perspective of noncompliance, the principles of autonomy, beneficence, nonmaleficence, and justice may be violated in relation to patients, healthcare professionals, and the general public. When organizational schemes have the potential to harm patients without their knowledge, autonomy is violated ethically, but also legally, in the form of the Patient Self-Determination Act of 1990. Hurting or injuring someone because of illegal or unethical schemes violates the principles of beneficence, nonmaleficence, and justice.

Compliance programs are not synonymous with ethics programs, yet organizations tend to use compliance programs as a way of addressing ethical issues (Pearson et al., 2003). These two programs, compliance and ethics, are needed and can complement each other if appropriately structured. Ethics programs focus on the values of an organization, pursuing virtue, and delivering ethical patient care, whereas compliance programs focus on obedience to legal and required details of performance and have enforcement capability. Today, compliance programs are mandatory, not optional. Some leaders of organizations, however, see compliance

BOX 12.3 ETHICAL FORMATIONS: BEST PRACTICES FOR EFFECTIVE COMPLIANCE AND ETHICS PROGRAMS

- Oversight of the organization by an administrator or officer
- Proper and detailed attention in the delegation of substantial discretionary authority
- Effective communication to people on all levels of the organization
- Reasonable steps to accomplish compliance for monitoring, auditing, and reporting suspicious wrongdoing without fear of retaliation
- Consistent attention and reinforcement of compliance standards, which includes disciplinary criteria
- Reasonable steps to respond to and prevent offenses and violations.

Source: Desio, P. (2010). An overview of the organizational guidelines. *U. S. sentencing guidelines.* Retrieved from http://www.ussc.gov/Education_and_Training/Guidelines_Educational_Materials/Organizational_Guidelines.cfm

programs more as a vehicle for protecting themselves rather than as a means to instill important ethical values.

Occupational Fraud and Abuse

Occupational fraud and abuse is defined as "the use of one's occupation for personal enrichment through the deliberate misuse or misapplication of the employment organization's resources or assets" (Association of Certified Fraud Examiners [ACFE], 2010, p. 6) Three types of occupational fraud and abuse have been identified by the ACFE:

- Asset misappropriations—stealing and misusing an organization's resources, such as skimming cash receipts, falsifying expense reports, or forging company checks
- Corruption—employees' use of their influences in a manner that violates the duty owed to the employer for personal gain, such as bribery, extortion, or a conflict of interest
- Financial fraud statement—a deliberate misstatement or omission of material information in an organization's financial report, such as documenting fictitious revenues, concealing expenditures and obligations, or reporting inflated assets

Occupational fraud and abuse has been a major priority with the Federal Bureau of Investigation (FBI, 2006) for a number of years. In 2008, asset misappropriation accounted for the majority (89.8%) of reported cases of fraud in the United States. The total cost for all three categories of occupational fraud and abuse, for those cases from 2008 that were reported in the ACFE (2010) study, was $18 billion.

There are numerous schemes that fall within the aforementioned categories of occupational fraud and abuse. Covered in this section are conflicts of interest and health care fraud, along with the related issue of whistleblowing.

Conflicts of Interest

Conflicts of interest, from the standpoint of ethics, are referred to as **conflicts of commitment**. Commitment conflicts are complex because the decision to engage in a conflict of interest involves loyalties, concerns, and emotions in relationships that collide with the organizational and public interests. There are various ways that conflicts of commitment can result in an ethical violation of the organization's code of conduct. Ritvo, Ohlsen, and Holland (2004) emphasized the conflict that executives experience when they feel compelled to choose job commitments over the expectations of home and family life. Often a person's ethical obligations to fulfill job commitments can interfere with the time available for family or others; for example, should an executive, who is also a father, tell his superior that his daughter's out-of-town soccer game takes priority over his attendance at a critical meeting with the hospital's executive board members?

BOX 12.4 ETHICAL FORMATIONS: SAVANNAH'S ETHICAL AND LEGAL VIOLATION AT HER WORKPLACE

Savannah, a registered nurse in charge of direct patient care, attended a party the night before a scheduled 12-hour work day, overindulged in cocktails, went to bed around 3 a.m., and came to work the next morning at 6:45 a.m. with a hangover and alcohol still on her breath. This situation placed Savannah in ethical violation of the organization's values and *The Code of Ethics for Nurses*, as well as a legal violation of the state board of nursing. If alcohol is on a person's breath, it is still in the bloodstream, which could alter Savannah's judgment in patient care, result in unsafe patient care and treatments.

- Discuss the ethical implications of Savannah's partying before work. Please explain your rationale.
- Explore specific ethical violations in Savannah's case in terms of her personal behavior, the hospital's ethics and values, patient safety, the American Nurses Association's (ANA) *Code of Ethics*, and the state board of nursing.
- Can you think of other options that Savannah should consider other than going to work in an altered state of mind? Make a list of the pros and cons of at least two other alternatives Savannah could have chosen.
- Describe and justify how you would have handled this situation had you been Savannah. Justify your strategies by using an ethical framework: theory, approach, or principle.
- Do you believe that the nursing supervisor should take action against Savannah? Why or why not? If you believe that the supervisor should take action against Savannah, describe the specific options for disciplinary action based on your general knowledge of institutional and state board of nursing disciplinary protocol. For this particular answer, you could search the Web for general institutional disciplinary protocols and your state board of nursing's disciplinary actions if you need more knowledge on this topic. Explain your rationale.
- Do you believe that the supervisor should report Savannah's behavior to the state board of nursing? Why or why not? Explain your rationale.

Morrison (2006) mentioned other types of ethical conflicts of commitment. One is when an individual's personal behavior conflicts with the organization's ethics, such as overindulgence of alcohol or use of other drugs. Because patient safety and competent care are critical to the viability of a healthcare organization, personal behavior outside the organization is extremely important, as is personal behavior inside the organization. Nurses, in particular, are open to scrutiny by the public and by hospital officials because of standards mandated by their nursing license and their direct care of patients. In Box 12.4, there is a scenario of an ethical violation that could be more common than people would like to admit.

Cooper (2006) framed a **conflict of interest** as a legal matter:

> [Conflicts of interest are] situations where our own personal interests are at odds with our obligations as a public official or our professional values. There may be combinations of conflicting roles and tensions between sources of authority, but more typically these occasions simply present us with an opportunity to use our public office for the sake of our private gain or to the private gain of our friends or relatives. (p. 129)

The main ethical issue involved in conflicts of interest is breach of trust to the public. Whatever activities an executive leader or board member engages in also affect the organization's public image. These types of activities present legal conflicts between the person's position of authority in an organization and self-interest or between a person's accountability toward an organization and personal profit. An example of a moderate-sized legal conflict of interest by a chief nursing executive in a hospital is illustrated in Box 12.5.

Compliance officers, or others in charge of overseeing ethical and legal issues, need to develop clear policies regarding conflicts of interest and conduct formal reviews of actions. Maintaining a clear focus on behaviors within and outside the organization helps to bring impending conflicts of interest to the forefront. Just like in fraud situations, employees and the public need to have an avenue for safe reporting of potential or alleged conflicts of interest.

It is essential that executives disclose all significant facts and arrangements of any proposed transaction to the board or another executive of higher authority (Cooper, 2006). When a board of trustees becomes aware that an executive's proposed transactions are not fully disclosed or the activities and timelines seem vague or fuzzy, the board should confront the person and allow for an explanation through deliberation; the board should then take disciplinary action toward the person if there was not a satisfactory explanation. If a board member is the one who

BOX 12.5 ETHICAL FORMATIONS: BETTY'S CONFLICT OF INTEREST AT HER WORKPLACE

Betty, the chief nursing executive, needed to make a decision about buying 340 new hospital beds for patient rooms. After she interviewed nurse managers at the units where the beds were going to be placed, Betty compiled her findings and decided to contact a well-known equipment company to obtain prices and a bid. No bids from other companies were obtained. The equipment company's executive salesperson, Jim, discussed options at length with her and invited her and her significant other to an upcoming all-expenses-paid, lavish junket at a five-star hotel in Hawaii to see demonstrations of the beds and to experience a comprehensive sales program. Betty thought, "We badly need some relaxation and stress relief. Hawaii would be so much fun. Would it be wrong for us to go?"

- If you were Betty, what should you do? Give your rationale. Justify your answer with an ethical framework: theory, approach, or principle.
- Discuss the ethical principles at stake. What breaches are possible?
- Do you consider this situation a conflict of interest? Why or why not? Give your rationale.
- Speculate how Betty would handle this case if she believed she needed to seek advice from someone in a higher authority. With whom would she discuss this issue?
- Discuss the policies that should be in place regarding this scenario.

has breached that trust, the other board members should exclude that member from meetings and deliberations until a time comes for confrontation. If money or luxury gifts are a source of the breach of trust, the state of affairs then becomes complicated. These types of breaches are difficult to prove and sometimes fall into a grey area of ethical wrongdoing. If board members cannot find solid evidence of a breach on their own, they must determine if legal fees and time are worth the effort of a trial that may never result in a conviction for that board member.

Health Care Fraud

Health care fraud is defined as "an intentional deception or misrepresentation made by a person with the knowledge that the deception could result in some unauthorized benefit to himself or some other person" (Stockdale, 2010, p. 3). In the revisions of the U.S. Sentencing Commission's Guidelines (2004), the U.S. Department of Justice (USDOJ) mandated that organizations continuously improve their ethics and compliance programs by intermittently assessing for the risk of criminal conduct and taking steps to alleviate the violations (Perkins, 2010). Since the 1990s, the USDOJ and the U.S. Department of Health and Human Services (USDHHS) began investigating and prosecuting abuse and fraud cases in healthcare organizations in significantly greater numbers (UDSHHS, 2006). The criminality in healthcare organizations, especially defrauding federal government programs such as Medicare, became apparent as the percentage of cases continually increased each year.

The FBI investigates all health care fraud for federal, state, and local levels of government and for private insurance and other programs. A significant trend that has concerned the FBI is the willingness for medical professionals to commit schemes that risk patients' health and cause potential patient harm, some of which include unnecessary and harmful surgeries, prescriptions for dangerous drugs, and substandard care practices. The FBI (2006) stated that high technology and computers have contributed to the increase in the number of fraudulent schemes. The effects of fraudulent schemes result in acts of malfeasance in terms of personal injury, wrongful death, and sometimes class action suits for the involved patients.

As the U.S. population grows older, more Medicare services are needed. This rise in Medicare usage serves as a temptation for an increased incidence of corporate-driven schemes and systematic abuse. Health care fraud events in 2005 were committed through various means throughout all segments of the healthcare system. Categories of fraudulent schemes that were reported by the FBI in 2006 are highlighted in Box 12.6.

Nurses may be involved unknowingly in other similar arrangements, such as assisting with keeping the records for providers of care who are operating secret fraudulent schemes. In these cases, proving the innocence of involved nurses in a court of law would be difficult. One such unethical practice in which nurses could

BOX 12.6 ETHICAL FORMATIONS: TYPES OF HEALTH CARE FRAUD REPORTED BY THE FBI IN 2006

- **Billing for services not rendered**: The provider submits a bill even when no medical service of any kind was provided, the service described in the claim for payment was not the service provided, or the service was previously billed and the claim already had been paid.
- **Upcoding of services**: The provider submits a bill using a procedure code that yields a higher payment than the code for the actual service rendered. Cases of upcoding include a routine follow-up doctor's office visit being billed instead as an initial or comprehensive office visit, group therapy being billed as individual therapy, unilateral procedures being billed as bilateral procedures, and 30-minute sessions being billed as 50 minutes or more.
- **Upcoding of items**: The provider delivers basic equipment to a patient, such as a manually propelled wheelchair, but instead bills for the more expensive motorized version of the wheelchair.
- **Duplicate claims**: The provider files two claims on the same service or item, but usually changes the date or some other portion on the second claim.
- **Unbundling**: The provider submits bills in a fragmented fashion to maximize the reimbursement for various tests or procedures that are required to be billed together at a reduced cost. For example, clinical laboratory tests are ordered individually or in a panel (e.g., lipid profile), but the provider will bill within each panel as if the tests had been done separately on different days.
- **Excessive services**: The provider bills for excessive services beyond the patient's actual needs, such as a medical care supplier billing for 30 wound care kits per week for a nursing home patient who only requires a dressing change once a day, or a provider billing for daily medical office visits when only monthly visits are needed.
- **Medically unnecessary services**: The provider bills for services not needed or unjustified based on the patient's medical condition, diagnosis, or progress, such as a provider who bills for an electrocardiogram (EKG) for a patient with no signs or symptoms that justify the test.
- **Kickbacks**: The provider or other staff in the system engages in a scheme to receive an illegal compensation, such as when money or gifts are accepted in exchange for the referral of a patient for healthcare services paid by Medicare or Medicaid. Gifts can include everything from money to jewelry to free paid vacations.

Source: Largely quoted from Federal Bureau of Investigation. (2006). FBI 2006 financial crimes report to the public: Health care fraud. Retrieved from http://www.fbi.gov/stats-services/publications/fcs_report2006/

be involved, unintentionally or otherwise, is in the billing and maintenance of fraudulent records on ambulance transfers of patients. There are many cases of fraudulent billing, but in one particular case, Tracie Gieger, a licensed practical nurse and wife of Jeffery Gieger, who owned an ambulance transfer company, was knowingly and actively involved in the billing fraud. After reviewing her case, the Mississippi Board of Nursing revoked her license in October 1998 based on her felony conviction. See more detail of the Giegers' ambulance fraud in Box 12.7.

BOX 12.7 ETHICAL FORMATIONS: AN EXAMPLE OF BILLING FRAUD: *UNITED STATES OF AMERICA V. JEFFERY W. GIEGER & TRACIE L. GIEGER*

On February 27, 1998, in the Southern District of Mississippi, the owners of Gieger Transfer Services, an ambulance company, were sentenced to 80 months in prison and ordered to pay restitution of $228,917 and a $12,500 fine (and 3 years of supervised release after the prison sentence was complete). The defendants (Tracie & Jeffery Gieger) billed Medicare $400 per ambulance trip, claiming that patients taken on nonemergency ambulance trips were bed confined when, in fact, many could walk and had no need for ambulance transportation. A substantial portion of the money paid to the United States under the agreement was derived from the forced sale of beachfront properties purchased by the owners following the sale of their company in September 1997. The forced sale of the properties resulted from a $2.25 million civil settlement with the owners and the company formerly owned by them. (U.S. Department of Justice, 1998)

The Giegers were electronically billing the cases. While Tracie was still an LPN, the Giegers founded the Gieger Transfer Service, Inc./Gieger Ambulance Service (GAS) and began transporting emergency and nonemergency patients. The company expanded quickly, and by 1997 GAS operated more than 40 ambulances in 12 counties in rural southeastern Mississippi.

A large number of their ambulance transfers were elders on Medicare. After they founded GAS, the Giegers began billing Medicare by filing all of their nonemergency transfers as bed-confined patients, a misrepresentation that sparked the FBI investigation in 1996. They directed their paramedics and emergency medical technicians (EMTs) not to use the word "ambulatory" on the patient transfer report. The Giegers were indicted on 57 counts, which included charges of Medicare fraud, conspiracy to submit false claims, money laundering, transmitting money instruments or funds derived from specified unlawful activities, and a number of other similar charges. In 1997, the Giegers were tried on 46 of the 57 counts of the indictment. The jury returned a Count 1 guilty verdict—a conspiracy to submit false claims to Medicare. However, the sentencing of the Giegers was increased because they abused a position of trust and the conspiracy involved vulnerable victims (related to the patients' ages).

On September 24, 1999, the Giegers filed an appeal but the appellate court upheld the convictions with the exception of the enhancement of the "vulnerable victim" provision. The Giegers' prison term was completed in 2004.

Source: U.S. Department of Justice. (1998). *Health care fraud report—Fiscal year 1998. Selected cases.* Retrieved from http://www.justice.gov/dag/pubdoc/health98.htm; Mississippi State Board of Nursing. (1998, October). *Disciplinary summary.* Retrieved from http://www.msbn.state.ms.us/pdf/dis1098.PDF; United States v. Jeffery W. Gieger & Tracie L. Gieger, 190 F.3d 661 (5th Cir. 1999).

Nurses can be involved in many other potentially unethical situations. Sometimes nurse practitioners or other providers are unaware of their own acts of health care fraud. One instance is when they accept gifts or possibly money from pharmaceutical companies in exchange for prescribing that company's medications. Nurses' involvement in the ordering of supplies from medical suppliers and other vendors can pose similar situations.

BOX 12.8 ETHICAL FORMATIONS: TWO CASES OF HEALTH CARE FRAUD SCHEMES REPORTED IN 2005

HealthSouth Corporation, Birmingham, Alabama, 2005

This corporation paid the U.S. government $327 million to settle allegations of fraud against Medicare and other federally insured healthcare programs. The government alleged that the rehabilitative services of HealthSouth engaged in three health care fraud schemes to cheat the government. The first scheme, requiring a $170 million settlement, involved alleged false claims for outpatient physical therapy services that were not properly supported by certified plans of care, were not administered by licensed physical therapists, or were not for one-on-one therapy as the corporation represented in the billing. The second scheme, requiring a $65 million settlement, involved alleged accounting fraud that resulted in overbilling Medicare on hospital cost reports and home office cost statements. The third scheme, requiring a $92 million settlement, involved allegedly billing Medicare for a range of unallowable costs, such as luxury entertainment and travel expenses for the annual administrators' meeting at Disney World, among many other incurred expenses. The remaining $76 million settlement involved four ***qui tam* lawsuits**, also known as whistleblowing lawsuits. (The term *qui tam* is an abbreviation of a Latin phrase that means "he who sues for the king as well as for himself." *Qui tam* lawsuits are filed by private citizens, who sue on behalf of the federal government by alleging fraud against those organizations that received government funding. The private citizen who filed the lawsuit receives a portion of the recovery money if the case is successful, and the government receives the major portion of recovered funds.)

Eisenhower Medical Center, Rancho Mirage, California, 2005

This corporation paid the U.S. government $8 million to settle allegations of overbilling federal health insurance programs. A former employee also filed a *qui tam* lawsuit. The allegation was that the healthcare financial advisors helped the hospital to seek reimbursement for unallowable costs, and specifically that the advisors prepared two cost reports—an inflated one submitted to Medicare and one designed for internal use only that reflected accurately the amount of reimbursement the hospital should have received.

Source: U.S. Department of Health and Human Services and the Department of Justice. (2006, August). *Health care fraud and abuse control program annual report for FY 2005.* Retrieved from http://oig.hhs.gov/publications/docs/hcfac/hcfacreport2005.pdf

Hospital-associated health care fraud is a tremendous problem in the United States. Two cases from 2005 are highlighted in Box 12.8. One case involved HealthSouth Corporation, whose central office is located in Birmingham, Alabama, and is the largest provider of integrated healthcare services in the country, with numerous locations across the United States; the other case was at Eisenhower Medical Center in Rancho Mirage, California. These two cases and the Gieger case are good examples of the cases that occur each year throughout the United States.

To reduce or prevent fraudulent schemes, Pearson et al. (2003) offered an exemplary list of broad normative ethical obligations for organizations. Although these obligations refer to organizations as a whole and not the individual leaders, providers of care and corporate leaders must make an effort to uphold these ethical obligations. Refer to Box 12.9, for a list of these ethical obligations.

BOX 12.9 ETHICAL FORMATIONS: EXEMPLARY ETHICAL OBLIGATIONS FOR ORGANIZATIONS

An exemplary ethical organization must:

1. Hold a set of values that emphasizes care of the sick and the promotion of health.
2. Involve key stakeholders to identify values in managing conflicts.
3. Clearly communicate the organization's set of ethical values to all employees and to the public.
4. Recognize that the full range of activities influences the ethical quality of patient care.
5. Stay alert to conflicts that could threaten the values.
6. Avoid making the same mistakes as in previous situations.
7. Ensure that it acts on its values: It "walks the walk" as well as "talks the talk."
8. Partner only with others who live by compatible values.

Source: Pearson, S. D., Sabin, J. E., & Emanuel, E. J. (2003). *No margin, no mission: Health-care organizations and the quest for ethical excellence* (p. 33). Oxford, UK: Oxford University Press.

Prevention strategies are the most effective and efficient ways to deter financial loss through fraud. For example, there is a supportive website by Blue Cross Blue Shield where people can access information regarding facts, statistics, and types of fraud (http://www.bcbs.com/report-healthcare-fraud/). To report a suspicious case of Medicare fraud or seek further directions on reporting, call the Medicare hotline at 1-800-447-8477. Nurses or others who suspect fraud of any kind should call 1-877-327-2583 to report their observations. Most defrauded companies will never recover their monetary losses; and they could be out of business literally in months, even days, if organizations do not put prevention measures in place. When organizations create a fraud prevention program, administrators or outside consultants need to assess the state of affairs within the organization. Strategies in the assessment phase include:

- The CEO or the board should consider hiring an external consultant to conduct the assessment.
- Answering the question: "What are the current fraud risks?"
- Interviews with stakeholders, which will usually reveal the organization's risks for fraud.
- An independent agent performing an internal audit.
- Setting benchmarks for measuring best practices to prevent fraud.

Adams, Campbell, Campbell, and Rose (2006) included a sample questionnaire for assessing risks of fraud in organizations. The questions yield quantitative and qualitative data. Executives or a consultant could adapt the following questions for their organization's survey and have key people complete it:

- How frequently (e.g., weekly, monthly, quarterly, or yearly) does management review key performance indicators?
- Have the board and members of the management team delineated specific responsibilities relating to the oversight and management of fraud risks with the organization?
- What is the fraud risk management budget in dollars? In full-time equivalent resources?
- How frequently (e.g., every 6, 12, 24, or 36 months) is the fraud risk management strategy updated?
- How frequently are organizational charts reviewed to ensure proper segregation of duties?
- Is an anonymous process available at any time for employees to use in reporting improprieties or breaches of ethics?
- Is the anonymous reporting process also available to customers and suppliers?
- Do you have a formal code of ethics or conduct for the board or senior management?
- Please list what you think are the top three fraud business risks that your organization faces. How would you assess your risk of exposure to each of these? (p. 58)

A new prevention program should be initiated or an existing one improved based on the assumptions that arise from the assessment data. Some of the necessary components of the program include an ethics educational program for all employees, a code of ethical conduct, and a hotline program. Once the program is in place, ongoing monitoring and training are necessary. Nurses need to serve in key positions to spot or report health care fraud in hospitals, clinics, or agencies. Refer to Box 12.10 to complete an analysis of the three cases already presented on health care fraud.

Leadership Ethics

A **leader** influences a group or organization by engaging in relationships to further the shared goals of the other leaders and followers. At the center of leadership is ethics. Leaders face extreme moral demands on a daily basis while they strive to provide direction and shape the ethical climate and culture of the organization. Best said by "Buzz" McCoy (2007), the definition of a **successful leader** is an **ethical leader** who

> attempts to align the values of the enterprise with those of the individuals who form it, striving to facilitate a sense of deep meaning and commitment in their work. A precondition is a heightened degree of sensitivity on the part of the leader to the values of society, the enterprise, and the individuals who constitute it. (p. 2)

BOX 12.10 ETHICAL FORMATIONS: AN ANALYSIS OF THE THREE CASES ON FRAUD

These three cases involve the Giegers and the two hospital cases that were highlighted in Boxes 12.7 and 12.8. Please review the cases and then refer to the exemplary ethical obligations for organizations as outlined by Pearson et al. (2003) and presented in Box 12.9.

The Gieger Case

- Based on the jury's rationale for sentencing, make a list of the exemplary ethical obligations that the Giegers, paramedics, and EMTs did not uphold.
- Do you believe that, as a paramedic working for the Giegers, your role would be to see that unethical practice was not committed? Why or why not? Give your rationale based on an ethical framework–theory, approach, or principle.
- If you had been a paramedic working for the Giegers, jot down ways that you could have acted to alleviate or arrest these problems. Keep your ethical framework in mind as you compose your strategies.

The Two Hospitals' Cases

- Describe the feelings of conflict you might experience if you were working as a registered nurse in some area of either of these two organizations when the lawsuits were filed and became public knowledge.
- Make a list of the exemplary ethical obligations that these two hospitals did not uphold.
- Explain actions you would take in light of the charges against your place of employment. Give your rationale based on one ethical framework–theory, approach, or principle.

Rost (1995; as cited in Griffith, 2007) offered two ways of analyzing the ethical nature of leadership. The first way is related to the process and performance of leadership. To analyze the ethical perspectives of process and performance, a question needs to be answered: "Is the leadership being done in a way that is ethical at the moment?" To answer this question, a person needs to examine the degree and nature of the influence relationship between the leaders and followers. For the process and performance to be regarded as ethical, people in the leader–follower relationship should be using a variety of nonforced measures to influence people and develop a collaborative agreement that reflects shared purposes. Griffith (2007) proposed that a prerequisite to analyzing the process and performance of leadership is to search for an ethical meaning in the very existence of influence relationships by answering such questions as: "Is it ethical for leaders to influence the values and purposes of followers?" and "Does the influence relationship deprive the followers of their free will?" The second way of analyzing the ethical nature of leadership is to determine whether the shared and intended change in the community or organization is ethical. Important to this second analysis is to scrutinize what the community or organization is proposing.

The goals must be genuinely communal and shared by everyone in the community as a whole.

Normative Leadership Theories

Leaders who are mindful of ethics motivate others to act in ethical ways. Ethics as praxis requires that leaders must first rethink their values on a personal level and then move from a personal ethics to a collective way of thinking. To lead with **ethics as praxis** means that a person clarifies, reflects on, makes sense of, practices, and embodies a leadership theory. At the foundation of normative leadership theories are the norms of ethical behavior, or how people ought to act, which originate from the classical ethical theories. Comprehending ethical theory contributes to a leader's expertise in leader and follower behaviors.

The ethical perspectives of three theories will be the focus of this section. Leadership theories selected for this section are not representative of all leadership theories, but these three—servant leadership, transformational leadership, and authentic leadership—have an emphasis in higher morality, ethical reasoning, altruism, caring, and the common good. These attributes are important for nursing leaders if they are to lead with ethics as praxis and have a greater influence on organizational outcomes.

Servant Leaders

Robert Greenleaf coined the term "servant leader" in his 1977 book, *Servant Leadership*. A **servant leader** consistently makes decisions to further the good of the group of followers over any decisions that satisfy self-interests. Servant leaders engage others and search for ethically meaningful ways to make decisions. In fact, Griffith (2007) identified servant leadership as the ultimate level of ethicality. Servant leaders exemplify the values of moral sensitivity, altruism, caring, empathy, and ongoing development. The characteristics of servant leadership vary from author to author, but Johnson (2012) identified five attributes he believed as most central to servant leadership:

- Stewardship: Acting on behalf of others and being an agent of the followers
- Obligation: Taking seriously the responsibilities to the followers and the organization
- Partnership: Viewing followers as partners, not subordinates
- Emotional healing: Being empathetic, an active listener, and instilling a sense of wholeness
- Elevating purpose: Striving for a high moral purpose and understanding the roles of followers and of oneself as a leader

Some people link weakness to any type of service and believe that servant leadership is an unrealistic and weak theory that does not work in many situations. However, the behavior of those being served must be the measurement for the extent to which servant leaders are successful. Greenleaf (1977/2002) stated that the test of servant leader success is to evaluate whether those served grow as persons: "do they, while being served, become healthier, wiser, freer, more autonomous, more likely themselves to become servants? And, what is the effect on the least privileged in society; will they benefit, or, at least, not be further deprived?" (p. 27). With the rapid changes away from traditional leadership theories, people are moving toward servant leadership theory as a simplistic yet ideal and ethical way of being in relationships with other leaders and followers.

Transformational Leaders

Ethical obligations, relationships, and deontology are at the center of transformational leadership. James McGregor Burns (1978) distinguished transformational leaders from transactional leaders, with a **transformational leader** focusing on raising the moral benchmark on human behaviors of both leaders and followers, internalizing a sense of commitment, facilitating the higher-order needs and creativity of followers, placing importance on relationships and shared goals, and striving for follower empowerment to promote transformation (Burns, 1978). They strive for change in the culture of an organization rather than working within the status quo and are measured by the degree of transformation demonstrated by the followers.

While Bernard Bass (1995; as cited in Johnson, 2012) researched and expanded the work of Burns, he promoted the idea that a transformational leader can also exhibit transactional leadership qualities. Transactional leaders focus on the management processes and controls facilitated by the values of responsibility, fairness, and honesty, but they persuade followers to conform by exercising their power. By using an approach that is utilitarian, transactional leaders evaluate the "morality of actions based on their outcomes" (p. 190).

Through research, four components of transformational leadership were identified (Bass, 2008):

- Idealized influence: A solid ground of high morality exists with ideals of trust and authenticity.
- Inspirational motivation: The personality traits and charisma of the transformational leaders inspire followers to commit to and search for meaning in their work toward achieving shared values and goals.
- Intellectual stimulation: Transformational leaders encourage followers to think freely and be creative with ways to connect to the leader and achieve shared goals.
- Individual consideration: Individuals are boosted by the transformational leader's focus on each person as an individual who has a need for self-actualization, growth, and opportunities. The leader's mentoring and teaching enhance the continued growth and success of the followers.

Other features of transformational leaders include seeing the big picture in detailed matters, role modeling, networking, and flexibility (Taylor, 2009). There are pseudotransformational leaders who claim they are transformational but are unethical in their relationships and actions (Bass, 1995; as cited in Johnson, 2012). The unethical behaviors of pseudoleaders result from their own self-interests and personal goals instead of the collective benefit for all. In contrast, the high moral standards of transformational leaders serve as the guiding principles in relationships and decision making.

Authentic Leaders

Servant leadership, transformational leadership, and authentic leadership have many commonalities, but a distinguishing feature of authentic leaders is that they are deeply anchored in relational transparency (honesty and openness) in their sense of self and their sense of right and wrong (Shirley, 2006). An **authentic leader** finds true identity in the self by retrieving and developing the soul; through an authentic presence, they inspire and encourage well-being and thriving (eudaimonia) in their followers. Leaders with **authentic presence** are people-focused leaders who are true to themselves and are deeply aware of who they are and how others perceive them. They epitomize Shakespeare's words, "This, above all: Unto thine own self be true." Being true to self translates to being powerful, and with that power, an authentic leader serves as a moral compass for, a facilitator to, and a supporter of followers striving to reach their high values and purposes. Many people say that when people encounter an authentic person, they know it because there is real genuine presence. According to Irvine and Reger (2006), the eight characteristics of authentic presence are clarity, courage, integrity, service, trust, humility, compassion, and vulnerability. Advantages of authentic leaders are that they are highly effective and unite their followers; disadvantages are that authenticity is overstated and sometimes is indistinguishable because various interpretations of the term exist (Johnson, 2012).

Leader Challenges

Donley (2005) stated, "Health care is undergoing a violent revolution that has disrupted traditional healthcare practices and undermined trust in the health professions. Business values have replaced or crowded out healthcare norms and many professional values" (Section 9).

Nurse leaders confront many ethical issues as a result of this aggressive healthcare environment, and when these issues are combined, they create extreme stress in nurses who are only trying to manage these challenges and stay balanced. One reason for this stress is the clash in values among people involved in decision making. In this environment, stress is evidenced in all relationships, not just in the usual difficult and uncivil relationships that nurses encounter in horizontal or vertical violence, but also in relationships that are generally more pleasant under normal circumstances.

Another reason for high stress is a toxic or destructive leader displaying unethical behaviors. Kellerman (2004) explained that people should not overlook bad leadership or link all leadership with good leadership because "it is confusing . . . misleading . . . and does a disservice" (p. 12). There are seven classifications of bad leaders, as identified by Kellerman: incompetent leaders, rigid leaders, intemperate leaders, callous leaders, corrupt leaders, insular leaders, and evil leaders. Followers' behaviors mirror leader behaviors.

Some of the issues that Hendren (2011), Thompson (2008), and Huston (2008) identified as what they perceive as the biggest challenges and needs that nursing faces in this intense environment, both now and in the future, are:

- Maintaining a high degree of patient safety and quality, improved outcomes of care, and evidenced-based care and documentation
- Patient satisfaction
- Reimbursement and cost-cutting pressures to meet the expectations of good patient outcomes
- Retention, an uninterrupted and robust pipeline of nurses in the making, and the nursing shortage—a continued problem for the near future
- Excellent decision-making skills
- Clever political skills
- New healthcare delivery models and team building to enhance the judicious use of the workforce and decrease waste
- Acceptable channels for succession of nursing leaders at all levels of administration

Patsy Anderson, an expert in organizational behavior and a nurse educator, stated that nurse leaders in healthcare centers often have difficulty saying "no" to the demand that their nursing personnel meet or exceed the increasingly raised expectations for patient outcomes while absorbing extra work in light of streamlined organizational budgets that have less resource allocation for nursing positions (personal communication, December 5, 2011). When nurse leaders give in and accept the responsibility of doing more with less, serious issues are at stake—issues of patient satisfaction and safety, better health outcomes, and the provision of quality services to the public.

Ethical dilemmas arise because these challenges are not easily tackled in healthcare organizations. Forced overtime of nurses, increased workload, and burnout from stress and fatigue jeopardize the well-being of patients and nurses. Another consideration is whether the healthcare organization's monetary sustainability is enough to offer quality services to the public. In response to economic pressures and stakeholder concerns, CEOs often overrule nurse-leader decisions to preserve quality care in favor of budget-related changes. These decisions often result in an infringement in one or more bioethical principles—autonomy, beneficence, nonmaleficence, and justice.

- Autonomy: Freedom of choice
  - The difficulties faced by the profession as a whole in saying "no" to expanded nursing responsibilities without a corresponding increase in autonomy makes it harder for nurses to maintain quality standards in practice. Fatigue and stress are associated with higher workloads, more job responsibilities, and overtime.
- Beneficence: Promote good
  - The increased workloads limit the ability of individual nurses and the profession as a whole to fulfill the expectations of promoting good in practice and care of patients.
- Nonmaleficence: Do no harm
  - The risk of missed or substandard care and the risk of corresponding worsening patient outcomes increase as nurses must take on larger workloads with fewer resources.
- Justice: Fairness
  - Individual nurses, as well as the profession as a whole, suffer injustice when job opportunities are diminished as a result of medical centers being forced to decrease services or close their doors to patients due to financial instability.
  - It is unfair to nurses when healthcare centers, whether by increasing workloads or by financial instability, limit the ability of nurses to give competent nursing care.
  - Issues of social justice are raised when patients are limited in their ability to receive provision of services and access to care comparable to patients in other locations.

Using Power to Achieve Leader Success

Power is defined as influence that leaders have over their followers in order to achieve common goals. In almost every interaction within an organization, power is used in some way. When leaders use their power in a positive way to guide and direct, followers more easily develop ethical ways to work. If leaders stay centered in ethics, they will use their power to create pragmatic solutions to achieve the organization's shared goals, even when they are faced with daily temptations to do otherwise. In 1959, French and Raven identified five bases of power. Leaders can use each power base alone or in combination with the other four bases.

- Legitimate power: Power that originates from the leader's title or position and from the belief by followers that the title gives the leader a right to that power over them.
- Referent power: Power that is created when followers believe the leader has admirable qualities they want to possess.

- Expert power: Power that develops when followers believe that the leader has expertise in the knowledge or skills related to the task or job.
- Reward power: Power that develops when leaders offer followers certain rewards for completion of tasks or for good behaviors, combined with the belief of followers that the leader will follow through with the rewards.
- Coercive power: Power that is based on the belief by followers that the leader has the ability to discipline or impose a penalty when the followers do not follow the required behaviors; leaders need to use caution in exercising this type of power.

Often, power is negatively equated with evilness and corruption, as evidenced by the many past moral failures in the history of leadership. If the leader abuses power for self-interest motives and personal gain instead of following through with good intentions, the result is wrongdoing. In a letter to Mandell Creighton on April 5, 1887, Lord Acton stated, "Power tends to corrupt and absolute power corrupts absolutely." Lord Acton, an English magistrate, became a moral judge as he held the best-known men to a historical standard or precedence (Acton Institute, 2011).

It is a well-known fact that power can corrupt a person in authority, and leadership is a complex, power-based relationship. Leaders must build strong, positive power bases to influence others. There are several ways for leaders to use power positively to promote success, but in this section three ways are covered—collaboration, quality, and leadership succession planning.

Collaboration

Principled leaders use their power to make collaborative decisions for best possible patient and organizational outcomes. For leaders to engage in **collaboration,** they must listen to new perspectives on what could be done to ensure best practices and confront difficulties within the organization. They seek open dialogue from wise people outside the organization and at all levels within the organization. A written ethical guide for leaders is the *Code of Ethics for Nurses with Interpretive Statements* (ANA, 2001).

Quality

Quality means that a leader uses power to strive for excellence in the delivery of care. The leaders are responsible for implementing quality throughout every process of the organization. Leaders who are ethical know that their obligation to the organization and community at large is to (1) focus on quality at all levels, (2) use benchmarking to denote successes and failures, and (3) use innovations to heighten quality. Organizations can improve their image if leaders use common sense judgments about ensuring quality and cutting wastes in organizational time and spending. The ANA *Code of Ethics for Nurses with Interpretive Statements*

(2001) clearly indicates the need for nursing leaders, as well as all nurses, to be accountable for quality in standards of care.

Leader Succession Planning

Leader succession planning is a way for leaders to allow and enable other leaders to surface within an organization so that successors have an opportunity to develop and use their leadership skills. Once people emerge as leader candidates, the existing leaders need to mentor them for future succession without fear of territorial loss. Ethical leaders realize the critical nature of having leaders in the making through a strong leadership succession program for the long-term success of the organization.

Good, ethical leaders are hard to find, but when an organization finds that leader, it must invest in that leader for the sake of the organization. People often place significant value on the trustworthiness and authenticity of the leader. Nurse leaders are often confronted with moral indecision. Ethical leadership has become an essential part of organizational leadership, largely because of the past leadership failures that have occurred in big business and healthcare organizations throughout the world. These failures have led to character-driven leadership styles such as the three leadership theories presented in this chapter. For guidance, leaders and staff nurses can refer to the American Nurses Association's *Code of Ethics for Nurses with Interpretative Statements* (2001) (see Box 12.11 for the essential aspects of ethical leadership).

BOX 12.11 ETHICAL FORMATIONS: ESSENTIAL ASPECTS FROM THE *CODE OF ETHICS FOR NURSES WITH INTERPRETIVE STATEMENTS* FOR FORMING ETHICAL LEADERSHIP

- All nurses, regardless of role, have a responsibility to create, maintain, and contribute to environments of practice that support nurses fulfilling their ethical obligations (6.2, p. 21).
- Organizational structures, role description . . . contribute to environments that can either present barriers or foster ethical practice and professional fulfillment (6.2, p. 21).
- Nurse administrators have a particular responsibility to assure that employees are treated fairly . . . (6.3, p. 21).
- Nurses should not remain employed in facilities that routinely violate patient rights or require nurses to severely and repeatedly compromise standards of practice or personal morality (6.3, p. 21).
- Organizational changes are difficult to accomplish and may require persistent efforts over time (6.3, p. 21).
- The nurse as administrator or manager must establish, maintain, and promote conditions of employment that enable nurses within that organization or community setting to practice in accord with accepted standards of nursing practice (7.1, pp. 22–23).

KEY POINTS

- An organization's relationship to its environment and the organization's interpretation of reality, truth, human nature, and human relationships represent the ethical dimensions that shape the organizational culture.
- Each organizational culture—adaptability, mission, clan, and bureaucratic—has the potential to be successful if the strategic plans that relate to the desired culture are accomplished and maintained.
- Organizational ethics is a way of acting that includes culture, processes, outcomes, and character.
- The ethical climate refers to the organizational members' shared perceptions on the values of power, trust, and interactions on how ethical decisions are made.
- Trust is the multifaceted, essential ingredient that serves as a lubricant for all operations and values in organizations. Without trust in organizations and among people, organizational values and relationships erode and crumble.
- Unethical and illegal behaviors committed by people ultimately shape the ambiance and character of the organization.
- Regulators of organizations and the government mandated the development of compliance programs to prevent unlawful behaviors and to promote conformity to regulations involving legal actions.
- In 2006 alone, health care fraud, which is reported separately from corporate fraud, increased dramatically. The FBI uncovered billions of dollars in losses with a total of 588 indictments and 534 convictions. Many other cases are still pending.
- Nurses are at an increased risk of participating, knowingly or unknowingly, in health care fraud cases. They need to develop a sharp perception for spotting dubious fraudulent cases in their workplace and report their suspicions to the fraud hotline.
- A leader, whose leadership is centered in ethics, influences a group or organization by engaging in relationships to further the shared goals of other leaders and the followers.
- Ethics as praxis means that a leader clarifies, reflects on, makes sense of, practices, and embodies a leadership theory.
- Some theories that are considered normative leadership theories include servant leadership, transformative leadership, and authentic leadership. These theories place a higher emphasis on morality, ethical reasoning, altruism, caring, and the common good.
- Leader challenges in today's healthcare system include maintaining patient safety, quality care, and satisfaction; issues of cost-cutting and reimbursement for services; nurse retention; political issues; and decision-making and team building skills.
- Nurse leaders use their power to influence followers in a positive, ethical way.

References

Acton Institute for the Study of Religion & Liberty. (2011). *About the Acton Institute.* Retrieved from http://www.acton.org/index/about

Adams, G. W., Campbell, D. R., Campbell, M., & Rose, M. P. (2006, January). Fraud prevention: An investment no one can afford to forego. *The CPA Journal,* pp. 56–59. Retrieved from http://www.nysscpa.org/cpajournal/2006/106/essentials/p56.htm

American Nurses Association. (2001). *Code of ethics for nurses with interpretive statements.* Silver Spring, MD: Author.

Association of Certified Fraud Examiners. (2004). *2004 report to the nations on occupational fraud and abuse.* Retrieved from http://www.acfe.com/uploadedFiles/ACFE_Website/Content/documents/2004RttN.pdf

Association of Certified Fraud Examiners. (2010). *Report to the nations on occupational fraud and abuse: 2010 global fraud study.* Retrieved from http://www.sacpasociety.com/docs/default-document-library/2011/09/15/Fraud_Report_2010.pdf?Status=Master

Bass, B. M. (1995). The ethics of transformational leadership. In J. Ciulla (Ed.), *Ethics: The heart of leadership* (pp. 169–192). Westport, CT: Praeger.

Bass, B. M. (with Bass, R.) (2008). *The Bass handbook of leadership: Theory, research and managerial applications* (4th ed.). New York, NY: Free Press/A Division of Simon & Schuster.

Boyle, P. J., DuBose, E. R., Ellingson, S. J., Guinn, D. E., & McCurdy, D. B. (2001). *Organizational ethics in health care: Principles, cases, and practical solutions.* San Francisco, CA: Jossey-Bass/John Wiley & Sons.

Brown, M. T. (2006). *Corporate integrity: Rethinking organizational ethics and leadership.* New York, NY: Cambridge University Press.

Burns, J. M. (1978/1982). *Leadership.* New York, NY: Harper & Row.

Cooper, T. L. (2006). *The responsible administrator: An approach to ethics for the administrative role* (5th ed.). San Francisco, CA: Jossey-Bass/John Wiley & Sons.

Daft, R. L. (2004). *Organizational theory and design* (8th ed.). Mason, OH: South-Western.

Desio, P. (2010). An overview of the organizational sentencing guidelines. *U.S. Sentencing Commission.* Retrieved from http://www.ussc.gov/Education_and_Training/Guidelines_Educational_Materials/Organizational_Guidelines.cfm

Donley, Sr. R. (2005). Challenges for nursing in the 21st century. *Nursing Economics, 23*(6), 312–318. Retrieved from http://www.medscape.com/viewarticle/521379

Federal Bureau of Investigation. (2006). *FBI 2006 financial crime report: Health care fraud.* Retrieved from http://www.fbi.gov/stats-services/publications/fcs_report2006/financial-crimes-report-to-the-public-fiscal-year-2006

French, J. R. P., & Raven, B. (1959). The bases of social power. In D. Cartwright (Ed.), *Studies in social power* (pp. 150–167). Ann Arbor, MI: University of Michigan Press.

Greenleaf, R. K. (1977/2002). *Servant leadership.* Mahwah, NJ: Paulist Press.

Griffith, S. D. (2007, July). Servant leadership, ethics and the domains of leadership. *Servant leadership research roundtable.* Regent University. Retrieved from http://www.regent.edu/acad/global/publications/sl_proceedings/2007/griffith.pdf

Gutmann, A. (1995). The virtues of democratic self-constraint. In A. Etzioni (Ed.), *New communitarian thinking: Persons, virtues, institutions, and communities* (pp. 154–169). Charlottesville, VA: University of Virginia Press.

Hendren, R. (2011, November). Top 5 challenges facing nursing in 2012. *Healthleadersmedia.* Retrieved from http://www.healthleadersmedia.com/print/NRS-273338/Top-5-Challenges-Facing-Nursing-in-2012

Huston, C. (2008). Preparing nurse leaders for 2020. *Journal of Nursing Management, 16*, 905–911.

Irvine, D., & Reger, J. (2006). *The authentic leader: It's about presence, not position.* Sanford, FL: DC Press/A Division of the Diogenes Consortium.

Jennings, M. M. (2006). *The seven signs of ethical collapse: How to spot moral meltdowns in companies...before it's too late.* New York, NY: St. Martin's Press.

Johnson, G. E. (2007). *Ethics in the workplace: Tools and tactics for organizational transformation.* Los Angeles, CA: Sage.

Johnson, G. E. (2012). *Meeting the ethical challenges of leadership: Casting light or shadow* (4th ed.). Los Angeles, CA: Sage.

Kellerman, B. (2004). *Bad leadership: What it is, how it happens, and why it happens (Leadership for the common good).* Boston, MA: Harvard Business School Press.

Knights, D., & O'Leary, M. (2006). Leadership, ethics and responsibility to the other. *Journal of Business Ethics, 67*, 125–137.

Kovanic, N., & Johnson, K. D. (2004). *Lies and truths: Leadership ethics in the 21st century.* Terre Haute, IN: Rule of Thumb.

Kramer, M., & Schmalenberg, C. (2002). Staff nurses identify essentials of magnetism. In M. McClure & A. Hinshaw (Eds.), *Magnet hospitals revisited* (pp. 25–59). Washington, DC: American Nurses.

Laschinger, H., Shamian, J., & Thomson, D. (2001). Impact of magnet hospital characteristics on nurses' perceptions of trust, burnout, quality of care and work satisfaction. *Nursing Economics, 19*, 209–219.

McCoy, B. H. (2007). *Living into leadership: A journal in ethics.* Stanford, CA: Stanford Business Book—Stanford University Press.

Mississippi State Board of Nursing. (1998, October). Disciplinary summary. Retrieved from http://www.msbn.state.ms.us/pdf/dis1098.PDF

Morrison, E. E. (2006). *Ethics in health administration: A practical approach for decision makers.* Sudbury, MA: Jones and Bartlett.

Pearson, S. D., Sabin, J. E., & Emanuel, E. J. (2003). *No margin, no mission: Health-care organizations and the quest for ethical excellence.* Oxford, UK: Oxford University Press.

Perkins, K. L. (2010, September 22). *Statement before the senate judiciary committee, Washington, D.C.: The FBI's efforts to combat significant financial crimes.* Federal Bureau of Investigation. Retrieved from http://www.fbi.gov/news/testimony/the-fbis-efforts-to-combat-significant-financial-crimes

Ritvo, R. A., Ohlsen, J. D., & Holland, T. P. (2004). *Ethical governance in health care: A board leadership guide for building an ethical culture.* Chicago, IL: Health Forum.

Rost, J. (1995). Leadership: A discussion about ethics. *Business Ethics Quarterly, 5*(1), 129–142.

Shirley, M. R. (2006). Authentic leaders creating healthy work environments for nursing practice. *American Journal of Critical Care, 15*, 266–267.

Shore, D. A. (2007). The (sorry) state of trust in the American healthcare enterprise. In D. A. Shore (Ed.), *The trust crisis in healthcare: Causes, consequences, and cures* (pp. 3–20). Oxford, UK: Oxford University Press.

Stockdale, H. (2010, March 15). Medicare program integrity: Activities to protect Medicare from payment errors, fraud, and abuse. *Congressional Research Service.* Retrieved from http://aging.senate.gov/crs/medicare18.pdf

Taylor, R. (2009). Leadership theories and the development of nurses in primary health care. *Primary Health Care, 19*(9), 40–45.

Thompson, P. A. (2008). Key challenges facing American nurse leaders. *Journal of Nursing Management, 16*(8), 912–914.

United States v. Jeffery W. Gieger & Tracie L. Gieger, 190 F.3d 661 (5th Cir. 1999).

U.S. Department of Health and Human Services and the Department of Justice. (2006, August). *Health care fraud and abuse control program annual report for fiscal year 2005.* Retrieved from http://oig.hhs.gov/publications/docs/hcfac/hcfacreport2005.pdf

U.S. Department of Justice. (1998). *Health care fraud report—Fiscal year 1998. Selected cases.* Retrieved from http://www.justice.gov/dag/pubdoc/health98.htm

Victor, B., & Cullen, J. B. (1987). A theory and measure of ethical climates in organizations. In W. C. Frederick (Ed.), *Research in corporate social performance and policy* (pp. 51–71). Greenwich, CT: JAI Press.

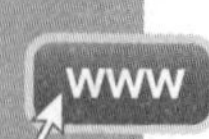

For a full suite of assignments and additional learning activities, use the access code located in the front of your book to visit this exclusive website: http://go.jblearning.com/butts. If you do not have an access code, you can obtain one at the site.

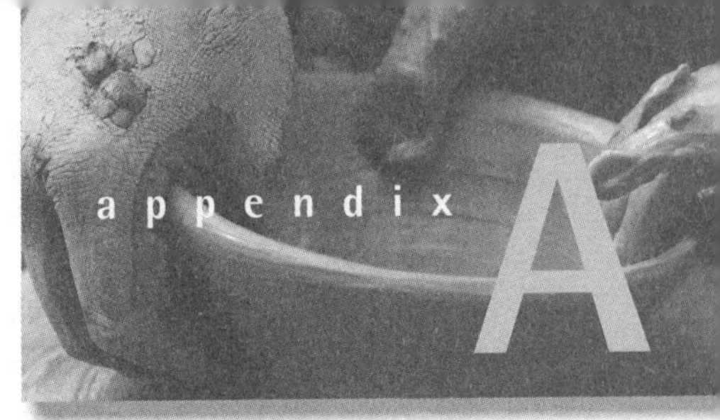

Code of Ethics for Nurses with Interpretive Statements

Preface

Ethics is an integral part of the foundation of nursing. Nursing has a distinguished history of concern for the welfare of the sick, injured and vulnerable and for social justice. This concern is embodied in the provision of nursing care to individuals and the community. Nursing encompasses the prevention of illness, the alleviation of suffering, and the protection, promotion and restoration of health in the care of individuals, families, groups and communities. Nurses act to change those aspects of social structures that detract from health and well-being. Individuals who become nurses are expected not only to adhere to the ideals and moral norms of the profession but also to embrace them as a part of what it means to be a nurse. The ethical tradition of nursing is self-reflective, enduring, and distinctive. A code of ethics makes explicit the primary goals, values, and obligations of the profession.

The Code of Ethics for Nurses serves the following purposes:

- It is a succinct statement of the ethical obligations and duties of every individual who enters the nursing profession.
- It is the profession's nonnegotiable ethical standard.
- It is an expression of nursing's own understanding of its commitment to society.

There are numerous approaches for addressing ethics; these include adopting or ascribing to ethical theories, including humanist, feminist, and social ethics, adhering to ethical principles, and cultivating virtues. The Code of Ethics for

Nurses reflects all of these approaches. The words "ethical" and "moral" are used throughout the Code of Ethics. "Ethical" is used to refer to reasons for decisions about how one ought to act, using the above mentioned approaches. In general, the word "moral" overlaps with "ethical" but is more aligned with personal belief and cultural values. Statements that describe activities and attributes of nurses in this Code of Ethics are to be understood as normative or prescriptive statements expressing expectations of ethical behavior.

The Code of Ethics uses the term *patient* to refer to recipients of nursing care. The derivation of this word refers to "one who suffers," reflecting a universal aspect of human existence. Nevertheless, it is recognized that nurses also provide services to those seeking health as well as those responding to illness, to students and to staff, in health care facilities as well as in communities. Similarly, the term *practice* refers to the actions of the nurse in whatever role the nurse fulfills, including direct patient care provider, educator, administrator, researcher, policy developer, or other. Thus, the values and obligations expressed in this Code of Ethics applies to nurses in all roles and settings.

The Code of Ethics for Nurses is a dynamic document. As nursing and its social context change, changes to the Code of Ethics are also necessary. The Code of Ethics consists of two components: the provisions and the accompanying interpretive statements. There are nine provisions. The first three describe the most fundamental values and commitments of the nurse; the next three address boundaries of duty and loyalty, and the last three address aspects of duties beyond individual patient encounters. For each provision, there are interpretive statements that provide greater specificity for practice and are responsive to the contemporary context of nursing. Consequently, the interpetive statements are subject to more frequent revision than are the provisions. Additional ethical guidance and detail can be found in ANA or constituent member association position statements that address clinical, research, administrative, educational or public policy issues.

Code of Ethics for Nurses with Interpretive Statements provides a framework for nurses to use in ethical analysis and decision-making. The Code of Ethics establishes the ethical standard for the profession. It is not negotiable in any setting nor is it subject to revision or amendment except by formal process of the House of Delegates of the ANA. The Code of Ethics for Nurses is a reflection of the proud ethical heritage of nursing, a guide for nurses now and in the future.

Code of Ethics for Nurses with Interpretive Statements

1 ***The nurse, in all professional relationships, practices with compassion and respect for the inherent dignity, worth and uniqueness of every individual, unrestricted by considerations of social or economic status, personal attributes, or the nature of health problems.***

1.1 Respect for human dignity

A fundamental principle that underlies all nursing practice is respect for the inherent worth, dignity, and human rights of every individual. Nurses take into account the needs and values of all persons in all professional relationships.

1.2 Relationships to patients

The need for health care is universal, transcending all individual differences. The nurse establishes relationships and delivers nursing services with respect for human needs and values, and without prejudice. An individual's lifestyle, value system and religious beliefs should be considered in planning health care with and for each patient. Such consideration does not suggest that the nurse necessarily agrees with or condones certain individual choices, but that the nurse respects the patient as a person.

1.3 The nature of health problems

The nurse respects the worth, dignity and rights of all human beings irrespective of the nature of the health problem. The worth of the person is not affected by disease, disability, functional status, or proximity to death. This respect extends to all who require the services of the nurse for the promotion of health, the prevention of illness, the restoration of health, the alleviation of suffering, and the provision of supportive care to those who are dying.

The measures nurses take to care for the patient enable the patient to live with as much physical, emotional, social, and spiritual well-being as possible. Nursing care aims to maximize the values that the patient has treasured in life and extends supportive care to the family and significant others. Nursing care is directed toward meeting the comprehensive needs of patients and their families across the continuum of care. This is particularly vital in the care of patients and their families at the end of life to prevent and relieve the cascade of symptoms and suffering that are commonly associated with dying.

Nurses are leaders and vigilant advocates for the delivery of dignified and humane care. Nurses actively participate in assessing and assuring the responsible and appropriate use of interventions in order to minimize unwarranted or unwanted treatment and patient suffering. The acceptability and importance of carefully considered decisions regarding resuscitation status, withholding and withdrawing life-sustaining therapies, forgoing medically provided nutrition and hydration, aggressive pain and symptom management and advance directives are increasingly evident. The nurse should provide interventions to relieve pain and other symptoms in the dying patient even when those interventions entail risks of hastening death. However, nurses may not act with the sole intent of ending a patient's life even though such action may be motivated by compassion, respect for autonomy and quality of life considerations. Nurses have invaluable experience, knowledge, and insight into care at the end of life and should be actively involved in related research, education, practice, and policy development.

1.4 The right to self-determination

Respect for human dignity requires the recognition of specific patient rights, particularly, the right of self-determination. Self-determination, also known as autonomy, is the philosophical basis for informed consent in health care. Patients have the moral and legal right to determine what will be done with their own person; to be given accurate, complete, and understandable information in a manner that facilitates an informed judgment; to be assisted with weighing the benefits, burdens, and available options in their treatment, including the choice of no treatment; to accept, refuse, or terminate treatment without deceit, undue influence, duress, coercion or penalty; and to be given necessary support throughout the decision-making and treatment process. Such support would include the opportunity to make decisions with family and significant others and the provision of advice and support from knowledgeable nurses and other health professionals. Patients should be involved in planning their own health care to the extent they are able and choose to participate.

Each nurse has an obligation to be knowledgeable about the moral and legal rights of all patients to self-determination. The nurse preserves, protects, and supports those interests by assessing the patient's comprehension of both the information presented and the implications of decisions. In situations in which the patient lacks the capacity to make a decision, a designated surrogate decision-maker should be consulted. The role of the surrogate is to make decisions as the patient would, based upon the patient's previously expressed wishes and known values. In the absence of a designated surrogate decision-maker, decisions should be made in the best interests of the patient, considering the patient's personal values to the extent that they are known. The nurse supports patient self-determination by participating in discussions with surrogates, providing guidance and referral to other resources as necessary, and identifying and addressing problems in the decision-making process. Support of autonomy in the broadest sense also includes recognition that people of some cultures place less weight on individualism and choose to defer to family or community values in decision making. Respect not just for the specific decision but also for the patient's method of decision making is consistent with the principle of autonomy.

Individuals are interdependent members of the community. The nurse recognizes that there are situations in which the right to individual self-determination may be outweighed or limited by the rights, health and welfare of others, particularly in relation to public health considerations. Nonetheless, limitation of individual rights must always be considered a serious deviation from the standard of care, justified only when there are no less restrictive means available to preserve the rights of others and the demands of justice.

1.5 Relationships with colleagues and others

The principle of respect for persons extends to all individuals with whom the nurse interacts. The nurse maintains compassionate and caring relationships with colleagues and others with a commitment to the fair treatment of individuals, to integrity-preserving compromise, and to resolving conflict. Nurses function in many roles, including direct care provider, administrator, educator, researcher and consultant. In each of these roles, the nurse treats colleagues, employees, assistants, and students with respect and compassion. This standard of conduct precludes any and all prejudicial actions, any form of harassment or threatening behavior, or disregard for the effect of one's actions on others. The nurse values the distinctive contribution of individuals or groups, and collaborates to meet the shared goal of providing quality health services.

2 The nurse's primary commitment is to the patient, whether an individual, family, group or community.

2.1 Primacy of the patient's interests

The nurse's primary commitment is to the recipient of nursing and health care services—the patient—whether the recipient is an individual, a family, a group, or a community. Nursing holds a fundamental commitment to the uniqueness of the individual patient; therefore, any plan of care must reflect that uniqueness. The nurse strives to provide patients with opportunities to participate in planning care, assures that patients find the plans acceptable and supports the implementation of the plan. Addressing patient interests requires recognition of the patient's place in the family or other networks of relationship. When the patient's wishes are in conflict with others, the nurse seeks to help resolve the conflict. Where conflict persists, the nurse's commitment remains to the identified patient.

2.2 Conflict of interest for nurses

Nurses are frequently put in situations of conflict arising from competing loyalties in the workplace, including situations of conflicting expectations from patients, families, physicians, colleagues, and in many cases, health care organizations and health plans. Nurses must examine the conflicts arising between their own personal and professional values, the values and interests of others who are also responsible for patient care and health care decisions, as well as those of patients. Nurses strive to resolve such conflicts in ways that ensure patient safety, guard the patient's best interests and preserve the professional integrity of the nurse.

Situations created by changes in health care financing and delivery systems, such as incentive systems to decrease spending, pose new possibilities of conflict between economic self-interest and professional integrity. Bonuses, sanctions, and incentives tied to financial targets are examples of features of health care systems that may present such conflict. Conflicts of interest may arise in any domain of nursing activity including clinical practice, administration, education or research. Advance practice nurses who bill directly for services and nursing executives with budgetary responsibilities must be especially cognizant of the potential for conflicts of interest. Nurses should disclose to all relevant parties (e.g., patients, employers, colleagues) any perceived or actual conflict of interest and in some situations should withdraw from further participation. Nurses in all roles must seek to ensure that employment arrangements are just and fair and do not create an unreasonable conflict between patient care and direct personal gain.

2.3 Collaboration

Collaboration is not just cooperation, but it is the concerted effort of individuals and groups to attain a shared goal. In health care, that goal is to address the health needs of the patient and the public. The complexity of health care delivery systems requires a multi-disciplinary approach to the delivery of services that has the strong support and active participation of all the health professions. Within this context, nursing's unique contribution, scope of practice, and relationship with other health professions needs to be clearly articulated, represented and preserved. By its very nature, collaboration requires mutual trust, recognition, and respect among the health care team, shared decision making about patient care, and open dialogue among all parties who have an interest in and a concern for health outcomes. Nurses should work to assure that the relevant parties are involved and have a voice in decision-making about patient care issues. Nurses should see that the questions that need to be addressed are asked and that the information needed for informed decision-making is available and provided. Nurses should actively promote the collaborative multi-disciplinary planning required to ensure the availability and accessibility of quality health services to all persons who have needs for health care.

Intra-professional collaboration within nursing is fundamental to effectively addressing the health needs of patients and the public. Nurses engaged in non-clinical roles, such as administration or research, while not providing direct care, nonetheless are collaborating in the provision of care through their influence and direction of those who do. Effective nursing care is accomplished through the interdependence of nurses in differing roles—those who teach the needed skills, set standards, manage the environment of care, or expand the boundaries of knowledge used by the profession. In this sense, nurses in all roles share a responsibility for the outcomes of nursing care.

2.4 Professional boundaries

When acting within one's role of a professional, the nurse recognizes and maintains boundaries that establish appropriate limits to relationships. While the nature of nursing work has an inherently personal component, nurse-patient relationships and nurse-colleague relationships have, as their foundation, the purpose of preventing illness, alleviating suffering, and protecting, promoting, and restoring the health of patients. In this way, nurse-patient and nurse-colleague relationships differ from those that are purely personal and unstructured, such as friendship. The intimate nature of nursing care, the involvement of nurses in important and sometimes highly stressful life events, and the mutual dependence of colleagues working in close concert all present the potential for blurring of limits to professional relationships. Maintaining authenticity and expressing oneself as an individual, while remaining within the bounds established by the purpose of the relationship, can be especially difficult in prolonged or long-term relationships. In all encounters, nurses are responsible for retaining their professional boundaries. When these boundaries are jeopardized, the nurse should seek assistance from peers or supervisors or take appropriate steps to remove her/himself from the situation.

3 The nurse promotes, advocates for, and strives to protect the health, safety, and rights of the patient.

3.1 Privacy

The nurse safeguards the patient's right to privacy. The need for health care does not justify unwanted intrusion into the patient's life. The nurse advocates for an environment that provides for sufficient physical privacy, including auditory privacy for discussions of a personal nature and policies and practices that protect the confidentiality of information.

3.2 Confidentiality

Associated with the right to privacy, the nurse has a duty to maintain confidentiality of all patient information. The patient's well-being could be jeopardized and the fundamental trust between patient and nurse destroyed by unnecessary access to data or by the inappropriate disclosure of identifiable patient information. The rights, well-being, and safety of the individual patient should be the primary factors in arriving at any professional judgment concerning the disposition of confidential information received from or about the patient, whether oral, written or electronic. The standard of nursing practice and the nurse's responsibility to provide quality care require that relevant data be shared with those members of the health care team who have a need to know. Only information pertinent to a patient's treatment and welfare is disclosed, and only to those directly involved with the patient's care. Duties of confidentiality, however, are not absolute and may need to be modified in order to protect the patient, other innocent parties, and in circumstances of mandatory disclosure for public health reasons.

Information used for purposes of peer review, third-party payments, and other quality improvement or risk management mechanisms may be disclosed only under defined policies, mandates, or protocols. These written guidelines must assure that the rights, well-being, and safety of the patient are protected. In general, only that information directly relevant to the task or specific responsibility should be disclosed. When using electronic communications, special effort should be made to maintain data security.

3.3 Protection of participants in research

Stemming from the right to self-determination, each individual has the right to choose whether or not to participate in research. It is imperative that the patient or legally authorized surrogate receive sufficient information that is material to an informed decision, to comprehend that information, and to know how to discontinue participation in research without penalty. Necessary information to achieve an adequately informed consent includes the nature of participation, potential harms and benefits, and available alternatives to taking part in the research. Additionally, the patient should be informed of how the data will be protected. The patient has the right to refuse to participate in research or to withdraw at any time without fear of adverse consequences or reprisal.

Research should be conducted and directed only by qualified persons. Prior to implementation, all research should be approved by a qualified review board to ensure patient protection and the ethical integrity of the research. Nurses should be cognizant of the special concerns raised by research involving vulnerable groups, including children, prisoners, students, the elderly, and the poor. The nurse who participates in research in any capacity should be fully informed about both the subject's and the nurse's rights and obligations in the particular research study and in research in general. Nurses have the duty to question and, if necessary, to report and to refuse to participate in research they deem morally objectionable.

3.4 Standards and review mechanisms

Nursing is responsible and accountable for assuring that only those individuals who have demonstrated the knowledge, skill, practice experiences, commitment, and integrity essential to professional practice are allowed to enter into and continue to practice within the profession. Nurse educators have a responsibility to ensure that basic competencies are achieved and to promote a commitment to professional practice prior to entry of an individual into practice. Nurse administrators are responsible for assuring that the knowledge and skills of each nurse in the workplace are assessed prior to the assignment of responsibilities requiring preparation beyond basic academic programs.

The nurse has a responsibility to implement and maintain standards of professional nursing practice. The nurse should participate in planning, establishing, implementing, and evaluating review mechanisms designed to safeguard patients and nurses, such as peer review processes or committees, credentialing processes, quality improvement initiatives, and ethics committees. Nurse administrators must ensure that nurses have access to and inclusion on institutional ethics committees. Nurses must bring forward difficult issues related to patient care and/or institutional constraints upon ethical practice for discussion and review. The nurse acts to promote inclusion of appropriate others in all deliberations related to patient care.

Nurses should also be active participants in the development of policies and review mechanisms designed to promote patient safety, reduce the likelihood of errors, and address both environmental system factors and human factors that present increased risk to patients. In addition, when errors do occur, nurses are expected to follow institutional guidelines in reporting errors committed or observed to the appropriate supervisory personnel and for assuring responsible disclosure of errors to patients. Under no circumstances should the nurse participate in, or condone through silence, either an attempt to hide an error or a punitive response that serves only to fix blame rather than correct the conditions that led to the error.

3.5 Acting on questionable practice

The nurse's primary commitment is to the health, well-being, and safety of the patient across the life span and in all settings in which health care needs are addressed. As an advocate for the patient, the nurse must be alert to and take appropriate action regarding any instances of incompetent, unethical, illegal, or impaired practice by any member of the health care team or the health care system or any action on the part of others that places the rights or best interests of the patient in jeopardy. To function effectively in this role, nurses must be knowledgeable about the Code of Ethics, standards of practice of the profession, relevant federal, state and local laws and regulations, and the employing organization's policies and procedures.

When the nurse is aware of inappropriate or questionable practice in the provision or denial of health care, concern should be expressed to the person carrying out the questionable practice. Attention should be called to the possible detrimental effect upon the patient's well-being or best interests as well as the integrity of nursing practice. When factors in the health care delivery system or health care organization threaten the welfare of the patient, similar action should be directed to the responsible administrator. If indicated, the problem should be reported to an appropriate higher authority within the institution or agency, or to an appropriate external authority.

There should be established processes for reporting and handling incompetent, unethical, illegal, or impaired practice within the employment settings so that such reporting can go through official channels, thereby reducing the risk of reprisal against the reporting nurse. All nurses have a responsibility to assist those who identify potentially questionable practice. State nurses associations should be prepared to provide assistance and support in the development and evaluation of such processes and reporting procedures. When incompetent, unethical, illegal or impaired practice is not corrected within the employment setting and continues to jeopardize patient well-being and safety, the problem should be reported to other appropriate authorities such as practice committees of the pertinent professional organizations, the legally constituted bodies concerned with licensing of specific categories of health workers and professional practitioners, or the regulatory agencies concerned with evaluating standards of practice. Some situations may warrant the concern and involvement of all such groups. Accurate reporting and factual documentation, and not merely opinion, undergird all such responsible actions. When a nurse chooses to engage in the act of responsible reporting about situations that are perceived as unethical, incompetent, illegal or impaired, the professional organization has a responsibility to provide the nurse with support and assistance and to protect the practice of those nurses who choose to voice their concerns. Reporting unethical, illegal, incompetent, or impaired practices, even when done appropriately, may present substantial risks to the nurse; nevertheless, such risks do not eliminate the obligation to address serious threats to patient safety.

3.6 Addressing impaired practice

Nurses must be vigilant to protect the patient, the public and the profession from potential harm when a colleague's practice, in any setting, appears to be impaired. The nurse extends compassion and caring to colleagues who are in recovery from illness or when illness interferes with job performance. In a situation where a nurse suspects another's practice may be impaired, the nurse's duty is to take action designed both to protect patients and to assure that the impaired individual receives assistance in regaining optimal function. Such action should usually begin with consulting supervisory personnel and may also include confronting the individual in a supportive manner and with the assistance of others or helping the individual to access appropriate resources. Nurses are encouraged to follow guidelines outlined by the profession and policies of the employing organization to assist colleagues whose job performance may be adversely affected by mental or physical illness or by personal circumstances. Nurses in all roles should advocate for colleagues whose job performance may be impaired to ensure that they receive appropriate assistance, treatment and access to fair institutional and legal processes. This includes supporting the return to practice of the individual who has sought assistance and is ready to resume professional duties.

If impaired practice poses a threat or danger to self or others, regardless of whether the individual has sought help, the nurse must take action to report the individual to persons authorized to address the problem. Nurses who advocate for others whose job performance creates a risk for harm should be protected from negative consequences. Advocacy may be a difficult process and the nurse is advised to follow workplace policies. If workplace policies do not exist or are inappropriate—that is, they deny the nurse in question access to due legal process or demand resignation—the reporting nurse may obtain guidance from the professional association, state peer assistance programs, employee assistance program or a similar resource.

4 The nurse is responsible and accountable for individual nursing practice and determines the appropriate delegation of tasks consistent with the nurse's obligation to provide optimum patient care.

4.1 Acceptance of accountability and responsibility

Individual registered nurses bear primary responsibility for the nursing care that their patients receive and are individually accountable for their own practice. Nursing practice includes direct care activities, acts of delegation, and other responsibilities such as teaching, research, and administration. In each instance the nurse retains accountability and responsibility for the quality of practice and for confirmity with standards of care.

Nurses are faced with decisions in the context of the increased complexity and changing patterns in the delivery of health care. As the scope of nursing practice changes, the nurse must exercise judgment in accepting responsibilities, seeking consultation, and assigning activities to others who carry out nursing care. For example, some advanced practice nurses have the authority to issue prescription and treatment orders to be carried out by other nurses. These acts are not acts of delegation. Both the advanced practice nurse issuing the order and the nurse accepting the order are responsible for the judgments made and accountable for the actions taken.

4.2 Accountability for nursing judgment and action

Accountability means to be answerable to oneself and others for one's own actions. In order to be accountable, nurses act under a code of ethical conduct that is grounded in the moral principles of fidelity and respect for the dignity, worth, and self-determination of patients. Nurses are accountable for judgments made and actions taken in the course of nursing practice, irrespective of health care organizations' policies or providers' directives.

4.3 Responsibility for nursing judgment and action

Responsibility refers to the specific accountability or liability associated with the performance of duties of a particular role. Nurses accept or reject specific role demands based upon their education, knowledge, competence, and extent of experience. Nurses in administration, education and research also have obligations to the recipients of nursing care. Although nurses in administration, education and research have relationships with patients that are less direct, in assuming the responsibilities of a particular role, they share responsibility for the care provided by those whom they supervise and instruct. The nurse must not engage in practices prohibited by law or delegate activities to others that are prohibited by the practice acts of other health care providers.

Individual nurses are responsible for assessing his or her own competence. When the needs of the patient are beyond the qualifications and competencies of the nurse, consultation and collaboration must be sought from qualified nurses, other health professionals, or other appropriate sources. Educational resources should be sought by nurses and provided by institutions to maintain and advance the competence of nurses. Nurse educators act in collaboration with their students to assess the learning needs of the student, the effectiveness of the teaching program, the identification and utilization of appropriate resources, and the support needed for the learning process.

4.4 Delegation of nursing activities

Since the nurse is accountable for the quality of nursing care given to patients, nurses are accountable for the assignment of nursing responsibilities to other nurses and the delegation of nursing care activities to other health care workers. While delegation and assignment are used here in a generic moral sense, it is understood that individual states may have a particular legal definition of these terms.

The nurse must make reasonable efforts to assess individual competency when assigning selected components of nursing care to other health care workers. This assessment involves evaluating the knowledge, skills, and experience of the individual to whom the care is assigned, the complexity of the assigned tasks, and the health status of the patient. The nurse is also responsible for monitoring the activities of these individuals and evaluating the quality of the care provided. Nurses may not delegate responsibilities such as assessment and evaluation; they may delegate tasks. The nurse must not knowingly assign or delegate to any member of the nursing team a task for which that person is not prepared or qualified. Employer policies or directives do not relieve the nurse of responsibility for making judgments about the delegation and assignment of nursing care tasks.

Nurses functioning in management or administrative roles have a particular responsibility to provide an environment that supports and facilitates appropriate assignment and delegation. This includes providing appropriate orientation to staff, assisting less experienced nurses in developing necessary skills and competencies, and establishing policies and procedures that protect both the patient and nurse from the inappropriate assignment or delegation of nursing responsibilities, activities, or tasks.

Nurses functioning in educator or preceptor roles may have less direct relationships with patients. However, through assignment of nursing care activities to learners they share responsibility and accountability for the care provided. It is imperative that the knowledge and skills of the learner be sufficient to provide the assigned nursing care and that appropriate supervision be provided to protect both the patient and the learner.

*5 **The nurse owes the same duties to self as to others, including the responsibility to preserve integrity and safety, to maintain competence, and to continue personal and professional growth.***

5.1 Moral self-respect

Moral respect accords moral worth and dignity to all human beings irrespective of their personal attributes or life situation. Such respect extends to oneself as well; the same duties that we owe to others we owe to ourselves. Self-regarding duties refer to a realm of duties that primarily concern oneself and include professional growth and maintenance of competence, preservation of wholeness of character, and personal integrity.

5.2 Professional growth and maintenance of competence

Though it has consequences for others, maintenance of competence and ongoing professional growth involves the control of one's own conduct in a way that is primarily self-regarding. Competence affects one's self-respect, self-esteem, professional status, and the meaningfulness of work. In all nursing roles, evaluation of one's own performance, coupled with peer review, is a means by which nursing practice can be held to the highest standards. Each nurse is responsible for participating in the development of criteria for evaluation of practice and for using those criteria in peer and self-assessment.

Continual professional growth, particularly in knowledge and skill, requires a commitment to lifelong learning. Such learning includes, but is not limited to, continuing education, networking with professional colleagues, self-study, professional reading, certification, and seeking advanced degrees. Nurses are required to have knowledge relevant to the current scope and standards of nursing practice, changing issues, concerns, controversies, and ethics. Where the care required is outside the competencies of the individual nurse, consultation should be sought or the patient should be referred to others for appropriate care.

5.3 Wholeness of character

Nurses have both personal and professional identities that are neither entirely separate, nor entirely merged, but are integrated. In the process of becoming a professional, the nurse embraces the values of the profession, integrating them with personal values. Duties to self involve an authentic expression of one's own moral point-of-view in practice. Sound ethical decision making requires the respectful and open exchange of views between and among all individuals with relevant interests. In a community or moral discourse, no one person's view should automatically take precedence over that of another. Thus the nurse has a responsibility to express moral perspectives, even when they differ from those of others, and even when they might not prevail.

This wholeness of character encompasses relationships with patients. In situations where the patient requests a personal opinion from the nurse, the nurse is generally free to express an informed personal opinion as long as this preserves the voluntariness of the patient and maintains appropriate professional and moral boundaries. It is essential to be aware of the potential for undue influence attached to the nurse's professional role. Assisting patients to clarify their own values in reaching informed decisions may be helpful in avoiding unintended persuasion. In situations where nurses' responsibilities include care for those whose personal attributes, condition, lifestyle, or situation is stigmatized by the community and are personally unacceptable, the nurse still renders respectful and skilled care.

5.4 Preservation of integrity

Integrity is an aspect of wholeness of character and is primarily a self-concern of the individual nurse. An economically constrained health care environment presents the nurse with particularly troubling threats to integrity. Threats to integrity may include a request to deceive a patient, to withhold information, or to falsify records, as well as verbal abuse from patients or coworkers. Threats to integrity may also include an expectation that the nurse will act in a way that is inconsistent with the values or ethics of the profession, or more specifically a request that is in direct violation of the Code of Ethics. Nurses have a duty to remain consistent with both their personal and professional values and to accept compromise only to the degree that it remains an integrity-preserving compromise. An integrity-preserving compromise does not jeopardize the dignity or well-being of the nurse or others. Integrity-preserving compromise can be difficult to achieve, but is more likely to be accomplished in situations where there is an open forum for moral discourse and an atmosphere of mutal respect and regard.

Where nurses are placed in situations of compromise that exceed acceptable moral limits or involve violations of the moral standards of the profession, whether in direct patient care or in any other forms of nursing practice, they may express their conscientious objection to participation. Where a particular treatment, intervention, activity, or practice is morally objectionable to the nurse, whether intrinsically so or because it is inappropriate for the specific patient, or where it may jeopardize both patients and nursing practice, the nurse is justified in refusing to participate on moral grounds. Such grounds exclude personal preference, prejudice, convenience or arbitrariness. Conscientious objection may not insulate the nurse against formal or informal penalty. The nurse who decides not to take part because of conscientious objection must communicate this decision in appropriate ways. Whenever possible, such a refusal should be made known in advance and in time for alternate arrangements to be made for patient care. The nurse is obliged to provide for the patient's safety, to avoid abandonment, and to withdraw only when assured that alternative sources of nursing care are available to the patient.

Where patterns of institutional behavior or professional practice compromise the integrity of all its nurses, nurses should express their concern or conscientious objection collectively to the appropriate body or committee. In addition, they should express their concern, resist, and seek to bring about a change in those persistent activities or expectations in the practice setting that are morally objectionable to nurses and jeopardize either patient or nurse well being.

6 ***The nurse participates in establishing, maintaining and improving health care environments and conditions of employment conducive to the provision of quality health care and consistent with the values of the profession through individual and collective action.***

6.1 Influence of the environment on moral virtues and values

Virtues are habits of character that predispose persons to meet their moral obligations; that is, to do what is right. Excellences are habits of character that predispose a person to do a particular job or task well. Virtues such as wisdom, honesty, and courage are habits or attributes of the morally good person. Excellences such as compassion, patience, and skill are habits of character of the morally good nurse. For the nurse, virtues and excellences are those habits that affirm and promote the values of human dignity, well-being, respect, health, independence, and other values central to nursing. Both virtues and excellences, as aspects of moral character, can be either nurtured by the environment in which the nurse practices or they can be diminished or thwarted. All nurses have a responsibility to create, maintain, and contribute to environments that support the growth of virtues and excellences and enable nurses to fulfill their ethical obligations.

6.2 Influence of the environment on ethical obligations

All nurses, regardless of role, have a responsibility to create, maintain, and contribute to environments of practice that support nurses in fulfilling their ethical obligations. Environments of practice include observable features, such as working conditions, and written policies and procedures setting out expectations for nurses, as well as less tangible characteristics such as informal peer norms. Organizational structures, role descriptions, health and safety initiatives, grievance mechanisms, ethics committees, compensation systems, and disciplinary procedures all contribute to environments that can either present barriers or foster ethical practice and professional fulfillment. Environments in which employees are provided fair hearing of grievances, are supported in practicing according to standards of care, and are justly treated allow the realization of the values of the profession and are consistent with sound nursing practice.

6.3 Responsibility for the health care environment

The nurse is responsible for contributing to a moral environment that encourages respectful interactions with colleagues, support of peers, and identification of issues that need to be addressed. Nurse administrators have a particular responsibility to assure that employees are treated fairly and that nurses are involved in decisions related to their practice and working conditions. Acquiescing and accepting unsafe or inappropriate practices, even if the individual does not participate in the specific practice, is equivalent to condoning unsafe practice. Nurses should not remain employed in facilities that routinely violate patient rights or require nurses to severely and repeatedly compromise standards of practice or personal morality.

As with concerns about patient care, nurses should address concerns about the health care environment through appropriate channels. Organizational changes are difficult to accomplish and may require persistent efforts over time. Toward this end, nurses may participate in collective action such as collective bargaining or workplace advocacy, preferably through a professional association such as the state nurses association, in order to address the terms and conditions of employment. Agreements reached through such action must be consistent with the profession's standards of practice, the state law regulating practice, and the Code of Ethics for Nursing. Conditions of employment must contribute to the moral environment, the provision of quality patient care, and professional satisfaction for nurses.

The professional association also serves as an advocate for the nurse by seeking to secure just compensation and humane working conditions for nurses. To accomplish this, the professional association may engage in collective bargaining on behalf of nurses. While seeking to assure just economic and general welfare for nurses, collective bargaining, nonetheless, seeks to keep the interests of both nurses and patients in balance.

7 The nurse participates in the advancement of the profession through contributions to practice, education, administration, and knowledge development.

7.1 Advancing the profession through active involvement in nursing and in health care policy

Nurses should advance their profession by contributing in some way to the leadership, activities, and the viability of their professional organizations. Nurses can also advance the profession by serving in leadership or mentorship roles or on committees within their places of employment. Nurses who are self-employed can advance the profession by serving as role models for professional integrity. Nurses can also advance the profession through participation in civic activities related to health care or through local, state, national, or international initiatives. Nurse educators have a specific responsibility to enhance students' commitment to professional and civic values. Nurse administrators have a responsibility to foster an employment environment that facilitates nurses' ethical integrity and professionalism, and nurse researchers are responsible for active contribution to the body of knowledge supporting and advancing nursing practice.

7.2 Advancing the profession by developing, maintaining, and implementing professional standards in clinical, administrative, and educational practice

Standards and guidelines reflect the practice of nursing grounded in ethical commitments and a body of knowledge. Professional standards and guidelines for nurses must be developed by nurses and reflect nursing's responsibility to society. It is the responsibility of nurses to identify their own scope of practice as permitted by professional practice standards and guidelines, by state and federal laws, by relevant societal values, and by the Code of Ethics.

The nurse as administrator or manager must establish, maintain, and promote conditions of employment that enable nurses within that organization or community setting to practice in accord with accepted standards of nursing practice and provide a nursing and health care work environment that meets the standards and guidelines of nursing practice. Professional autonomy and self-regulation in the control of conditions of practice are necessary for implementing nursing standards and guidelines and assuring quality care for those whom nursing serves.

The nurse educator is responsible for promoting and maintaining optimum standards of both nursing education and of nursing practice in any settings where planned learning activities occur. Nurse educators must also ensure that only those students who possess knowledge, skills and the competencies that are essential to nursing graduate from their nursing programs.

7.3 Advancing the profession through knowledge development, dissemination, and application to practice

The nursing profession should engage in scholarly inquiry to identify, evaluate, refine, and expand the body of knowledge that forms the foundation of its discipline and practice. In addition, nursing knowledge is derived from the sciences and from the humanities. Ongoing scholarly activities are essential to fulfilling a profession's obligations to society. All nurses working alone or in collaboration with others can participate in the advancement of the profession through the development, evaluation, dissemination, and application of knowledge in practice. However, an organizational climate and infrastructure conducive to scholarly inquiry must be valued and implemented for this to occur.

8 The nurse collaborates with other health professionals and the public in promoting community, national, and international efforts to meet health needs.

8.1 Health needs and concerns

The nursing profession is committed to promoting the health, welfare, and safety of all people. The nurse has a responsibility to be aware not only of specific health needs of individual patients, but also of broader health concerns such as world hunger, environmental pollution, lack of access to health care, violation of human rights, and inequitable distribution of nursing and health care resources. The availability and accessibility of high-quality health services to all people require both inter-disciplinary planning and collaborative partnerships among health professionals and others at the community, national, and international levels.

8.2 Responsibilities to the public

Nurses, individually and collectively, have a responsibility to be knowledgeable about the health status of the community and existing threats to health and safety. Through support of and participation in community organizations and groups, the nurse assists in efforts to educate the public, facilitates informed choice, identifies conditions and circumstances that contribute to illness, injury and disease, fosters healthy life styles, and participates in institutional and legislative efforts to promote health and meet national health objectives. In addition, the nurse supports initiatives to address barriers to health, such as poverty, homelessness, unsafe living conditions, abuse and violence, and lack of access to health services.

The nurse also recognizes that health care is provided to culturally diverse populations in this country and in all parts of the world. In providing care, the nurse should avoid imposition of the nurse's cultural values upon others. The nurse should affirm human dignity and show respect for the values and practices associated with different cultures and use approaches to care that reflect awareness and sensitivity.

9 ***The profession of nursing, as represented by associations and their members, is responsible for articulating nursing values, for maintaining the integrity of the profession and its practice, and for shaping social policy.***

9.1 Assertion of values

It is the responsibility of a professional association to communicate and affirm the values of the profession to its members. It is essential that the professional organization encourages discourse that supports critical self-reflection and evaluation within the profession. The organization also communicates to the public the values that nursing considers central to social change that will enhance health.

9.2 The profession carries out its collective responsibility through professional associations

The nursing profession continues to develop ways to clarify nursing's accountability to society. The contract between the profession and society is made explicit through such mechanisms as (a) The Code of Ethics for Nurses, (b) the standards of nursing practice, (c) the ongoing development of nursing knowledge derived from nursing theory, scholarship, and research in order to guide nursing actions, (d) educational requirements for practice, (e) certification, and (f) mechanisms for evaluating the effectiveness of professional nursing actions,

9.3 Intraprofessional integrity

A professional association is responsible for expressing the values and ethics of the profession and also for encouraging the professional organization and its members to function in accord with those values and ethics, Thus, one of its fundamental responsibilities is to promote awareness of and adherence to the Code of Ethics and to critique the activities and ends of the professional association itself. Values and ethics influence the power structures of the association in guiding, correcting, and directing its activities. Legitimate concerns for the self-interest of the association and the profession are balanced by a commitment to the social goods that are sought. Through critical self-reflection and self-evaluation, associations must foster change within themselves, seeking to move the professional community towards its stated ideals.

9.4 Social reform

Nurses can work individually as citizens or collectively through political action to bring about social change. It is the responsibility of a professional nursing association to speak for nurses collectively in shaping and reshaping health care within our nation, specifically in areas of health care policy and legislation that affect accessibility, quality, and the cost of health care, Here, the professional association maintains vigilance and takes action to influence legislators, reimbursement agencies, nursing organizations, and other health professions, In these activities, health is understood as being broader than delivery and reimbursement systems, but extending to health-related sociocultural issues such as violation of human rights, homelessness, hunger, violence and the stigma of illness.

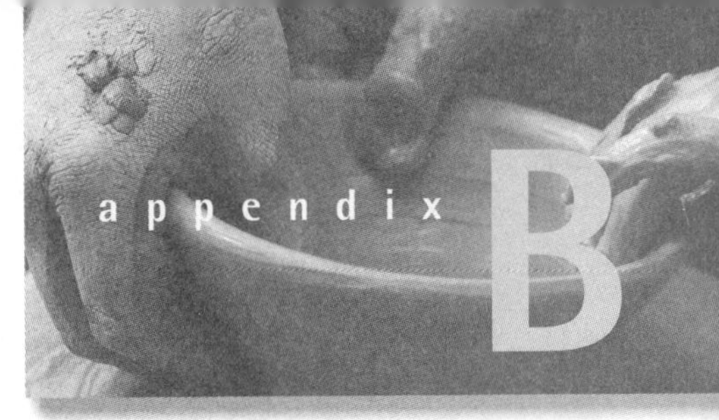

The ICN Code of Ethics for Nurses

The ICN Code of Ethics for Nurses

An international code of ethics for nurses was first adopted by the International Council of Nurses (ICN) in 1953. It has been revised and reaffirmed at various times since, most recently with this review and revision completed in 2005.

Preamble

Nurses have four fundamental responsibilities: to promote health, to prevent illness, to restore health and to alleviate suffering. The need for nursing is universal.

Inherent in nursing is respect for human rights, including cultural rights, the right to life and choice, to dignity and to be treated with respect. Nursing care is respectful of and unrestricted by considerations of age, colour, creed, culture, disability or illness, gender, sexual orientation, nationality, politics, race or social status. Nurses render health services to the individual, the family and the community and co-ordinate their services with those of related groups.

The ICN Code

The *ICN Code of Ethics for Nurses* has four principal elements that outline the standards of ethical conduct.

Elements of the Code

1. Nurses and People

The nurse's primary professional responsibility is to people requiring nursing care. In providing care, the nurse promotes an environment in which the human rights, values, customs and spiritual beliefs of the individual, family and community are respected.

The nurse ensures that the individual receives sufficient information on which to base consent for care and related treatment.

The nurse holds in confidence personal information and uses judgement in sharing this information.

The nurse shares with society the responsibility for initiating and supporting action to meet the health and social needs of the public, in particular those of vulnerable populations.

The nurse also shares responsibility to sustain and protect the natural environment from depletion, pollution, degradation and destruction.

2. Nurses and Practice

The nurse carries personal responsibility and accountability for nursing practice, and for maintaining competence by continual learning.

The nurse maintains a standard of personal health such that the ability to provide care is not compromised.

The nurse uses judgement regarding individual competence when accepting and delegating responsibility.

The nurse at all times maintains standards of personal conduct which reflect well on the profession and enhance public confidence.

The nurse, in providing care, ensures that use of technology and scientific advances are compatible with the safety, dignity and rights of people.

3. Nurses and the Profession

The nurse assumes the major role in determining and implementing acceptable standards of clinical nursing practice, management, research and education.

The nurse is active in developing a core of research-based professional knowledge.

The nurse, acting through the professional organisation, participates in creating and maintaining safe, equitable social and economic working conditions in nursing.

4. Nurses and Co-workers

The nurse sustains a co-operative relationship with co-workers in nursing and other fields.

The nurse takes appropriate action to safeguard individuals, families and communities when their health is endangered by a coworker or any other person.

Suggestions for Use of the *ICN Code of Ethics for Nurses*

The *ICN Code of Ethics for Nurses* is a guide for action based on social values and needs. It will have meaning only as a living document if applied to the realities of nursing and health care in a changing society.

To achieve its purpose the *Code* must be understood, internalised and used by nurses in all aspects of their work. It must be available to students and nurses throughout their study and work lives.

Applying the Elements of the *ICN Code of Ethics for Nurses*

The four elements of the *ICN Code of Ethics for Nurses*: nurses and people, nurses and practice, nurses and the profession, and nurses and co-workers, give a framework for the standards of conduct. The following chart will assist nurses to translate the standards into action. Nurses and nursing students can therefore:

- Study the standards under each element of the *Code*.
- Reflect on what each standard means to you. Think about how you can apply ethics in your nursing domain: practice, education, research or management.
- Discuss the *Code* with co-workers and others.
- Use a specific example from experience to identify ethical dilemmas and standards of conduct as outlined in the *Code*. Identify how you would resolve the dilemmas.
- Work in groups to clarify ethical decision making and reach a consensus on standards of ethical conduct.
- Collaborate with your national nurses' association, co-workers, and others in the continuous application of ethical standards in nursing practice, education, management and research.

ELEMENT OF THE CODE # 1: NURSES AND PEOPLE

Practitioners and Managers

Provide care that respects human rights and is sensitive to the values, customs and beliefs of all people.

Provide continuing education in ethical issues.

Provide sufficient information to permit informed consent and the right to choose or refuse treatment.

Use recording and information management systems that ensure confidentiality.

Develop and monitor environmental safety in the workplace.

Educators and Researchers

In curriculum include references to human rights, equity, justice, solidarity as the basis for access to care.

Provide teaching and learning opportunities for ethical issues and decision making.

Provide teaching/learning opportunities related to informed consent.

Introduce into curriculum concepts of privacy and confidentiality.

Sensitise students to the importance of social action in current concerns.

National Nurses' Associations

Develop position statements and guidelines that support human rights and ethical standards.

Lobby for involvement of nurses in ethics review committees.

Provide guidelines, position statements and continuing education related to informed consent.

Incorporate issues of confidentiality and privacy into a national code of ethics for nurses.

Advocate for safe and healthy environment.

ELEMENT OF THE CODE # 2: NURSES AND PRACTICE

Practitioners and Managers

Establish standards of care and a work setting that promotes safety and quality care.

Establish systems for professional appraisal, continuing education and systematic renewal of licensure to practice.

Monitor and promote the personal health of nursing staff in relation to their competence for practice.

Educators and Researchers

Provide teaching/learning opportunities that foster life long learning and competence for practice.

Conduct and disseminate research that shows links between continual learning and competence to practice.

Promote the importance of personal health and illustrate its relation to other values.

National Nurses' Associations

Provide access to continuing education, through journals, conferences, distance education, etc.

Lobby to ensure continuing education opportunities and quality care standards.

Promote healthy lifestyles for nursing professionals.

Lobby for healthy workplaces and services for nurses.

ELEMENT OF THE CODE # 3: NURSES AND THE PROFESSION

Practitioners and Managers

Set standards for nursing practice, research, education and management.

Foster workplace support of the conduct, dissemination and utilisation of research related to nursing and health.

Promote participation in national nurses' associations so as to create favourable socio-economic conditions for nurses.

Educators and Researchers

Provide teaching/learning opportunities in setting standards for nursing practice, research, education and management.

Conduct, disseminate and utilise research to advance the nursing profession.

Sensitise learners to the importance of professional nursing associations.

National Nurses' Associations

Collaborate with others to set standards for nursing education, practice, research and management.

Develop position statements, guidelines and standards related to nursing research.

Lobby for fair social and economic working conditions in nursing. Develop position statements and guidelines in workplace issues.

ELEMENT OF THE CODE #4: NURSES AND CO-WORKERS

Practitioners and Managers

Create awareness of specific and overlapping functions and the potential for interdisciplinary tensions.

Develop workplace systems that support common professional ethical values and behaviour.

Develop mechanisms to safeguard the individual, family or community when their care is endangered by health care personnel.

Educators and Researchers

Develop understanding of the roles of other workers.

Communicate nursing ethics to other professions.

Instill in learners the need to safeguard the individual, family or community when care is endangered by health care personnel.

National Nurses' Associations

Stimulate co-operation with other related disciplines.

Develop awareness of ethical issues of other professions.

Provide guidelines, position statements and discussion fora related to safeguarding people when their care is endangered by health care personnel.

Dissemination of the *ICN Code of Ethics for Nurses*

To be effective the *ICN Code of Ethics for Nurses* must be familiar to nurses. We encourage you to help with its dissemination to schools of nursing, practising nurses, the nursing press and other mass media. The Code should also be disseminated to other health professions, the general public, consumer and policy-making groups, human rights organisations and employers of nurses.

Glossary of Terms Used in the *ICN Code of Ethics for Nurses*

Co-worker Other nurses and other health and non-health related workers and professionals.

Co-operative relationships A professional relationship based on collegial and reciprocal actions, and behaviour that aim to achieve certain goals.

Family A social unit composed of members connected through blood, kinship, emotional or legal relationships.

Nurse shares with society A nurse, as a health professional and a citizen, initiates and supports appropriate action to meet the health and social needs of the public.

Personal health Mental, physical, social and spiritual wellbeing of the nurse.

Personal information Information obtained during professional contact that is private to an individual or family, and which, when disclosed, may violate the right to privacy, cause inconvenience, embarrassment, or harm to the individual or family.

Related groups Other nurses, health care workers or other professionals providing service to an individual, family or community and working toward desired goals.

International Council of Nurses
3, place Jean-Marteau
1201 Geneva, Switzerland
Tel. +41 (22) 908 01 00
Fax +41 (22) 908 01 01
email: icn@icn.ch
Web site: www.icn.ch
• CONSEIL INTERNATIONAL DES INFIRMIÈRES • CONSEJO INTERNACIONAL DE ENFERMERAS • INTERNATIONAL COUNCIL OF NURSES

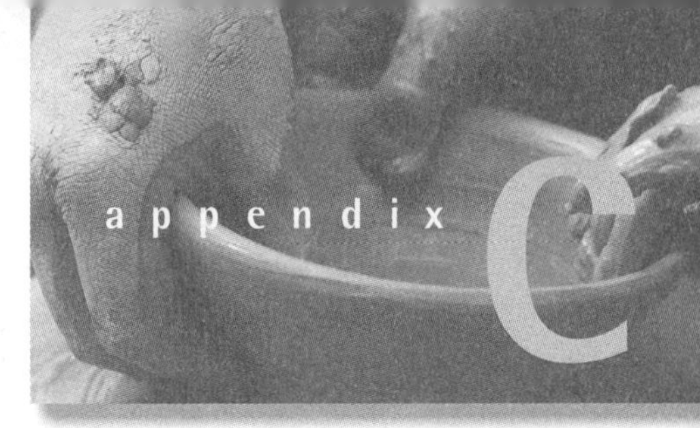

American Hospital Association: The Patient Care Partnership

Understanding Expectations, Rights, and Responsibilities

What to expect during your hospital stay:

- High-quality hospital care
- A clean and safe environment
- Involvement in your care
- Protection of your privacy
- Help when leaving the hospital
- Help with your billing claims

When you need hospital care, your doctor and the nurses and other professionals at our hospital are committed to working with you and your family to meet your health care needs. Our dedicated doctors and staff serve the community in all its ethnic, religious, and economic diversity. Our goal is for you and your family to have the same care and attention we would want for our families and ourselves.

The sections explain some of the basics about how you can expect to be treated during your hospital stay. They also cover what we will need from you to care for you better. If you have questions at any time, please ask them. Unasked or unanswered questions can add to the stress of being in the hospital. Your comfort and confidence in your care are very important to us.

What to Expect during Your Hospital Stay

High-Quality Hospital Care

Our first priority is to provide you the care you need, when you need it, with skill, compassion, and respect. Tell your caregivers if you have concerns about your care or if you have pain. You have the right to know the identity of doctors, nurses, and others involved in your care, and you have the right to know when they are students, residents, or other trainees.

A Clean and Safe Environment

Our hospital works hard to keep you safe. We use special policies and procedures to avoid mistakes in your care and keep you free from abuse or neglect. If anything unexpected and significant happens during your hospital stay, you will be told what happened, and any resulting changes in your care will be discussed with you.

Involvement in Your Care

You and your doctor often make decisions about your care before you go to the hospital. Other times, especially in emergencies, those decisions are made during your hospital stay. When decision making takes place, it should include:

Discussing your medical condition and information about medically appropriate treatment choices.

To make informed decisions with your doctor, you need to understand:

- The benefits and risks of each treatment.
- Whether your treatment is experimental or part of a research study.
- What you can reasonably expect from your treatment and any long-term effects it might have on your quality of life.
- What you and your family will need to do after you leave the hospital.
- The financial consequences of using uncovered services or out-of-network providers.

Please tell your caregivers if you need more information about treatment choices.

Discussing your treatment plan. When you enter the hospital, you sign a general consent to treatment. In some cases, such as surgery or experimental treatment, you may be asked to confirm in writing that you understand what is planned and agree to it. This process protects your right to consent to or refuse a treatment. Your doctor will explain the medical consequences of refusing recommended treatment. It also protects your right to decide if you want to participate in a research study.

Getting information from you. Your caregivers need complete and correct information about your health and coverage so that they can make good decisions about your care. That includes:

- Past illnesses, surgeries, or hospital stays.
- Past allergic reactions.
- Any medicines or dietary supplements (such as vitamins and herbs) that you are taking.
- Any network or admission requirements under your health plan.

Understanding your health care goals and values. You may have health care goals and values or spiritual beliefs that are important to your well-being. They will be taken into account as much as possible throughout your hospital stay. Make sure your doctor, your family, and your care team know your wishes.

Understanding who should make decisions when you cannot. If you have signed a health care power of attorney stating who should speak for you if you become unable to make health care decisions for yourself, or a "living will" or "advance directive" that states your wishes about end-of-life care, give copies to your doctor, your family, and your care team. If you or your family need help making difficult decisions, counselors, chaplains, and others are available to help.

Protection of Your Privacy

We respect the confidentiality of your relationship with your doctor and other caregivers, and the sensitive information about your health and health care that are part of that relationship. State and federal laws and hospital operating policies protect the privacy of your medical information. You will receive a Notice of Privacy Practices that describes the ways that we use, disclose, and safeguard patient information and that explains how you can obtain a copy of information from our records about your care.

Preparing You and Your Family for When You Leave the Hospital

Your doctor works with hospital staff and professionals in your community. You and your family also play an important role in your care. The success of your treatment often depends on your efforts to follow medication, diet, and therapy plans. Your family may need to help care for you at home.

You can expect us to help you identify sources of follow-up care and to let you know if our hospital has a financial interest in any referrals. As long as you agree that we can share information about your care with them, we will coordinate our activities with your caregivers outside the hospital. You can also expect to receive information and, where possible, training about the self-care you will need when you go home.

Help with Your Bill and Filing Insurance Claims

Our staff will file claims for you with health care insurers or other programs such as Medicare and Medicaid. They also will help your doctor with needed documentation. Hospital bills and insurance coverage are often confusing. If you have questions about your bill, contact our business office. If you need help understanding your insurance coverage or health plan, start with your insurance company or health benefits manager. If you do not have health coverage, we will try to help you and your family find financial help or make other arrangements. We need your help with collecting needed information and other requirements to obtain coverage or assistance.

While you are here, you will receive more detailed notices about some of the rights you have as a hospital patient and how to exercise them. We are always interested in improving. If you have questions, comments, or concerns, please contact: American Hospital Association.

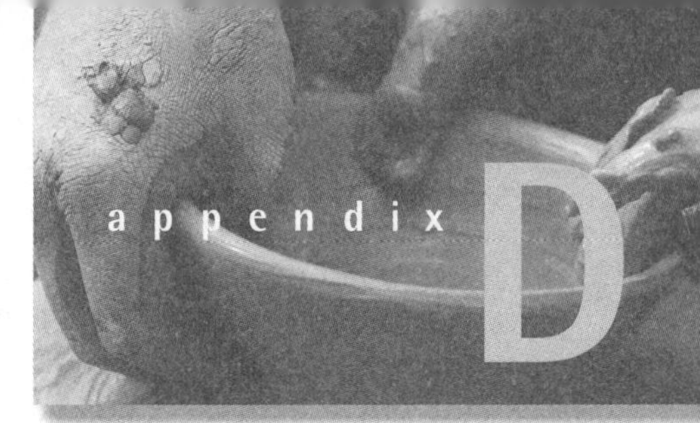

Patient Self-Determination Act

Mississippi Advance Health-Care Directive

Introduction

You have the right to make health care decisions, including decisions about nursing home care, for yourself. Under the law, a patient must consent to any treatment or care received. Generally, if you are a competent adult, you can give this consent for yourself. For you to give this consent, you should be told what the recommended procedure is, why it is recommended, what risks are involved with the procedure, and what the alternatives are.

If you are not able to make your own health care decisions, your advance directives can be used. An "advance directive" can be an Individual Instruction or a Power of Attorney for Health Care.

An "Individual Instruction" is a directive concerning a health care decision. An Individual Instruction can be written or oral. No specific format is required for Individual Instructions.

A "Power of Attorney for Health Care" ("PAHC") is a document through which you designate someone as your agent to make health care decisions for you if you are unable to make such decisions. The PAHC comes into play when you cannot make a health care decision, either because of a permanent or temporary illness or injury. The PAHC must specifically authorize your agent to make health care decisions for you and must contain the standard language set out in the law. This language is included in the form of the PAHC contained in the Form section at the back of this document. Otherwise, the PAHC can contain any instructions which you wish.

If you are unable to make a decision and have not given or prepared individual instructions or a PAHC, you may designate an adult of your choice, called a surrogate, to make health care decisions for you. If you do not appoint a surrogate, the members of your family may make decisions for you.

The law on making health care decisions and advance directives is discussed in this [document] in detail.

Please read the entire document.

Your Right Under Mississippi Law to Make Decisions Concerning Health Care

The Patient Self-Determination Act of 1990 (The "PSDA") is a federal law which imposes on the state and providers of health care—such as hospitals, nursing homes, hospices, home health agencies, and prepaid health care organizations—certain requirements concerning advance directives and an individual's rights under state law to make decisions concerning medical care. This [document] will discuss your rights under state law to make health care decisions and set out a description of the Mississippi law on advance directives.

- **What Are My Rights to Accept or Refuse Treatment or Care?**
  In general, you have the right to make health care decisions, including decisions about nursing home care, for yourself if you are 18 or older and are competent.

- **What Information Must I Be Told to Give My Consent?**
  The physician should explain to you the pertinent facts about your illness and the nature of the treatment in nontechnical terms which are understandable to you.

  The physician also should explain to you why the proposed treatment is recommended.

  The physician should inform you of all reasonable risks and material consequences or "side effects" associated with the proposed treatment.

  Finally, the physician must tell you about any other types of treatment which you could undergo instead. The nature, purpose, and reasonable risks and consequences of these treatments should be explained to you.

  With this information, you can then make your health care decision.

- **What If I Am Unable to Make These Decisions?**
  If you cannot make a health care decision because of incapacity, your advance directive, such as an Individual Instruction or Power of Attorney for Health Care, can be used. If you have not signed an advance directive, you may designate an adult of your choice, called a surrogate, to make the decision. If you do not have

an advance directive and you have not designated a surrogate, a family member may make the decision for you. If you do not have an advance directive, have not designated a surrogate, and do not have a family member available to make a health care decision for you, then an adult who shows care and concern and who is familiar with your values may make health care decisions for you. If you do not have advance directives and do not have anyone to make health care decisions for you, then a court might have to make the decision for you.

- **What Is an Advance Directive?**

The PSDA defines an "advance directive" as a written instruction, such as an Individual Instruction or Power of Attorney for Health Care, recognized under State law and relating to the provision of health care when the individual is incapacitated. Two types of advance directives are statutorily recognized in Mississippi: Individual Instruction and Power of Attorney for Health Care.

Individual Instruction

- **What Is an Individual Instruction?**

An Individual Instruction means an individual's direction concerning a health care decision for the individual. The instruction may be oral or written. The instruction may be limited to take effect only if a specified condition arises.

- **What Must the Individual Instruction Say?**

Mississippi law does not prescribe any particular format for individual instructions. However, the law does specify an acceptable format for those instructions which deal with End-of-Life Decisions, Artificial Nutrition and Hydration, and Relief from Pain. This form is Part 2 of the form at the back of this document.

- **Where Should I Keep My Individual Instruction?**

You should provide a copy of your Individual Instruction to anyone you designate to make health care decisions for you and to your health care provider. Your Individual Instruction should not be filed with the Mississippi Department of Health.

- **How Can My Individual Instruction Be Revoked?**

The Individual Instruction is valid until revoked. You may revoke an Individual Instruction in any manner that indicates an intent to revoke.

- **Will My Individual Instruction Be Followed?**

Your Individual Instruction must be honored by your agent, family, surrogate or health care provider.

For reasons of conscience, a physician, hospital, nursing home or other provider has the right to refuse to follow your Individual Instruction; but a provider not honoring your Individual Instruction must cooperate in your transfer to another provider who will follow your Individual Instruction.

Upon admission, you should receive a copy of the facility's policies concerning advance directives. You should review these policies and determine whether the facility will follow your Individual Instruction.

- **Should I Give My Physician a Copy of My Individual Instruction?**
  Yes. If you have a written Individual Instruction, you should give a copy to the physician who has primary responsibility for your health care. A copy also should be given to any other provider, such as a hospital, home health agency, or nursing home, from which you are receiving care.

Power of Attorney for Health Care

- **What Is a Power of Attorney for Health Care?**
  You may designate an individual or agent to make health care decisions for you if you are unable to make such a decision because of a permanent or temporary illness or injury. The document authorizing this action is the Power of Attorney for Health Care (PAHC).

- **What Must the PAHC Contain?**
  The PAHC must be properly witnessed, must specifically authorize your agent to make health care decisions for you, and must contain the standard language set out in the law. This language is included in the form of PAHC contained in the Form section at the back of this document.
  Otherwise, the PAHC can contain any instructions which you wish.

- **What Should I Do with the PAHC?**
  The PAHC does not need to be filed with the Mississippi Department of Health or any court. You should keep the PAHC for yourself and give a copy to the agent you named in the PAHC.

  A copy should also be given to your physician to make a part of your medical records. You should also give a copy to any other provider from which you are receiving care, such as a nursing home, hospital, or a home health agency. You might also want to provide a copy to your clergy, family members, and friends who are not named in the documents.

- **Who Will Decide that I Cannot Act and My Agent Should Act for Me?**
  Unless otherwise specified in the PAHC, the physician designated by you or your agent to have primary responsibility for your health care will make this determination. In making this determination, your physician will act in accordance with "generally accepted health care standards."

- **Who Can Act as My Agent?**
  Unless related to you by blood, marriage, or adoption, your agent may not be an owner, operator, or employee of a residential long term care institution at

which you are receiving care. Otherwise, any person, such as a family member or a friend, may act as the agent. The agent does not need to be a lawyer.

- **What Are the Powers of My Agent?**
  Your agent has whatever power you give in the PAHC to make health care decisions for you. "Making health care decisions" means a decision regarding your health care, including the selection and discharge of health care providers and institutions; approval and disapproval of diagnostic tests, surgical procedures, medications, and orders not to resuscitate; and direction to provide, withhold, or withdrew artificial nutrition and hydration.

- **Are There Limitations on the Power of My Agent?**
  Your agent has a duty to act according to what you put in the PAHC or as you otherwise have made known to him or her. If your desires are unknown, he or she must act in your best interest. Your agent cannot make a particular health care decision for you if you are able to make that decision.

- **What If Someone Other than the Agent Wants to Make Health Care Decisions for Me?**
  Unless the PAHC says otherwise, your agent has priority over any other person to act for you.

- **Will a Health Care Provider Recognize My Agent's Authority?**
  In general, yes.

  Upon admission, you should receive a copy of the facility's policies on advance directives. You should review these policies and determine whether the facility will follow your PAHC.

- **Can My PAHC Be Changed?**
  You can change your agent by a signed writing, or you can revoke the authority for your agent to make decisions by personally informing your primary physician or the health care provider who has undertaken primary responsibility for your health care.

General

- **What If I Have an Individual Instructions or PAHC I Signed When Living in Another State?**
  To be binding, these documents must meet Mississippi law. Many out-of-state documents will not meet these requirements. The safest route is to execute new documents following the Mississippi statute.

- **Do I Need Both an Individual Instruction and PAHC?**
  No. You may include Individual Instructions in your PAHC.

- **What Other Documents Should Be Considered?**
  Individual Instructions and PAHC are the only documents recognized in Mississippi by statute. However, depending upon particular circumstances, the state may recognize other health care directives or indications of your desires concerning health care. You also should discuss these options with your lawyer.
- **Can I Let My Family Make These Decisions?**
  Members of your family may make decisions for you if you are unable to do so and have not left Individual Instructions or PAHC. Family members, however, might disagree among themselves or with the physician. In such instances, Individual Instructions or PAHC can help to clarify the decisions and who can make them.
- **When Will a Court Make This Decision?**
  As a last resort, if someone authorized to consent for you has refused or declined to do so and no other person known to be available is authorized to consent, a court may order treatment for you if you are not able to do so.

Advance Health Care Directive

Explanation

You have the right to give instructions about your own health care. You also have the right to name someone else to make health care decisions for you. This form lets you do either or both of these things. It also lets you express your wishes regarding the designation of your primary physician. If you use this form, you may complete or modify all or any part of it. You are free to use a different form.

Part 1 of this form is a power of attorney for health care. Part 1 lets you name another individual as agent to make health care decisions for you if you become incapable of making your own decisions or if you want someone else to make those decisions for you now, even though you are still capable. You may name an alternate agent to act for you if your first choice is not willing, able, or reasonably available to make decisions for you. Unless related to you, your agent may not be an owner, operator, or employee of a residential long term health care institution at which you are receiving care.

Unless the form you sign limits the authority of your agent, your agent may make all health care decisions for you. This form has a place for you to limit the authority of your agent. You need not limit the authority of your agent if you wish to rely on your agent for all health care decisions that may have to be made. If you choose not to limit the authority of your agent, your agent will have the right to:

- Consent or refuse consent to any care, treatment, service, or procedure to maintain, diagnose, or otherwise affect a physical or mental condition;
- Select or discharge health care providers and institutions;

- Approve or disapprove diagnostic tests, surgical procedures, programs of medication, and orders not to resuscitate; and
- Direct the provision, withholding, or withdrawal of artificial nutrition and hydration and all other forms of health care.

Part 2 of this form lets you give specific instructions about any aspect of your health care. Choices are provided for you to express your wishes regarding the provision, withholding, or withdrawal of treatment to keep you alive, including the provision of artificial nutrition and hydration, as well as the provision of pain relief. Space is provided for you to add to the choices you have made or for you to write out any additional wishes.

Part 3 of this form lets you designate a physician to have primary responsibility for your health care.

Part 4 of this form lets you authorize the donation of your organs at your death, and declares that this decision will supersede any decision by a member of your family.

After completing this form, sign and date the form at the end and have the form witnessed by one of the two alternative methods listed below. Give a copy of the signed and completed form to your physician, to any other health care providers you may have, to any health care institution at which you are receiving care, and to any health care agents you have named. You should talk to the person you have named as agent to make sure that he or she understands your wishes and is willing to take the responsibility.

You have the right to revoke this advance health care directive or replace this form at any time.

Part 1

Power of Attorney for Health Care

(1) *Designation of Agent:* I designate the following individual as my agent to make health care decisions for me.

____

(Name of individual you choose as agent)

____

(Address) (City) (State) (Zip code)

____

(Home phone) (Work phone)

Optional: If I revoke my agent's authority or if my agent is not willing, able or reasonably available to make a health care decision for me, I designate as my first alternate agent:

____

(Name of individual you choose as first alternate agent)

____

(Address) (City) (State) (Zip code)

____

(Home phone) (Work phone)

Optional: If I revoke the authority of my agent and first alternate or if neither is willing, able or reasonably available to make a health care decision for me, I designate as my second alternate agent:

____

(Name of individual you choose as second alternate agent)

____

(Address) (City) (State) (Zip code)

____

(Home phone) (Work phone)

(2) *Agent's Authority*: My agent is authorized to make all health care decisions for me, including decisions to provide, withhold, or withdraw artificial nutrition and hydration and all other forms of health care to keep me alive, except as I state here:

____

____

____

(add additional sheets if needed)

(3) *When Agent's Authority Becomes Effective*: My agent's authority becomes effective when my primary physician determines that I am unable to make my own health care decisions unless I mark the following box. If I mark this box [ ], my agent's authority to make health care decisions for me takes effect immediately.

(4) *Agent's Obligation*: My agent shall make health care decisions for me in accordance with this Power of Attorney for Health Care, any instructions I give in Part 2 of this form, and my other wishes to the extent known to my agent. To the extent my wishes are unknown, my agent shall make health care decisions for me in accordance with what my agent determines to be in my best interest. In determining my best interest, my agent shall consider my personal values to the extent known to my agent.

(5) *Nomination of Guardian*: If a guardian of my person needs to be appointed for me by a court, I nominate the agent designated in this form. If that agent is not willing, able, or reasonably available to act as guardian, I nominate the alternate agents whom I have named, in the order designated.

Part 2

Instructions for Health Care

If you are satisfied to allow your agent to determine what is best for you in making end-of-life decisions, you need not fill out this part of the form. If you do fill out this part of the form, you may strike any wording you do not want.

(6) *End-of-life Decisions*: I direct that my health care providers and others involved in my care provide, withhold, or withdraw treatment in accordance with the choice I have marked below:

[ ] (a) Choice Not To Prolong Life
I do not want my life to be prolonged if (i) I have an incurable and irreversible condition that will result in my death within a relatively short time, (ii) I become unconscious and, to a reasonable degree of medical certainty, I will not regain consciousness, or (iii) the likely risks and burdens of treatment would outweigh the expected benefits, or

[ ] (b) Choice to Prolong Life

I want my life to be prolonged as long as possible within the limits of generally accepted health care standards.

(7) *Artificial Nutrition and Hydration*: Artificial nutrition and hydration must be provided, withheld or withdrawn in accordance with the choice I have made in paragraph (6) unless I mark the following box. If I mark this box [ ], artificial nutrition and hydration must be provided regardless of my condition and regardless of the choice I have made in paragraph (6).

(8) *Relief from Pain:* Except as I state in the following space, I direct that treatment for alleviation of pain or discomfort be provided at all times, even if it hastens my death:

____

____

(9) *Other Wishes:* (If you do not agree with any of the optional choices above and wish to write your own, or if you wish to add to the instructions you have given above, you may do so here.):
I direct that:

____

____

(Add any additional sheets if needed.)

Part 3

Primary Physician

(Optional)

(10) *I designate the following physician as my primary physician*:

____
(Name of physician)

____
(Address) (City) (State) (Zip code)

____
(Phone) (Phone)

Optional: If the physician I have designated above is not willing or reasonably available to act as my primary physician, I designate the following physician as my primary physician:

____
(Name of physician)

____
(Address) (City) (State) (Zip code)

____
(Phone) (Phone)

(11) *Effect of Copy*: A copy of this form has the same effect as the original.

(12) *Signatures:* Sign and date the form here:

____
(Date) (Sign your name)

____
(Address) (Print your name)

____
(City) (State)

Part 4

Certificate of Authorization for Organ Donation

(Optional)

I, the undersigned, this ____________day of ___________, 20__, desire that my ________________________________organ(s) be made available after my demise for:

(a) Any licensed hospital, surgeon or physician, for medical education, research, advancement of medical science, therapy or transplantation to individuals;

(b) Any accredited medical school, college or university engaged in medical education or research, for therapy, educational research or medical science purposes or any accredited school or mortuary science;

(c) Any person operating a bank or storage facility for blood, arteries, eyes, pituitaries, or other human parts, for use in medical education, research, therapy or transplantation to individuals;

(d) The donee specified below, for therapy or transplantation needed by him or her, do donate my _________ for that purpose to ______________ (name) at ____ (address).

I authorize a licensed physician or surgeon to remove and preserve for use my ______________________________________ for that purpose.

I specifically provide that this declaration shall supersede and take precedence over any decision by my family to the contrary.

Witnessed this ________ day of_____________________, 20______.

____

(donor)

____

(address)

____

(telephone)

____

(witness)

____

(witness)

(13) *Witnesses*: This Power of Attorney will not be valid for making health care decisions unless it is either (a) signed by two (2) qualified adult witnesses who are personally known to you and who are present when you sign or acknowledge your signature; or (b) acknowledged before a notary public in the state.

Alternative No. 1

Witness:

I declare under penalty of perjury pursuant to Section 97-9-61, Mississippi Code of 1972, that the principal is personally known to me, that the principal signed or acknowledged this Power of Attorney in my presence, that the principal appears to be of sound mind and under no duress, fraud or undue influence, that I am not the person appointed as agent by this document, and that I am not a health care provider, nor an employee of a health care provider or facility. I am not related to the principal by blood, marriage or adoption, and to the best of my knowledge, I am not entitled to any part of the estate of the principal upon the death of the principal under a will now existing or by operation of law.

____

(Signature of witness) (Date)

____

(Printed name of witness)

____

(Street address City State Zip code)

Witness:

I declare under penalty of perjury pursuant to Section 97-9-61, Mississippi Code of 1972, that the principal is personally known to me, that the principal signed or acknowledged this Power of Attorney in my presence, that the principal appears to be of sound mind and under no duress, fraud or undue influence, that I am not the person appointed as agent by this document, and that I am not a health care provider, nor an employee of a health care provider or facility.

____

(Signature of witness) (Date)

____

(Printed name of witness) (Date)

____

(Street address City State Zip code)

Alternative No. 2

State of___________________________________

County of _________________________________

On this the _______day of __________, in the year___, before me, ________________________________ (insert name of notary public) appeared ____, personally known to me (or proved to me on the basis of satisfactory evidence) to be the person whose name is subscribed to this instrument, and acknowledged that he or she executed it. I declare under the penalty of perjury that the person whose name is subscribed to this instrument appears to be of sound mind and under no duress, fraud or undue influence.

Notary Seal:

____
(Signature of Notary Public)

Glossary

1981 Uniform Determination of Death Act: Legislation passed by the National Conference of Commissioners on Uniform State Laws to provide a comprehensive and consistent means for determining death.

Abortion: The death of a fetus, either via premature birth (miscarriage or spontaneous abortion) or the intentional termination of a pregnancy.

Act Utilitarians: Followers of utilitarianism who believe that the morality of actions are based on the specific circumstances in which they are performed and that an action should be chosen based on its likelihood of positive consequences in that particular situation. Compare with *rule utilitarians.*

Active euthanasia: Taking purposeful steps to end a life, such as the administration of certain drugs. One reason for inducing death in this manner might be a terminal illness.

Adaptation Theory: The idea that people adapt to the physical and social environment in which they live.

Adherence: The degree to which a patient follows a healthcare professional's prescribed treatment regimen. Adherence suggests a higher level of patient involvement and agreement than compliance. See *compliance.*

Adolescent development process: The physical, emotional, and cognitive changes that take place in children as they age; the process consists of 3 steps and takes place over a period of 11 years. See *early adolescence, middle adolescence,* and *late adolescence.*

Adolescents facing their own death: Adolescents with a terminal disease, who often struggle with issues of identity or worth because of their perceived lack of a future.

Advance directive: Written instructions for use in making medical decisions if a patient is rendered incompetent or is otherwise unable to express consent. See *living will, medical care directive, durable power of attorney,* and *psychiatric advance directive.*

Advocacy: Campaigning or working in support of a cause or person.

Ageism: Discrimination against/negative perceptions of older persons strictly on the basis of age.

Anorexia nervosa: An eating disorder that is not about food but is characterized by the extremely limited or nonexistent consumption of food in relation to an intense fear of weight gain. The person equates thinness with self-worth.

Assisted reproductive technology (ART): All types of fertility treatments in which both eggs and sperm are handled.

Attentive listening: Actively paying attention to what is being said; techniques include focusing on the speaker, not interrupting the speaker, and re-stating the speaker's thoughts to ensure that there has been no misunderstanding.

Authentic leader: A leader who places great importance on things such as openness, honesty, and transparency in relationships with his/her followers; a deeply-rooted sense of right and wrong; and his/her own self identity.

Authentic presence: Being true to oneself.

Autonomy: The ability to make independent decisions for oneself and to have those decisions respected by others.

Baby Doe rules: Also known as the 1984 Child Abuse Prevention and Treatment Act Amendments; these rules prohibit parents or physicians from withholding treatment from impaired neonates, with institutions that do not follow these rules being punished with a reduction in federal funds.

BART behavioral intervention program: The Becoming A Responsible Teen program, which is a popular theory- and evidence-based, health-risk prevention education program for adolescents that draws from both Bandura's social learning theory and the information–motivation–behavioral skills model.

Basic dignity: The respect and equality due to all human beings.

Being a good citizen: Anticipating ethical dilemmas in relationships and engaging in dialogue with affected parties to resolve concerns.

Beneficence: The ethical principle of doing good. See *nonmaleficence*.

Best interests standard: A decision-making criterion used for patients who have never been competent and able to express their own autonomous wishes for health care (such as a child or mentally disabled adult). A surrogate makes a decision for the patient based on the surrogate's assessment of what would provide the most benefits and fewest burdens to the patient.

Bioethics: A branch of ethics specifically focused on issues related to health care/medicine.

Boundary crossing: Actions that go beyond the established limits of a relationship, which can cause harm to the person whose limits were not respected.

Bulimia: An eating disorder characterized by binging (consuming large amounts of food) and purging (intentional vomiting to empty the stomach).

Chronic illness: Any illness that lasts for an extended period of time, and sometimes permanently.

Claim rights: Also called positive rights; rights that a person can only express if another person/entity allows it to happen (either by providing assistance so that the claim is met, or by not interfering with the claim). See *liberty right*.

Collaboration: Working together to achieve common goals.

Common morality: Generally-accepted beliefs within a community regarding normative beliefs and behavior.

Community: A group of people with a shared interest in a common good and the ability to engage with each other to achieve common goals.

Compassion: An understanding and recognition of suffering, along with an honest desire to alleviate said suffering.

Compliance: An assumed agreement between a patient and a healthcare professional about a proposed treatment regimen, which is taken as an indication that the patient intends to follow the healthcare professional's care plan. Compliance suggests an unequal patient–provider relationship, with the patient essentially submitting to a treatment plan with which they may or may not agree. See *adherence*.

Compliance program: Also known as a risk-management program; an internal department at an organization charged with ensuring that the organization follows regulations and preventing unlawful conduct.

Concordance: An approach to medication wherein a patient and provider agree on a treatment regimen after a discussion of the patient's beliefs and wishes in regards to the medication (if, when, and how a medicine is used).

Confidentiality: The nondisclosure of information; preventing access to information by unapproved parties.

Conflicts of commitment: A conflict of interest as viewed from an ethical perspective. See *conflict of interest.*

Conflict of interest: When an individual's personal interests and desires are at odds with their public duties or values.

Controlled non-heart-beating donor: Organ donors who are maintained on mechanical ventilation prior to organ retrieval; these donors often have advance directives regarding organ donation.

Courage: The ability to confront those things that could be harmful or dangerous without fear.

Cultural relativism: The belief that morals are inseparable from the culture in which they develop, such that ideas or actions that are deemed "wrong" or "immoral" in one culture may not be viewed that way in a different culture.

Culturally-sensitive care: Providing care that understands and respects the beliefs, values, and customs of the person receiving the care.

Culture: A set of values, attitudes, customs, beliefs, and so on that are shared by a particular group. Culture can be defined on the basis of race, religion, nationality, ethnicity, and/or other personal, geographic, or social characteristics.

Dead donor rule: The guiding principle in regards to potential organ donors, consisting of two parts: that the donor must be declared dead before organ retrieval can begin, and that care or treatment must not be compromised in favor of potential organ recipients (i.e., the organ donor must not be allowed to die so that organs become available).

Death: The irreversible cessation of circulatory and respiratory, or neurologic, functions.

Death anxiety: An innate fear of death or nonbeing.

Decisional capacity: The ability to make what would generally be considered a reasonable choices.

Deontology: A branch of ethics that judges morality based on adherence to accepted rules and duties; literally, "the study of duty." (Compare with *virtue ethics.*)

Depression: Chronic feelings of sadness, anger, or low self-esteem that interfere with daily life and prevent enjoyment in previously pleasurable activities.

Descriptive ethics: A form of ethical inquiry concerned with describing and identifying, rather than understanding, a person's morals.

Disenfranchised grief: The sorrow that results when the grieving process is not allowed or cannot be done openly; the hidden nature of the grief often results in prolonging and intensifying the process.

Distributive justice: The concept of fair allocation of resources in a society.

Do not resuscitate (DNR) order: A written order kept in a patient's medical record to indicate that healthcare personnel are not to perform cardiopulmonary resuscitation (CPR) or other resuscitative measures on a patient.

Doctor–Nurse game: A term referring to the relationship between doctors and nurses that is founded on the belief that the doctor is superior and that open disagreements between nurse and doctor are to be avoided. This resulted in the need for nurses to be circumspect when providing guidance or suggestions to a doctor, so that the advice was not seen as challenging the doctor's perceived authority.

Donor cards: Legal documents, carried by people who agree to donate their organs, that give permission to others to use the organs after death.

Durable power of attorney: A legal document that designates a particular person to make healthcare decisions for an incapacitated patient.

Duty to warn: The need to disclose confidential information in instances where a clearly identifiable person is at risk of harm.

Early adolescence: The first stage of an adolescent's development; this step takes place between the ages of 10 and 14 years and is marked by a need for experimentation and discovery (usually connected to the onset of puberty).

Egg donation: A form of assisted reproduction where a woman donates her eggs; the eggs are artificially inseminated with the sperm from the prospective father, and the embryos are implanted into the prospective mother's uterus.

Embryo donation: A form of assisted reproduction where a couple with successful pregnancies donates embryos (usually those remaining after *in vitro* fertilization treatment) to another couple.

Emergency contraception (EC): Birth control measures taken after sexual intercourse to prevent pregnancy. Emergency contraception includes RU486 (mifepristone) and Plan B (the "morning-after pill").

Ethic of an organization: How an organization defines its core mission and values, as well as how it thinks about and implements said values.

Ethical climate: How an organization responds to ethical issues, as determined by its members' shared values.

Ethical leader: A leader who is able to influence others through non-coercive means and who works towards righteous goals.

Ethical objectivism: The belief that the concepts or principles of morality are universal.

Ethical relativism: The belief that differing ideas of morality between people and/or groups are acceptable.

Ethical subjectivism: A type of ethical relativism that does not believe in a universal morality; rather, ethical subjectivists believe that each individual creates his or her own morality based on personal feelings.

Ethics: The study of ideal human behavior and existence, focused on understanding the concepts of and distinguishing between right and wrong.

Ethics as praxis: The use of theory to think about, understand, and practice moral behavior.

Euthanasia: A good or painless death; the act of intentionally ending a life—often, though not always—with the goal of limiting or relieving pain and suffering.

Fear appeals: Persuasive messages that emphasize the negative consequence of a behavior or action in order to frighten the target audience into not performing the action (or into choosing a healthy action instead).

Fiduciary relationships: A relationship in which one party has a formal duty to uphold one's responsibilities and commitments and to act in the best interest of the other members of the relationship.

Freedom: The state of self-direction; not being confined or controlled by others.

Full moral status: The belief that an entity deserves certain privileges and rights (such as autonomy). The designation of full moral status can be based on any number of criteria, including sentience and concepts of personhood.

Futile: Something that is unable to be successful.

Futile treatments: Procedures that are unlikely to provide any benefit to a patient and that could, instead, cause substantial harm.

Gatekeepers: A suicide prevention program designed to train school nurses to recognize the warning signs of suicidal ideation and intervene as needed.

Gender selection: Using genetic testing to sex embryos, then selecting for implantation only those embryos of the desired sex.

Genetic screening: The use of professional counselors to discuss the potential for inheritable diseases, most often used for individuals or couples with a personal or family history of diseases caused by genetic defects.

Genuineness: A lack of pretense when engaging in interpersonal relationships; credibility and honesty when interacting with others.

Gestational surrogacy: A form of surrogacy where a woman carries a embryo to which she has no genetic relationship (the embryo is created from the egg and sperm of the prospective parents).

Giver of communication: An entity (such as a nurse) who is responsible for determining how, where, and what type of information is provided to a particular group.

Health care fraud: The intentional misuse or misappropriation of healthcare monies or equipment for personal gain.

Health disparities: The differences in health outcomes that can be attributed to inequalities in healthcare delivery.

Health risk behaviors: Actions and conduct that are dangerous to the health and well-being of the participants. Examples include drug and alcohol use, engaging in unsafe sex, and unhealthy eating habits.

Honesty: The quality of deliberate truthfulness and authenticity in one's actions and interactions; a lack of deception.

Horizontal violence: Abuse committed by nurses toward other nurses; conflict and anger occurring among nurses, as opposed to conflict coming from outside of the nursing community.

Imaginative dramatic rehearsal: Imagining an ideal scenario (such as an ideal death) in order to take meaning from the experience as well as shape how the scenario plays out in real life.

Infertility: The inability to conceive a child.

Informed consent: Agreement to a procedure or action based on an understanding of the facts and possible consequences of said procedure or action. The three basic elements of informed consent are (1) receipt of information, (2) voluntary (unforced) agreement to the conditions presented, and (3) competency of the person(s) providing consent.

Inheritable genetic modification (IGM): Changes made to a person's genetic material that would not only affect that person, but all of the person's descendents.

Integrity: Honest and just behavior; maintaining consistent, ethical values in actions and relationships.

Involuntary euthanasia: The intentional taking of one's life when the person could consent, but does not—for example, in cases of capital punishment.

Just generosity: Giving that reflects the needs of, rather than what is perceived to be owed to, the recipients; giving that is meaningful to the giver.

Justice: A moral concept of rightness based on fairness and equality.

Justified paternalism: The belief that beneficence overrules the need to respect autonomy in cases where a patient's autonomy is compromised and the planned interventions would be deemed acceptable by general consensus.

Kantian deontology: A specific type of deontology, formulated by Immanuel Kant (1724–1804), in which the morality of an action is based only on the dutifulness of the action itself, not on the action's consequences. In Kantian deontology, the ends can never justify the means, because people are an end in and of themselves and should never merely be used to attain some goal.

Late adolescence: The third and final stage of an adolescent's development; this step takes place between the ages of 18 and 20 years and is completed by the transition from adolescence to adulthood, demonstrated by the increased importance of the future.

Late-term abortion: An abortion performed in the third trimester.

Leader: One who is able to influence others.

Leader succession planning: Preparing and nurturing those with leadership skills and potential.

Libertarianism: A theory of entitlement that suggests that only those who contribute to the system should be able to receive the benefits of said system.

Liberty rights: Also called negative rights; rights that person has the freedom to express without the need for assistance from others. Freedom of speech and civil rights are examples of liberty rights. See *claim rights.*

Limits of confidentiality: The situations in which patient confidentiality can be breached, usually consisting of situations in which there is potential harm to a patient or others.

Living will: A formal legal document that outlines a person's desired medical care to be provided in specific circumstances; a type of advance directive.

Losing a loved one: The death of a close family member or friend.

Mandated choice: The requirement that competent individuals select an option (such as in regards to organ donation) on official documents (e.g., drivers' licenses, tax returns). This decision becomes binding unless written documentation to reverse the decision is provided.

Market justice: The belief that benefits and burdens should be distributed based on individual abilities and contributions (i.e., wealthy people should not have to shoulder burdens because of their success).

Maternal–fetal conflict: The conflict that arises when the interests of a pregnant woman (as defined by the woman) differ from the interests of the fetus (as defined by a physician).

Medical care directive: An informal (not legally-binding) document that provides instructions to a physician regarding the types of medical treatments a patient does/does not want, to be used in the event that the patient becomes incapacitated and unable to provide consent; a type of advance directive.

Medicalization: The transformation of human social conditions into medical diagnoses so that physicians then have the authority to prescribe treatments and preventive measures for the condition.

Meta-ethics: The study of the terminology of morality (e.g., good, wrong) to understand concepts and ideas related to moral behavior.

Middle adolescence: The second stage of an adolescent's development; this step takes place between the ages of 15 and 17 years and is dominated by peer influence and a need for peer acceptance and validation.

Moral agency: The ability to make decisions that can affect the well-being of oneself or others; taking responsibility for one's own thoughts, beliefs, and actions.

Moral community: A community formed by people who want to and work toward promoting a sense of well being for all members of said community.

Moral courage: The ability to act rightly in spite of opposition or constraints.

Moral distress: The feelings of anguish and/or frustration when the "right thing" is impossible to do.

Moral imagination: The use of creative thought processes, such as empathetic projection, to make moral decisions and become aware of new possibilities and answers to questions.

Moral integrity: Being in possession of characteristics (such as honesty and trustworthiness) that traditionally define a person with good character; following a framework of internal, consistent values in all actions or dealings.

Moral reasoning: The use of critical thinking to examine questions of right and wrong. See *reasoning.*

Moral rights: Inherent, universal privileges that cannot be taken away.

Moral self-government: A person's ethics, values, and direction, as linked to their ability to make decisions that are consistent with their personal worldview.

Moral space: The space in which people live their lives.

Moral suffering: Feelings of discomfort or anguish that come from the imperfectness of life, when there is no satisfactory outcome to a situation or when it is impossible to affect change in a negative situation.

Morals: Ethically derived thoughts and actions that are judged "good" or "bad" based on ethical reasoning; the goodness of how people actually behave.

Nonadherence: The degree to which a prescribed treatment regimen will not be followed; nonadherence can be intentional or caused by constraints outside of the patient's control.

Noncompliance: Not following a healthcare professional's suggested treatment regimen (i.e., not taking or incorrectly taking prescribed medications), either intentionally or otherwise.

Non-heart-beating donor (NHBD): A donor whose heart has stopped beating at the time of organ retrieval. See *Controlled* and *Uncontrolled non-heart-beating donor* for specifics.

Nonmaleficence: The ethical obligation to not cause harm. See *beneficence*.

Nonvoluntary euthanasia: The intentional taking of patient's life when the patient is unable to consent to the procedure—for example, after authorization by a surrogate decision maker.

Normative ethics: A form of ethical inquiry concerned with how humans should behave and act, based on ascribing the concepts of "right" and "wrong" to values and ways of being.

Nursing ethics: The study of moral issues related to, and through the lens of, nursing. Issues include those associated with the basic concepts of nursing, such as health and healing.

Obesity: The accumulation of excess body fat.

Observer evaluation: Quality-of-life judgments made by anyone other than the person whose life is under consideration.

Occupational fraud and abuse: The use of one's position of employment for personal gain, attained via unlawful or unethical actions.

Open system: An organization where relationships and interactions with external bodies are important.

Organ procurement: The act of obtaining an organ for transplantation via one of many programs or systems.

Organization: A group of people who work together to attain shared goals.

Organizational citizenship: The expectations that society has for open systems, specifically in terms of the relationships that organizations have with their communities.

Organizational culture: An organization's common philosophy, behavior, and focus, either in the past or as currently experienced.

Organizational ethics: The goodness of actions, character, and purpose of an organization, along with its culture.

Organizational integrity: The widespread valuing of honesty and right behavior across an organization's membership.

Organizational trust: The authenticity and dependability of an organization in regards to its interactions with others (individuals, other organizations, society as a whole).

Palliative care: Care that focuses on maintaining quality of life and relieving pain and suffering instead of a cure.

Partial-birth abortion: A nonmedical term that refers a procedure called intact dilation and extraction (intact D & E), used to perform abortions in the third trimester. See *late-term abortion.*

Passive euthanasia: Taking a life by the purposeful withdrawal or withholding of treatments or procedures used to prolong or sustain life.

Paternalism: The belief that the requirement to perform beneficence outweighs the need to respect a person's autonomy; the idea that people in positions of authority "know what's best" and that it is acceptable for said authority figures to make decisions on behalf of others.

Patient advocacy: Working to uphold the rights and needs of patients, via three core features: protecting patient autonomy, promoting patients' wishes, and effecting social justice in health care.

Persistent vegetative state (PVS): A state in which a person with severe brain damage has enough automatic function to survive with constant medical intervention (e.g., can breathe without a ventilator) but does not exhibit any awareness or higher brain function.

Personal dignity: The value a community places on an individual and his/her place in society.

Personal evaluation: In quality-of-life judgments, a person's rating of the value of her/his life.

Personal regard: Caring for one's own personal needs; considering oneself worthy of care.

Physician-assisted suicide: Taking one's own life via self-administration of physician-ordered drugs.

Poetic intimacy: A form of sexual education that emphasizes sensuality and graceful language as a way for adolescents to address and understand their sexual feelings.

Population: A group of people who share at least one defining characteristic but who do not necessarily have a shared interest in a common good. See *community*.

Power: The ability to successfully influence the actions of others.

Precautionary principle: The belief that action should be taken to prevent a future harm, even if there is no concrete evidence that future harm is inevitable.

Preimplantation genetic diagnosis (PGD): The use of genetic testing to screen embryos for multiple characteristics, including gender and potential genetic abnormalities.

Prenatal genetic diagnosis: Genetic testing performed on a fetus to screen for genetic disorders prior to birth.

Presumed consent: The automatic consent to a procedure or action, unless the person specifically indicates the opposite. Used in some countries as the approach to organ donation (i.e., persons are assumed to agree to organ donation unless they have stated otherwise).

PRISMS: An acronym of actions central to patient advocacy: Persuade, Respect, Intercede, Safeguard, Monitor, Support.

Privacy: The ability to remain hidden and secluded (including keeping information inaccessible).

Privilege: A legal status that protects certain individuals (such as medical professions) from having to disclose information in court proceedings; privilege is not guaranteed, and there are limits to the types of information that can be kept confidential.

Professional nursing boundaries: A set of limits that define the relationships between nurses and those with whom they interact. Boundaries establish a sense of mutual control and safe space.

Psychiatric advance direction (PAD): Written instructions regarding a patient's wishes regarding his/her psychiatric treatment, should the patient lose the ability to consent to treatment.

Pure autonomy standard: Using a previously autonomous (but now incapacitated) patient's own decisions and wishes to direct care.

Quality: Excellence and high standards with regard to a product or service.

Quality of life: A subjective and highly variable assessment of the worth of a life, specifically the level of satisfaction in the living situation, to determine the value of pursuing treatments or interventions to remain alive.

***Qui tam* lawsuits:** Also known as whistleblower lawsuits; lawsuits filed by private citizens, on behalf of the government, against recipients of federal money that are alleged to have committed wrongdoing.

Rational suicide: A type of voluntary, active euthanasia, in which a person takes his/her own life after careful consideration and for reasons that would seem understandable to outside parties.

Reasoning: The use of critical thinking to examine questions and reach sound, logical conclusions.

Right to autonomy: The belief that persons should be able to make their own decisions regarding their bodies or actions.

Right to die: The idea that an autonomous person has the prerogative to refuse life-saving or life-sustaining treatments.

Right to freedom: The belief that a person should not be restricted in their actions, behavior and life.

Right to privacy: The belief that a person's life, actions, and thoughts do not have to be made public.

Rule of double effect: A set of criteria used to determine the ethics of a decision that involves weighing the benefit of an action (the intended, expected, positive outcome) with its possible negative but foreseeable consequences or effects. The action is considered ethical if the action in and of itself is moral, if the actor intends only the positive outcome, or if the good outcome greatly outweighs the possible negatives.

Rule utilitarians: Followers of utilitarianism who believe that there are specific rules that should always be adhered to, as they usually (though not necessarily always) provide the most benefit for the largest number of people. Compare with *act utilitarians.*

Secret drinking: Hidden or underground consumption of alcohol.

Servant leader: A leader who puts the good of the group being led before his/her own personal desires or aggrandizement.

Sexual abstinence: Traditionally, not engaging in sexual intercourse (specifically, penis–vagina penetrative intercourse). However, because of the variety of alternative methods for demonstrating sexual intimacy that do not involve vaginal penetration and the rise in same-sex relationships among adolescents, a new definition is necessary.

Sexual abuse: Any form of unwanted sexual activity that is forced upon a person.

Slippery slope argument: An argument based around the proposition that a small action can have critical, unforeseen consequences at some point in the future. In some cases, the original action is morally justifiable, but the hypothetical potential outcomes are considered unethical or dangerous. Slippery slope arguments, because they deal with potential—not actual—outcomes, often are lacking in concrete supporting evidence.

Social justice: The belief in equality for all people.

Socialized power: The idea that power should be used to promote the well being of others.

Soft paternalism: See *weak paternalism.*

Sperm sorting: The use of genetic testing to select specific embryos for use in *in vitro* fertilization. See *preimplantation genetic diagnosis.*

Spirituality: A sense of a unification of self with the world, with or without a belief in a higher power; a highly personal and important part of a person's being.

Stigma: The association of individuals with certain characteristics (such as mental illness) with negative, shameful feelings.

Substituted judgment standard: When a surrogate makes choices for an incapacitated (but formerly competent) patient based on what the surrogate thinks the patient would most likely want (usually derived from previous communications with the patient).

Successful leader: A leader who works to ensure that the values of an organization align with those of its members.

Suffering: The feeling experienced when a person is unable to achieve personal fulfillment; a negative experience that permeates the entire being.

Suffering person: A tormented being, whose pain can be apparent to others.

Suicidal tendency: Behaviors, words, or actions that suggest a person is considering suicide.

Suicide: The taking of one's own life.

Surplus reproductive products: The sperm, eggs, and embryos that are left after a successful pregnancy. Because *in vitro* fertilization has a low success rate, multiple fertilized eggs may be created but remain unused.

Surrogacy: The use of a third party to carry a fetus to term.

Surrogate decision maker: Also known as a proxy; an individual who is chosen to act on behalf of a patient who is incapable of making decisions. Either the patient or the courts delegate this privilege.

Tall poppy syndrome: A subset of *horizontal violence* in which people are attacked or criticized because of their (perceived or actual) achievements and success.

Terminal sedation: Sedating a patient into unconsciousness, then withholding life-sustaining measures until the patient dies.

Theory: A fact-based explanation for how something works or why things happen a certain way.

Therapeutic privilege: A legal right for physicians to withhold information from patients based on the potential for said information to harm the patient. Acceptable ranges of harm range from the possibility of negative effects to serious consequences.

Traditional surrogacy: A form of surrogacy where the surrogate donates her eggs, which are artificially inseminated using sperm from the prospective father.

Transformational leader: A leader who emphasizes improving the well-being of his/her followers by changing the culture in which they all work or live.

Trust: The belief that others will not take advantage of one's vulnerabilities.

Trustworthiness: Authenticity related to how dependable and accountable for one's actions a person is.

Truthful sort: A concept formulated by Aristotle to describe a person who is inherently honest; one who is honest in all situations, regardless of the need for honesty.

Truthfulness: A lack of deception when interacting and speaking with others; when translated to "truthtelling" in the medical profession, an ethical obligation to provide accurate information combined with respecting a person's autonomy.

Unavoidable trust: Patients' dependent need to have confidence in health care professionals' integrity and competence before this confidence has been earned.

Uncontrolled non-heart-beating donor: An organ donor who experiences cardio-respiratory arrest outside of a medical setting and cannot be resuscitated, but is declared legally dead prior to organ retrieval.

Underage drinking: The consumption of alcohol by persons under the legal drinking age (i.e., younger than 21 years old in the United States).

Utilitarianism: A form of consequentialism in which actions and behavior should be judged by the usefulness of their outcomes (compare with *Kantian deontology*). Ethical behavior produces the most good or happiness and the least harm or unhappiness in a given situation.

Value: Something that is viewed as good, meaningful, desirable, and/or worthwhile.

Veil of ignorance: The idea that people would make impartial decisions regarding resource distribution if they were unable to know the social or economic positions of themselves or others; if a cover (veil) shielded people from seeing their place within society, this lack of knowledge (ignorance) would help them make unbiased decisions because they would not know if or how such decisions would (positively or negatively) affect their own situation.

Virtue ethics: A subset of ethical thought concerned with *being* good (having moral character—"How should I be?") rather than *doing* good (following rules or duties— "What should I do?"). Compare with *deontology*.

Virtues: Positive character traits and/or habits that persons develop by thinking about and paying close attention to their thoughts and actions.

Voluntary euthanasia: An autonomous patient makes the decision to end his/her life. See *physician-assisted suicide*.

Weak paternalism: Making decisions regarding what is best for a person when the person's ability to be autonomous (self-directing) is compromised in some way (when a person is unable to make rational decisions).

Wholeness of character (in nursing): The recognition, integration, and expression of the values of the nursing profession and one's own moral values.

Withholding or withdrawing treatment: Not providing, or removing, life-sustaining treatment.

Index

Boxes, figures, and tables are indicated by b, f, and t following page numbers.

Q

R

S

D